Basic
Adolescent Gynecology

Basic
Adolescent Gynecology
An Office Guide

edited by

Victor C. Strasburger, M.D.
Chief of Adolescent Medicine
The University of New Mexico School of Medicine
Albuquerque

with 18 contributors

Urban & Schwarzenberg
Baltimore-Munich

Urban & Schwarzenberg, Inc.
7 E. Redwood Street
Baltimore, Maryland 21202
USA

Urban & Schwarzenberg GmbH
Landwehrstrasse 61
D-8000 Müenchen 2
West Germany

Printed in the United States

Notices

The Editors (or Authors) and the Publisher of this work have made every effort to ensure that the drug dosage schedules herein are accurate and in accord with the standards accepted at the time of publication. The reader is strongly advised, however, to check the product information sheet included in the package of each drug he or she plans to administer to be certain that changes have not been made in the recommended dose or in the contraindications for administration.

The publishers have made an extensive effort to trace original copyright holders for permission to use borrowed material. If any have been overlooked, it will be corrected at the first reprint.

5	4	3	2	1
94	93	92	91	90

Library of Congress Cataloging-in-Publication Data

Basic adolescent gynecology : an office guide / edited by Victor C.
   Strasburger : with 18 contributors.
       p. cm.
   Includes bibliographical references.
   ISBN 0-8067-4001-9
   1. Adolescent gynecology. I. Strasburger, Victor C., 1949-
   [DNLM: 1. Contraception—in adolescence. 2. Genital Diseases,
   Female—in adolescence. WS 360 A2394]
   RJ478.A355 1990
   618.1'00835'2—dc20
   DNLM/DLC
   for Library of Congress   90-11977
                                                                       CIP

Sponsoring Editor: Charles W. Mitchell
Managing Editor: Kathleen C. Millet
Manuscript Editor: Andrea Clemente
Design and Production: Stony Run Publishing Services, Baltimore, Maryland
Compositor: Phototype America, Cedar Falls, Iowa
Printer: John D. Lucas Printing Company, Baltimore, Maryland

ISBN 0-8067-4001-9 Baltimore
ISBN 3-541-74001-9 Munich

Contents

Contributors   vii
Foreword   ix
Preface   xi
Acknowledgments   xiii

1   **Current Issues in Adolescent Sexuality**   1
    Victor C. Strasburger

2   **Prescribing Oral Contraceptives**   23
    Victor C. Strasburger

3   **Barrier Contraception**   45
    Samuel K. Parrish, Jr.

4   **Consent and Confidentiality:** Critical Issues in Providing Contraceptive Care   59
    Adele D. Hofmann

5   **A Color Guide to Gynecologic Problems**   75
    Paula K. Braverman

6   **Vulvovaginitis**   81
    Donald E. Greydanus, Kenneth Sladkin, and Robin Rosenstock

7   **Breast Disorders**   113
    Col. Manuel Schydlower, Lt. Col. Walter K. Imai,
    Maj. Elisabeth M. Stafford, and Maj. Alan G. Getts

8   **Menstrual Disorders**   141
    John W. Kulig

9   **Evaluation and Management of Abdominal and Pelvic Pain**   173
    Jerold C. Woodhead, Douglas W. Laube, Kevin M. Wood,
    Lynn C. Richman, Susan R. Johnson, Vera Loening-Baucke, and
    Wilbur L. Smith

Index   231

Color figures for Chapter 5 appear between pages 78 and 79. The credits for these figures are as follows:

Figures 5-8, 5-10, 5-55: Reprinted with permission of Laurie Katz, M.D.

Figure 5-9: Reprinted with permission of Sabine O'Laughlin, M.D.

Figures 5-13, 5-37, 5-38, 5-47, 5-59: Reprinted with permission of Elsevier Science Publishing Co., Inc. from Office Microscopic Examination of Sexually Transmitted Diseases, by Gilchrist MJ, Rauh JL: *Journal of Adolescent Health Care*, 6:311–320. Copyright 1985 by The Society for Adolescent Medicine.

Figures 5-15, 5-17 through 5-26, 5-40, 5-56: Reprinted with permission of Ortho Pharmaceutical Company.

Figures 5-29, 5-57: Reprinted with permission of Syntex Laboratories, Inc.

Figures 5-32, 5-33, 5-50: Reprinted with permission of Syva Company.

Figures 5-34, 5-41 through 5-44, 5-58: Reprinted with permission of Reed and Carnrick.

Figures 5-51, 5-52, 5-54: Reprinted with permission of Joseph S. Rauh, M.D.

Figure 5-53: Reprinted with permission of Thomas V. Sedlacek, M.D.

Contributors

Paula K. Braverman, M.D.
Ambulatory Pediatrics Building
St. Christopher's Hospital for Children
5th and Lehigh Avenues
Philadelphia, PA 19133

Maj. Alan G. Getts, M.D.
Adolescent Medicine Service
William Beaumont Army Medical
    Center
El Paso, TX 79920-5001

Donald E. Greydanus, M.D.
Department of Pediatrics
Iowa Methodist Medical Center
Des Moines, IA 50309

Adele D. Hofmann, M.D.
Children's Hospital of Orange County
455 South Main Street
Orange, CA 92668

Lt. Col. Walter K. Imai, M.D.
Adolescent Medicine Service
William Beaumont Army Medical
    Center
El Paso, TX 79920-5001

Susan R. Johnson, M.D.
Department of Obstetrics and
    Gynecology
University of Iowa Hospitals and Clinics
Iowa City, IA 52242

John W. Kulig, M.D.
750 Washington Street, Box 479
Boston, MA 02111

Douglas W. Laube, M.D.
Department of Obstetrics and
    Gynecology
University of Iowa Hospitals and Clinics
Iowa City, IA 52242

Vera Loening-Baucke, M.D.
Department of Pediatrics
University of Iowa Hospitals and Clinics
Iowa City, IA 52242

Samuel K. Parrish, Jr., M.D.
Adolescent Medicine Service
Medical College of Pennsylvania
Philadelphia, PA 19129

Lynn C. Richman, Ph.D.
Department of Pediatrics
University of Iowa Hospitals and Clinics
Iowa City, IA 52242

Robin Rosenstock, M.D.
Department of Pediatrics
Iowa Methodist Medical Center
Des Moines, IA 50309

Col. Manuel Schydlower, M.D.
Adolescent Medicine Service
William Beaumont Army Medical
    Center
El Paso, TX 79220-5001

Kenneth Sladkin, M.D.
Broadlawns Medical Center
Des Moines, IA

Wilbur L. Smith, M.D.
Department of Radiology
University of Iowa Hospitals and Clinics
Iowa City, IA 52242

Maj. Elisabeth M. Stafford, M.D.
Adolescent Medicine Service
William Beaumont Army Medical
    Center
El Paso, TX 79920-5001

Victor C. Strasburger, M.D.
Department of Pediatrics
University of New Mexico School of
    Medicine
Albuquerque, NM 87131

Kevin W. Wood, Ph.D.
Department of Pediatrics
University of Iowa Hospitals and Clinics
Iowa City, IA 52242

Jerold C. Woodhead, M.D.
Department of Pediatrics
University of Iowa Hospitals and Clinics
Iowa City, IA 52242

Foreword

Because adolescents mature earlier than in past decades and because their sexual behavior places them at risk of reproductive health conditions, pediatricians and other primary care providers are being challenged to deliver the most up-to-date reproductive health services to this population. Optimal preventive, diagnostic, and therapeutic adolescent gynecologic services are delivered to young people when the practitioner is knowledgeable about adolescent sexuality, prevention of pregnancy and sexually transmitted diseases, consent and confidentiality, and breast and menstrual disorders. We are painfully aware of the potential morbidity of adolescent sexual behavior when young people do not receive optimal counseling, guidance, and treatment: teenage pregnancy, untreated sexually transmitted diseases resulting in infertility for some, and possible exposure to the human immunodeficiency virus (HIV) through high-risk sexual and drug-abusing behaviors.

Thus this work, *Basic Adolescent Gynecology: An Office Guide,* is particularly timely. The need to educate practitioners about adolescent gynecology has never been as great. The uniqueness of this book is that it is written for primary care practitioners by specialists in adolescent medicine. The advantage of this approach is that the gynecologic needs of the adolescent who seeks services are placed in the context of adolescence as a developmental period, an understanding of which is vital to optimal prevention, diagnosis, and treatment of adolescent gynecologic concerns.

The authors are pediatricians who all have had extensive experience in adolescent medicine and adolescent gynecology. They combine their special expertise skillfully in a text that is easily readable. Dr. Strasburger is to be congratulated for assembling such knowledgeable authors and for developing this book.

Lest we be discouraged by the many challenges facing our young people, we should remember that there is much more we can do as concerned physicians to help our young people. A first step is to learn as much as we can about adolescent gynecology so that we can provide optimal services to adolescents; this book provides the state-of-the-art information we need!

Elizabeth R. McAnarney, M.D.
Chief, General Pediatrics/Adolescent Medicine
University of Rochester Medical Center

Preface

This book may represent the first volume on adolescent gynecology written exclusively by *pediatricians*. As such, it is designed to provide a practical (but authoritative and detailed) guide to the office practice of adolescent gynecology by both gynecologists and nongynecologists alike. It is *not* intended to be a comprehensive textbook that will cover every exigency in the field; rather, it may serve as a starting point or a guide to clinicians who are interested in doing more work with adolescent patients.

The fact that pediatricians authored this book should not lead the reader to think that we are making a territorial claim to the field. On the contrary, our gynecologist colleagues are extremely important to us. But teenagers are sometimes difficult to lure into the traditional, conservative American health care system; and asking them to see a pediatrician for their immunizations, a dermatologist for their acne, an orthopedist for their sports physical, and a gynecologist for their family planning needs may be overly optimistic. One-stop shopping—particularly in the pediatrician's or family practitioner's office—could go far in preventing much of the major morbidity of adolescence: teen pregnancy and sexually transmitted diseases.

Acknowledgments

Since this book may represent the first volume on adolescent gynecology written exclusively by *pediatricians,* it behooves me to mention and thank our gynecologic colleagues, to whom we are eager to defer when our abilities are surpassed. My thanks to the authors involved in this book, particularly Don Greydanus. All of them are excellent clinicians and teachers, each with their own unique style. Rather than homogenize their efforts, I have chosen instead to let the diversity of their styles shine through. I think that it will make for more interesting reading. My editor at Urban & Schwarzenberg, Charles Mitchell, deserves all the credit for making this project succeed. His enthusiasm and loyalty have been impressive. The enthusiasm and *generosity* of Mr. William Curnow of Ortho Pharmaceutical Corporation, who underwrote the cost of producing the superb color plates in this edition, have been equally impressive. Lastly, I would like to thank three warm and supportive physicians, without whom this book would never have been conceived or written: Dr. John Johnson, Chairman of Pediatrics at the University of New Mexico School of Medicine; Dr. Clark Hansbarger, Deputy Chairman; and Dr. Alison Reeve—my wife.

V.C.S.

To my father, Arthur C. Strasburger, a gentle man and a true
professional, who would have been very proud
*to see his son's book being published by a **Baltimore** publisher.*

Basic
Adolescent Gynecology

1

Current Issues in Adolescent Sexuality

Victor C. Strasburger

In 1990, teenage pregnancy remains the number one threat to the health and welfare of America's teenage females. This threat exists despite the advent and expansion of school-based health clinics, an increased public interest in sex education (due, primarily, to the fear of AIDS), a wider array of lower-dose oral contraceptives (OCs), and continued efforts to expand the availability of contraception for teenagers.

The United States has the highest rate of teenage pregnancy and abortion in the industrialized Western world, according to a 1985 Guttmacher report (Alan Guttmacher Institute, 1986; Trussell, 1988). Despite the fact that American teenagers are no more sexually active than their European peers, the pregnancy rate for American females 15–19 years old stands at 96 per 1,000, compared to a rate of 44 per 1,000 in Britain, 35 per 1,000 in Sweden, and 14 per 1,000 in the Netherlands. Overall, this amounts to more than one million teenage pregnancies in the United States annually, with 400,000 abortions and 470,000 live births (Henshaw and Van Vort, 1989). The majority of births are to unmarried teenagers, under the age of 18, and U.S. girls under age 15 are five times more likely to give birth than young girls in any other Western country surveyed. The report concluded that the lowest rates of teenage pregnancy could be found in countries that had:

1. Nonjudgmental attitudes towards sex
2. Easy access to contraceptive services for young people
3. Availability of contraceptives for free, or at a low cost, without the threat of parental notification
4. Comprehensive sex education programs

In 1987, after reviewing the relevant research and program experience, a National Academy of Sciences Panel on Adolescent Pregnancy and Childbearing published the following recommendations (Panel on Adolescent Pregnancy, 1987):

1. Prevention of teenage pregnancy should have the highest priority in the United States.
2. Sexually active teenagers, both male and female, need access to effective contraceptive methods and increased motivation to use them. Delaying the onset of sexual intercourse would also reduce the rate of teenage pregnancy, but little is known about how to achieve this. Consequently, increasing the availability of contraceptives for teenagers is the best current strategy for lowering the teenage pregnancy rate.

3. Society must learn to associate teenage males as being an equal part of the problem (and the solution).
4. Young people must be taught to make responsible decisions about their sexual behavior.
5. If priorities must be developed, then younger teenagers and those who are most socially and economically disadvantaged should be targeted first.

These studies should help to clarify the pediatrician's potential contributions to the problem into the 1990s. As one Dutch sociologist stated, "How can the richest country in the world allow a situation to continue that would not be tolerated in other countries?" (Dryfoos, 1985).

Adolescent Sexuality

Teenage Sexual Activity

An estimated 12 million of the 29 million young people between the ages of 13 and 19 in the United States have had sexual intercourse—7 million males and 5 million females (Alan Guttmacher Institute, 1981). These data were obtained from the pioneering surveys of Zelnik and Kantner, who surveyed 1,500–2,700 metropolitan teenagers in 1971, 1976, and 1979. Unfortunately, due to lack of funding, they have not continued their surveys in the 1980s. Zelnik and Kantner found that by age 17, 52% of males and 44% of females had experienced sexual intercourse (Zelnick and Kantner, 1980). While these data were alarming, they must still be placed in proper perspective (Strasburger, 1985a): A 15-year-old who had intercourse once and then abstained was classified as being as "sexually active" as a 17-year-old who had intercourse five times a week with multiple partners. In fact, their data revealed that nearly 42% of the sexually active teens had *not* had intercourse within the four weeks prior to being interviewed, and another 25% of the females had had intercourse only once or twice. Nearly one-half of the sexually experienced females reported having only a single partner, and nearly 85% reported no more than three partners (Zelnik, 1983).

Several studies have been conducted in the 1980s, although only one achieves the comprehensive nature of the Zelnik and Kantner surveys—a survey of over 36,000 Minnesota teenagers in 1986–1987 (Zelnik and Kantner, 1980; Coles and Stokes, 1985; Alan Guttmacher Institute, 1986; Harris and Associates, 1986; Hofferth et al., 1987; Mott and Haurin, 1988; Trussell, 1988; Blum, 1989). National studies do exist, but they suffer from small numbers, or the fact that their primary goal was acquisition of information other than about sexual activity. Often such studies fail to survey populations of younger adolescents. One national study used data derived from the National Survey of Family Growth (NSFG), conducted in 1982 (Hofferth et al, 1987). According to this study, certain trends approached but did not reach statistical significance: levels of sexual activity among white teenagers increased during the 1970s and leveled off between 1979 and 1982. For black teenagers, sexual activity levels rose during the early 1970s, leveled off between 1976 and 1979, and declined from 1979 until 1982. However, female teenagers 15 years and under seem to be initiating sexual intercourse at a steadily increasing rate.

In a second study, a representative sample of 1,000 American teenagers were surveyed by Louis Harris and Associates in the fall of 1986 (Harris and Associates, 1986). Of all the 12- to 17-year-olds, nearly 3 of 10 (28%) said they had had sexual intercourse, with the proportion rising steeply from 4% of 12-year-olds to 57% of 17-year-olds (Table 1–1). These data are consistent with the 1970s studies.

In 1986–1987, an intensive effort to collect health data from more than 36,000 Minnesota public school students was initiated by the University of Minnesota (Blum, 1989). Their findings amplified the Zelnik and Kantner surveys and found continued increases in rates of sexual activity among adolescents (Tables 1–2 and 1–3). Among their findings:

- By 12th grade, 55% of females and 70% of males have had intercourse.
- At every age, metropolitan teenagers are more likely to have had intercourse than their more rural counterparts.
- Of sexually active teens, one-third of males and one-fourth of females have initiated sexual relations by the age of 13.
- Teenagers who are sexually active report a pattern of irregular intercourse: 75% have had intercourse either rarely (a few times per year or less) or occasionally (1–4 times per month).

Table 1–1   Sexual Activity of Teenagers in the 1980s

Age total	Percent who had sexual intercourse		Mean
	Males	Females	
12	1	7	4
13	11	10	10
14	31	9	20
15	35	22	29
16	49	42	46
17	61	53	57

Adapted from Louis Harris and Associates, 1986.

Table 1–2   Minnesota Study: Percent Ever Having Had Sexual Intercourse by Grade, Gender, and Region

Gender and region	Grade (%)					
	7th	8th	9th	10th	11th	12th
Females						
Metro	11.2	16.3	26	40.5	45.2	55.2
Greater Minn	5.9	9.2	18.8	30.8	41.4	56.9
Males						
Metro	17.5	25.7	28.6	41.1	57	72.4
Greater Minn	6.6	14.6	18.7	35.9	51.8	70.9

Adapted from Blum, 1989.

Table 1–3   Age at First Sexual Intercourse

Age (years)	Females (%)	Males (%)
10–11	6.4	14.5
12–13	17.0	22.0
14–15	42.8	37.6
16–17	33.2	25.0
	Median age = 14.6 yr	Median age = 14.0 yr

Among adolescents ever having had sexual intercourse.
Adapted from Blum, 1989.

Taken together, the surveys give a picture of slow increases in rates of sexual intercourse among older adolescents and greater increases among younger adolescents (Table 1–4). While the numbers of sexually active 13-year-olds remains small, intercourse at such a young age places the teenager at tremendous health and psychological risk.

Why Do Teenagers Become Sexually Active?

Teenage sexual activity can be viewed from a variety of perspectives—as a normal developmental milestone, a transition-marking behavior, or a risk-taking behavior. Sexual relationships are most appropriate when people can appreciate the distinctions between love and lust, intimacy and sex, and can practice contraception appropriately, and when sexual intercourse occurs in the context of a committed, mature, emotional relationship. Ordinarily, this developmental milestone is achieved by late adolescence (18–21 years) or even later. In a 1985 Roper Poll, in which a national sample of 4,000 men and women aged 18 and older were surveyed, 50% of women and 40% of men believed that premarital sex is immoral, both groups opposed the sexual double standard, and only one of seven women and one of five men were happy with "the new morality," involving greater sexual freedom (Roper Organization, 1985).

Nevertheless, one of the endearing features of adolescence is teenagers' eagerness to cheerfully ignore their elders' sage advice about what is best for them. As Shakespeare noted in "The Winter's Tale": "I wish there were no age between ten and three-and-twenty, or that youth would sleep out the rest; for there is nothing in the between but getting wenches with child, wronging the ancientry, stealing, fighting." Teenagers simply do not need or ask for their parents' permission (or their physician's) before embarking on their initial sexual encounters.

There are numerous possible explanations for why teenagers engage in sexual intercourse (Strasburger, 1985c): 1) attaining more mature, "adult" status; 2) establishing a sense of autonomy and independence; 3) testing their newly developed bodies; 4) testing their capability for intimacy; 5) gaining a sense of physical attractiveness; and 6) rejecting social conventions. But are there specific determinants of early sexual activity? In the landmark study in this area, Jessor and Jessor (Jessor and Jessor, 1975) followed a group of 450 high school and 450 college students longitudi-

Table 1–4   Teenage Sexual Activity

		Age (%)					
		13		15		17	
	N	M	F	M	F	M	F
Zelnik and Kantner (1979)	1,717	14	2	35	19	52	44
NSFG (1982)	1,157	—	—	—	17	—	41
NLSY (1983)	10,846	—	—	18	8	48	33
Coles and Stokes (1985)	1,067	12	6	31	26	38	46
Harris (1986)	1,000	11	10	35	22	57	53
Minnesota (1989)	36,284	17	11	29	26	57	45

Adapted from Zelnik and Kantner, 1980; Coles and Stokes, 1985; Hofferth et al., 1987; Louis Harris and Associates, 1986; Mott and Haurin, 1988; and Blum, 1989.

NSFG, National Survey of Family Growth; NLSY, National Longitudinal Survey of Youth Labor Market Experience.

nally for 4 years to examine, prospectively, the transition from virginity to non-virginity. Characteristics of the group that became sexually active included:

1. They expected and valued achievement less.
2. They tended to be more tolerant of differences between themselves and others.
3. They were less religious.
4. They were more apt to have friends whose views differed from their parents' views.
5. They were more influenced by their peers.
6. They had parents who were less approving of nonconventional behavior and friends who were more approving of it.
7. They engaged in more nonconventional behavior themselves (e.g., lower school performance, less church-going, more use of alcohol and marijuana). A recent survey of over 12,600 young men and women, aged 14–22 years, confirmed the association between drug use and earlier onset of sexual intercourse, particularly for marijuana (Mott and Haurin, 1988). In this context, sexual behavior can be seen as a risk-taking or transitional behavior that may be appealing to certain teenagers for a number of psychological or family reasons.

Alternatively, the increasing number of early sexual relationships can be viewed as a barometer of the state of health of the American family. Adolescents have a special need for close relationships, and if that need is not fulfilled within the family, the adolescent may seek elsewhere or seek other means for satisfying this need. Divorce and poverty may be important contributory factors, according to several studies. In one, white teenagers in fatherless families were 60% more likely to be sexually active (Gordon et al., 1979). In another, daughters in white, female-headed households were more likely to begin sex before age 15 years and to have multiple partners (Akpom et al., 1976). And uniformly throughout the 1970s and 1980s, black teenagers have had higher rates of sexual activity and pregnancy than whites (Hofferth et al., 1987). Several studies also show that a teenager's unhappiness at home or feelings of alienation from one's mother correlates with an earlier age at first intercourse and with having more than two sexual partners (Table 1–5) (Fox, 1979). In a recent study, religious mothers who disapproved of premarital sex tended to have less sexually experienced teenagers (Thornton and Camburn, 1987). Conversely, rates of sexual experience increased among teens whose mothers had had a premarital pregnancy themselves, had married young, or had divorced and remarried (Thornton and Camburn, 1987).

Table 1–5   Sexually Active Teenagers and Their Perceived Relationships with Their Parents

Relationship	% sexually active
Mother + Father +	6.4
Mother − Father −	37.5
Mother + Father −	44.0
Mother − Father +	66.7

Adapted from Welches LJ: Adolescent sexuality. In Mercer R (Ed): *Perspectives on Adolescent Health Care*. JB Lippincott, Philadelphia, 1979.

Religion and conformity to "traditional values"—whether society's or parents'—may also play an important role. However, even conservative religious youth show surprisingly high rates of sexual activity: a 1987 study of 1,438 "born-again" teenagers from eight different religious denominations found that by age 18, 43% had engaged in sexual intercourse (Update, 1988). However, those who were irregular church attenders, not active in youth groups, or who reported that the Bible was not important in their daily lives *were* substantially more likely to have engaged in intercourse (Update, 1988).

Self-esteem has always been considered a major factor in sexual decision-making among adolescents, although it remains unclear whether this is actually true or merely adults' wishful thinking. Studies seem to indicate that success and academic performance correlate negatively with early sexual activity, while other risk-taking behaviors are positively correlated (Davis, 1989). But self-esteem and peer group factors may not be playing the central role here (Davis, 1989). One study of nearly 200 13 to 15-year-olds found that "school self-esteem"—but not "home self-esteem" or "peer self-esteem"—was higher among virgins than nonvirgins (Young, 1989). And a large national study of over 13,000 high school sophomores in 1980–1982 found that three measures alone could explain teenagers' willingness to consider having a child outside of marriage: 1) socioeconomic level, 2) academic ability, and 3) being raised in a single-mother household (Abrahamse et al, 1988).

The 1986 Harris Report confirmed many of these earlier findings (Louis Harris, 1986). Sexual activity was found to be highest among:

1. Teenagers whose parents were not college graduates
2. Teenagers whose school grades averaged C, D, or F
3. Black teenagers

These data may reflect the fact that sexual activity—and certainly, teenage pregnancy—could be socioeconomically predetermined, with more "upwardly mobile" teenagers choosing to delay onset of sexual intercourse. For those who did begin sexual intercourse early in the Harris Report, social pressure was cited as the main reason (73% females, 50% males), with peer pressure also frequently mentioned (28% females, 21% males).

Another crucial determinant of a teenager's decision when and with whom to initiate sexual intercourse may be television (Strasburger, 1985b,e, 1989a,b). With many parents reluctant to teach their children about sex, and many school programs varying in the quality of their health education programs, television has become the leading source of sex education in the United States today (Strasburger, 1985e). It shows teens the adult world to which they were not formerly privy (Meyrowitz, 1985)—a world that contains nearly 14,000 sexual references, innuendoes, and behaviors each year (Sprafkin and Silverman, 1981; Harris and Associates, 1988). Teenage females are particularly avid viewers of afternoon soap operas, where sex is frequently portrayed as being impersonal, emotionless, and exploitative (Sprafkin and Silverman, 1982). On soap operas, unmarried partners are eight times more likely to have sexual relationships than married partners, and 94% of all sexual encounters are between people not married to each other (Greenberg et al., 1981). The sexiest soap opera, "General Hospital," also commands the largest teenage audience (Nielson, 1984).

Interestingly, a sizeable minority of teenagers believe that TV gives a *realistic* picture of sexually transmitted diseases (45%), pregnancy and the consequences of intercourse (41%), use of birth control (27%), and people making love (24%). When

Table 1–6   Sex on Television: Adult vs. Adolescent Perceptions

	TV gives realistic picture (%)	TV gives exaggerated picture (%)	TV doesn't deal much (%)	Unsure (%)
Teenagers (N = 1,000)				
STD's	45	12	34	9
Risk of pregnancy	41	21	27	11
Birth control	28	14	44	13
Making love	24	53	14	10
Adults (N = 1,253)				
STD's	28	6	63	3
Risk of pregnancy	24	25	45	6
Birth control	17	9	68	6
Making love	18	68	11	3

Adapted from Louis Harris and Associates, 1986.

adults were surveyed in a 1985 Harris Poll, they were found to be far more skeptical about TV's portrayal of sexual matters (Table 1–6) (Harris and Associates, 1986).

Scientific evidence that television directly affects adolescent sexual behavior is suggestive but scanty (Strasburger, 1989b). The National Institute of Mental Health summary report on the effects of television on children noted that American teenagers rate the media just behind peers and parents as major influences on their attitudes and behavior (National Institute of Mental Health, 1982). In a 1978 survey, researchers found a significant correlation between the amount of sexually oriented TV watched and the probability of an adolescent having had intercourse (Center for Population Options, 1987). In a 1983 survey, researchers found that a preference for Music Television (MTV) correlated with increased sexual experience among 14- to 16-year-olds (Center for Population Options, 1987). As one former Federal Communications Commissioner noted, "There is no question that children learn from TV. The only question is, what are they learning?" (Strasburger, 1985d). One current television journalist agrees (Ellerbee, 1986):

> Children, if they watched *Dallas*, already have a working familiarity with lust. They learned about impotence from *Donahue*. *Love, Sidney* taught them about homosexuality, and, one hopes, tolerance. *Kojak* told them all about the street names for prostitution and prostitutes. Soap operas offer daily classes in frigidity, menopause, abortion, infidelity and loss of appetite. If they've watched more than one made-for-television movie, they know about rape. Johnny Carson gives graduate courses in divorce and Jerry Falwell has already spoiled all of it with his class—"An Overview of Sin 101." Parents should probably view television as a blessing; after all, it took television to finally get sex education out of the schools and back in the home, where it belongs. Call it educational TV.

Teenage Sexual Practices

While determining the numbers of sexually active teenagers at any one time may have some usefulness to an adult society that finds itself irritated by sexual activity among the young, trying to assess what other sexual practices they engage in besides intercourse holds little, if any, interest. Indeed, since the Kinsey Report was issued 40 years ago, it is difficult enough to find good data about adult sexual practices. A few small studies have tried to look at the range of adolescent sexual activity, and the Minnesota study adds some important information about sexual orientation and homosexuality.

In 1984, psychiatrist Robert Coles organized a survey of 1,067 teenagers nationwide that asked about their intimate sexual practices (Coles and Stokes, 1985). Exactly how representative the sample was is subject to question. Nevertheless, Coles did generate some interesting information about previously unresearched topics—approximately 20% of 13-year-olds, 40% of 15-year-olds, and 60% of 17-year-olds of both sexes had engaged in vaginal play; 41% of 17- to 18-year-old girls reported performing fellatio, and about one-third of 17- to 18-year-old boys reported performing cunnilingus (Coles and Stokes, 1985).

In a small study of 74 affluent 12th grade students and 172 inner-city youth attending an adolescent clinic (mean age for both groups was 17 years), a surprising 27% of the latter group reported having had anal intercourse. Only 7% of the affluent students reported having had anal intercourse. Most importantly, 70% of teenagers reported never using condoms during such intercourse (Jaffe et al., 1988).

A recent study of 366 San Francisco teenagers (mean age 17 years) found higher rates of oral sex: 80% of both sexes reported engaging in oral receptive sex, while 71% of females and 91% of males reported giving oral sex. Rates were highest among white teenagers. For anal sex, 20% of the females and 12% of the males reported at least one experience. While no males reported having had anal sex with another male, 7% of teenagers did report having had sexual relations with someone who had had a same-sex encounter (Broering et al., 1989).

In the Minnesota study—which represents the largest sampling of adolescents to date—90% of males and 83% of females viewed themselves as exclusively heterosexual, and only 1% of 12th grade males and less than 1% of 12th grade females viewed themselves as mostly or completely homosexual. Over 10% of teenagers were unsure about their sexual orientation (Blum, 1989).

Much more complete information is needed before intelligent prevention programs can be shaped; yet, in the Reagan-Bush era, such research seems highly unlikely on a national scale.

Teenage Contraceptive Practices

Although the subject of contraception for teenagers is, unfortunately, a controversial one, establishing a birth control clinic in every school and on every street corner in the United States would still not eradicate the problem of teenage pregnancy (Strasburger, 1985b,c). As a rule, teenage females do not usually think about using a medical means of birth control until after they have been sexually active for 6–12 months; yet, half of all teenage pregnancies occur in the first 6 months after initiation of intercourse, and 20% occur during the first month alone (Zabin et al., 1979). Nevertheless, significant inroads have been made in the past decade: According to the Alan Guttmacher Institute, contraceptive use averts 680,000 teenage pregnancies a year (Dryfoos, 1985).

Although they remain controversial, school-based health clinics (SBHCs) have made a dramatic impact on teenage pregnancy rates in certain schools—primarily, those clinics which offer comprehensive health services, on-site dispensing of contraceptives, and sex education in the classroom that is led by the clinic personnel. The ''gold standard'' for school-based health clinics—the one established in St. Paul,

Minnesota in the mid-1970s—has successfully cut the birth rate in multiple schools by 40%–50%, with a repeat pregnancy rate of only 1.4% within 2 years (Edwards et al., 1977; Dryfoos and Klerman, 1988). Baltimore's school-based project also shows evidence of success (Zabin et al., 1986; Hardy et al., 1987).

By 1990, there will be an estimated 200 SBHCs in the United States (Lovick, 1988). Not all are likely to be successful in lowering the teenage pregnancy rates in their communities. In most clinics, only 20%–30% of health visits are for family planning services (Lovick and Wesson, 1986). Some clinics operate only part-time, while others may not attract a majority of the school's sexually active population. But most importantly, only a handful of school clinics dispense contraceptives on-site. It is entirely possible that there is a direct correlation between the likelihood of using a medical method of contraception (and therefore, a lower rate of teen pregnancy) and the distance a teenager is forced to travel from a school clinic that does not dispense contraception to a local health facility that does. At present, all of the data available indicate that unless a full-scale approach like the one in St. Paul is adopted, the average SBHC will not have a significant impact on either teenage pregnancy rates or rates of sexual activity in its school (D. Kirby, personal communication, 1988).

Although contraceptives are more widely available than ever before, there is still considerable disparity between the initiation of sexual intercourse and the consistent use of reliable contraception. In the earliest surveys in the 1970s, use of contraceptives at first intercourse was shown to be heavily age-dependent, rising from less than 25% of under 15-year-olds to 41% of 15- to 17-year-olds and 55% of 18- to 19-year-olds (Baldwin, 1983). In their surveys, Zelnik and Kantner found that use of BCPs or an intrauterine device (IUD) actually decreased 40% at first intercourse by 1979, while withdrawal had doubled. At most recent intercourse, use of BCPs or IUDs had dropped 50%, while withdrawal increased 30% and use of the rhythm method increased 50% (Zelnik and Kanter, 1980). Data collected from the National Survey of Family Growth (NSFG) conducted in 1982, using a national sample of nearly 8,000 women 15–44 years of age, confirmed the fact that only 33%–50% of teenage women use a contraceptive at first intercourse and that age is the single most important predictor. Of those who practice contraception, 30%–40% use condoms, 20%–30% use withdrawal, and only 10%–20% use BCPs. The study also showed that the chances of using contraception at first intercourse increased with being white, having a mother who had more than a high school education, delaying first coitus until age 19 or later, and living within an intact family (Mosher and Bachrach, 1987). In a sample of black teenagers aged 13–19 in Chicago, the most important predictors of first-time use were social class, neighborhood quality, and parents' marital status (Hogan et al., 1985)—the first two of which may be reflections of the teens' upward mobility.

Again, the Minnesota study in 1986–1987 offers some impressive insights into adolescent contraception and perhaps the first encouraging news in a long time (Tables 1–7 and 1–8) (Blum, 1989):

- Overall, 77% of sexually active teenagers reported using some form of contraception.
- Use of contraception increased from 67% of 7th graders to nearly 90% of 11th-12th graders.
- Overall, condoms were the most popular form of contraception (41%), followed by oral contraceptives (30% of 11th-12th graders).
- Unfortunately, the use of withdrawal increased with age as well, doubling from 9% of 7th graders to 18% of 12th graders.

Table 1–7   Contraceptive Habits of Sexually Active Youth (Minnesota Study)

	Grades 7-8 (%)	Grades 9-10 (%)	Grades 11-12 (%)
Condom	33	20	12
Oral contraceptives	8	12	30
Withdrawal	9	17	18
Other	4	3	2
Don't use	46	48	39

Adapted from Blum, 1989.

Table 1–8   Frequency of Primary Contraception Use Among Sexually Active Teens Who Use Contraception (Minnesota Study)

	Grades 7–8 (%)	Grades 9–10 (%)	Grades 11–12 (%)
Oral contraception			
Always	54	77	87
Often/sometimes	26	16	10
Rarely	20	7	3
Condoms			
Always	49	55	57
Often/sometimes	27	29	33
Rarely	25	16	10
Withdrawal			
Always	26	27	23
Often/sometimes	29	25	23
Rarely	45	49	54

Adapted from Blum, 1989.

Not only do researchers know why certain teenagers use contraception, they know why others do not (Fig. 1–1) (Zelnik and Kantner, 1979; Alan Guttmacher Institute, 1981; Strasburger, 1985c). The idiosyncrasies of adolescent psychology seem to combine to conspire against successful contraception during early adolescence. Teenagers often see themselves egocentrically as being actors in their own personal fable, in which the normal rules (e.g., having unprotected sexual intercourse may cause an unwanted pregnancy) may apply to everyone but themselves (Elkind, 1978). Even though 70% of teenagers are able by age 16 to reach the final level of cognitive operational thought described by Piaget (Piaget, 1969)—sequential logical thinking (formal operations)—they may still suffer from what Elkind calls "pseudostupidity": "the capacity to conceive many different alternatives is not immediately coupled with the ability to assign priorities and to decide which choice is more or less appropriate than others" (Elkind, 1984).

What role sex education and communication within the family play in the teenager's decision whether to use contraception or not has been controversial for many years. Sex education has been controversial because conservative elements within the society have long held that it gives teenagers ideas that they otherwise would never have. Yet how can a one-semester course in sex education—no matter how graphic— compete with 10 or 15 years of parental, peer, media, and religious influences? All children receive sex education at home—watching whether their parents are affectionate with each other, observing their parents' reaction to sexy programs on television,

Why teenagers fail to use birth control

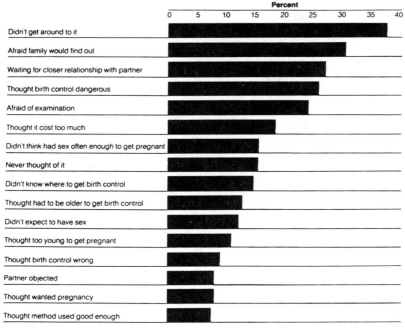

Percent of teenage clinic patients getting medical birth control help for the first time, citing reasons
for delaying the clinic visit, 1980. Percentages do not add to 100 because some patients gave more than one answer.

1–1   Percent of teenagers seeking birth control at their first clinic visit, citing
reasons why they delayed. Percentages do not add to 100 because some patients
gave more than one answer. (*Source: Teenage Pregnancy: The Problem That Hasn't
Gone Away*, p. 45, Figure 42. © 1981 The Alan Guttmacher Institute.)

listening to their parents' conversations with other adults, etc. According to every study
to date, those children who receive sex education at school are no more likely to become
sexually active than they are to become historians because they are taught history. Nor,
for the same reasons, are they likely to become sexually active at a later age than if they
had not been offered the course (Kirby, 1980; Furstenberg et al., 1985; Dawson, 1986;
Alan Guttmacher Institute, 1989; Stout and Rivara, 1989).

In 1988, the Alan Guttmacher Institute undertook a survey of state policies on
sex education (Fig. 1–2) (Alan Guttmacher Institute, 1989; Kenney et al, 1989).
Interestingly, they found considerable support for the concept of sex education in the
schools. However, the reason for such programs had little to do with teenage pregnancy
or contraception. Of the nearly $6.3 million states spent on sex education in
1987–1988, $5.1 million was designated specifically for AIDS education. In a related
study, nearly one-third of sex education teachers said their biggest problem was
pressure from parents and administrators, especially if they tried to deal with the issues
of homosexuality, condoms, or abortion (Forrest and Silverman, 1989). Only six states
allow explicit discussion about condoms. While 32 states require or encourage instruc-
tion about pregnancy prevention—and Alabama and Utah either discourage or prohibit
it—only Delaware and Georgia specifically deal with risks and benefits of all contraceptive methods (Kenney et al., 1989).

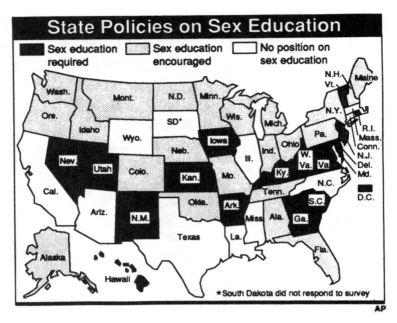

1–2 (Source: *Risk and Responsibility—Teaching Sex Education in America's Schools Today*, p. 2. © 1989 The Alan Guttmacher Institute.)

All of the available data point to the fact that sex education programs: 1) increase students' awareness and knowledge of human reproduction and methods of contraception, and 2) increase students' tolerance of others' sexual behavior (without any change in the values that regulate their own behavior). Whether such programs can actually increase students' use of contraception is still problematical. Zelnik and Kim's work showed no increased use after sex education in school (Zelnik and Kim, 1982). Later researchers may have uncovered the reason for this: a 1984 survey revealed that a large proportion of teenagers may be initiating sexual activity before they can even be exposed to a sex education course. Among teenage females who were sexually active, only 48% of 15-year-olds and 61% of 18-year-olds had received sex education in school. For sexually active males, only 26% of 15-year-olds and 52% of 18-year-olds took a course. Only among older sexually active teenage women was there a trend towards sex education causing increased use of contraception, and the trend was only slight (73% versus 64% among females not taking a program) (Marsiglio and Mott, 1986).

One persistent misconception (and barrier to the expansion of school-based health clinics, for example) is the notion that increased availability of contraceptives will make teenagers more sexually promiscuous. Not only do a variety of data indirectly disprove this hypothesis—e.g., the majority of adolescents seeking birth control at clinics are already sexually active (Reichelt, 1979; Zabin et al., 1979), and only 30% of teenagers use contraceptives at first intercourse (Louis Harris and Associates, 1986)—but also an early and frequently overlooked study looked specifically at this notion (Reichelt, 1978). Using a 1-year follow-up study of 213 teenage women receiving BCPs from a clinic in a midwestern city, Reichelt found that although there was some increase in frequency of coitus 1 year later, there was no increase in numbers of sexual partners (Tables 1–9 and 1–10) (Reichelt, 1978).

Table 1–9   Frequency of Intercourse Before and After Obtaining OCs

Frequency of intercourse/ month	Baseline (N = 196) (%)	1 year later (N = 207) (%)
0	15	11
1	23	14
2–4	35	26
5–7	9	15
8–10	8	15
11 +	10	19

Adapted from Reichelt, 1978.

Table 1–10   Number of Sexual Partners Before and After Obtaining OCs

Number of partners	Initial (N = 196) (%)	1 year later (N = 209) (%)
0	15	11
1	76	82
2	8	5
3	1	2

Adapted from Reichelt, 1978.

Role of the Physician

How Physicians and Teenagers Perceive Each Other

Adolescents are clearly ambivalent about seeing their family physician for contraceptive care. A Canadian survey revealed that teenagers are afraid that their family doctors will tell their parents (57%) or that the teens themselves will be embarrassed (53%) or not able to talk freely (28%) (Herold and Goodwin, 1979). In turn, many physicians—particularly pediatricians—are ambivalent about seeing teenage patients or prescribing contraceptives for them. A recent survey by Comerci (Comerci, 1983) showed that 20% of pediatricians responding did not want to see adolescents in their practice, and an additional 26% admitted that their knowledge of adolescent medicine was inadequate. Compared with gynecologists and family practitioners, pediatricians are the least likely to want to treat teenage patients (Chamie et al, 1982) (Table 1–11) and the least likely to prescribe BCPs to a sexually active 15-year-old female (Table 1–12) (Orr, 1984).

In the Harris Report (Harris and Associates, 1986) the following factors were highest ranked in evaluating teenagers' use or lack of use of family planning clinics versus their family physicians:

1. Guaranteeing confidentiality (78%)
2. Cost (75%)
3. Easy access (70%)

Confidentiality is clearly a key issue for most adolescents. However, another study has documented that middle-class teenagers, at least, would be willing and able to pay for physician services. In a survey of 165 middle-class teenagers in New York, 94% indicated that they would be able and willing to pay a fee: two-thirds could pay as much as $10, half could pay $15, and one-fifth could pay $20 or more (Fisher et al, 1985).

Table 1-11   Physician Specialties and Willingness to Treat Adolescent Patients

	Ob-Gyn (%)	F.P. (%)	Ped. (%)
Treat teenagers	99	92	48
Treat teens under age 18	99	87	45
Treat teens under age 18 and on own consent	81	62	36

Adapted from Chamie et al., 1982.
Ob-Gyn, obstetrician-gynecologist; F.P., family practitioner; Ped., pediatrician.

Table 1-12   How Different Specialists Would Treat a 15-Year-Old Seeking Contraceptives

Speciality	Serve (%)	Refer (%)	Do neither (%)
Ob-Gyn ($N=541$)	92	3	5
F.P. ($N=265$)	66	17	17
Pediatrician ($N=401$)	32	61	7

Adapted from Orr, 1984.

One important additional consideration may be the pelvic examination itself. In the Harris Report, 69% of teenage females said that this requirement frightened them away, and an equal percentage of those who had actually undergone a pelvic exam said that they still had a fear of them (Harris and Associates, 1986).

Even if physicians decide that they are unwilling to provide contraceptive services for teens, they must still learn to routinely ask "the sexual question" of any young woman they are asked to evaluate, particularly those with abdominal pains, vaginal symptoms, or dysuria (Demetriou et al., 1982; Braverman and Strasburger, 1989). With the incidence of pelvic inflammatory disease in 15- to 19-year-olds as high as 1 in 8 (Washington et al, 1985), obtaining a sexual history becomes absolutely crucial if, for example, unnecessary appendectomies are to be avoided. A Massachusetts pediatrician interviewed 244 young people coming to her office for a routine physical exam and asked them about their sexual activity and their previous health exams. Only 22% of the females and 4% of the males, all aged 13-18, said that their doctors had ever asked them about their sexual activity. And among the teenagers who were sexually active at the time of the initial interview, 62% had never been asked about it (Fine and Jacobson, 1986). A study of teenage females in the Stanford Hospital Emergency Room showed that a sexual history was elicited from 100% of minority females but only 44% of whites and only 27% of those under 15 years of age (Hunt and Litt, 1982). *No medical history of a teenager—male or female—is complete without a sexual history* (Braverman and Strasburger, 1989).

Physicians and the Law

One reason pediatricians may be loath to treat adolescents, particularly for contraceptive counseling, may be the fear of legal repercussions (analagous to the teenager's fear of parental repercussions). For example, a 1982 survey of Connecticut physicians showed that only 1 of 79 pediatricians could successfully answer a basic quiz on the legal aspects of treating teenagers in that state (Strasburger and Eisner, 1982).

Nearly two decades ago, the Rockefeller Commission on Population strongly recommended that teenagers be accorded free access to contraceptives. This finding was rejected by President Nixon as fostering immoral activities and destroying parental control of children (Blake, 1973). When California passed a statute allowing teenagers the right to consent for contraceptive care, Governor Ronald Reagan vetoed it, stating that the bill "represented the unwarranted intrusion into the prerogatives of parents . . . . and would endanger the traditional vital role of the family . . . . Birth control should begin with—prior to marriage—saying no" (Bodine, 1973).

Despite these pronouncements, the Supreme Court extended to minors the "right of privacy" regarding procreative decisions in a 1977 decision, *Carey v. Population Services International* (431 U.S. 693, 1977). More recently, a federal court of appeals in Michigan held in the case of *Doe v. Irwin* that a state-supported county clinic that counseled teenagers and prescribed birth control without parental consent or notification was under no obligation to do so against the wishes of the teenager. The Supreme Court refused to review the case (615 F. 2d. 1162, 6th Cir. 1980, cert. denied, 101 S. Ct. 95).

In January, 1983, President Reagan attempted to create a federal regulation that clinics receiving federal funds would have to notify, within 10 days, the parents of minors who had sought contraceptive services. The proposed regulation drew over 120,000 written comments to the Department of Health and Human Services—most of them unfavorable. The so-called "squeal rule" was overturned by rulings in federal courts of appeal in Washington and New York later that year, and in December 1983 the Reagan administration announced that it was giving up on its attempt (Associated Press, 1983) (*Planned Parenthood Federation of America v. Heckler*, 712 F. 2d 650 (D.C. Cir. 1983); *New York v. Heckler*, 719 F. 2d 1191 (2d Cir. 1983)).

Physicians need to familiarize themselves with the laws and rulings in their states that affect adolescent health care. But, in general, the following principles are uniform throughout the United States (Holder, 1985; Strasburger et al., 1985):

Parental Consent
1. When possible, it is always preferable to obtain parental consent, or at least inquire about the feasibility of obtaining it.

Mature Minors
1. By state statute in many states (Fig. 1–3) or by common law (judge-granted), a "mature minor" can consent to his or her own health care. Who qualifies as being "mature" is left to the judgment of the health professional, but most typically it is someone at least 15 years of age, who is capable of understanding the risks and benefits of medical treatment and, therefore, is able to give an informed consent.
2. In the past 20 years, there has not been a successful suit against a physician for treatment of a "mature minor" without parental consent, even in states without mature minor statutes (except in cases of nontherapeutic sterilization or organ/tissue donation).

Contraception
1. A physician who prescribes contraceptives to a mature minor without parental consent or notification faces little risk of liability.
2. However, the physician's record should document:
    a. that the patient is at risk of pregnancy and qualifies as a mature minor
    b. that inquiry about the feasibility of parental consent has been made

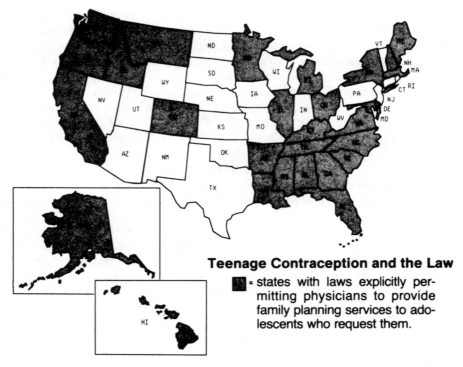

Teenage Contraception and the Law

█ = states with laws explicitly permitting physicians to provide family planning services to adolescents who request them.

1–3   From: Levine C: Beyond the squeal rule. *Medica 1*:21-23, 1984, with permission.

      c.   that a full medical and sexual history and appropriate physical and pelvic exams have been done

      d.   that the risks and benefits of the contraceptive method have been explained in detail and understood

3.   There is no history of a successful suit against a physician for prescribing birth control for a minor. One reason for this may be that a lawsuit is a matter of public record, and no parent wants their teenagers' sexual activities publicized in the local newspaper.

4.   The status of the immature minor remains very unclear. However, if a 13-year-old girl is sexually active, there is a high likelihood that her family is dysfunctional and that the mother is aware of her activities.

Abortion

1.   Several Supreme Court rulings (e.g., *H.L. v. Matheson* in 1981, *City of Akron v. Akron Center for Reproductive Health* in 1983) have reaffirmed that states may require, by statute, parental consent or notification before an abortion is performed on a minor. However, in such a situation, the minor must have access to an alternative to obtaining her parents' consent—typically, a court hearing in which she can demonstrate sufficient maturity to make the abortion decision herself. In such proceedings, the judge merely determines if the minor is "mature," or, if not, then whether the abortion would be in her "best interests." More recently, the U.S. Supreme Court permitted a 15-year-old Florida teenager to obtain an

abortion without parental consent (Associated Press, 1989). The Florida parental consent for abortions law had been declared unconstitutional by a state appeals court, since it did not conform with the judicial bypass system instituted by the Supreme Court in 1983.

2. If no state statute exists that restricts a minor's access to abortion, and she qualifies as a "mature minor," she can consent to an abortion as she would to any other medical treatment.

3. Under *no circumstances* should an abortion be performed when the patient herself refuses to give her consent, regardless of her degree of maturity or the wishes of her parents.

4. The impact of parental notification laws on adolescent abortions remains unclear, but two preliminary studies indicate that such laws do not decrease the number of adolescent abortions, do not increase communication with parents, and may simply force teenagers seeking abortions to go to court or travel out of state (Cartoof and Klerman, 1986; Blum et al., 1987).

Note: On July 3, 1989, the U.S. Supreme Court handed down its ruling in *Webster v. Reproductive Health Services.* A deeply divided Court (5-4) upheld a Missouri statute that prohibited state facilities and state employees from performing abortions in Missouri and mandated tests of viability in pregnancies beyond 20 weeks gestation (Carlson, 1989). The ruling itself may not have much practical, immediate impact on the ability of teenagers to obtain abortions, but the significance of the decision extends far beyond this. Clearly, four Justices are now ready to overturn *Roe v. Wade* and allow states greater discretion in regulating abortions, four want to keep the right to abortion intact, and Justice O'Connor sits squarely in the middle (Carlson, 1989). In addition, the decision may signal the beginning of a series of campaigns on a state-by-state level to implement legislation similar to Missouri's (Cassidy, 1989; Hoggart, 1989). This could conceivably have a "chilling effect" on teenagers' decisions to seek abortions. Finally, the Supreme Court has agreed to hear three additional cases in its Fall term beginning in October 1989. Two of the cases involve parental notification and the third would require abortion clinics to meet hospital-level guidelines. Any of the three could provide an opportunity to overturn *Roe* or allow the Court to make further in-roads into women's access to abortion.

Solutions

Physicians

Over 15 years ago, Dr. Adele Hofmann published an article in *Clinical Pediatrics* entitled, "Identifying and Counselling the Sexually Active Adolescent Is Every Physician's Responsibility." In it, she concluded (Hofmann, 1972):

> For an adolescent girl to have become pregnant because of ignorance about contraception, because she cannot bring herself to confide in parents, and because physicians have avoided their responsibility in taking the initiative in this area is indeed a harsh and cruel price for her and her consort to pay. It is time that all physicians and parents recognize the rights and needs of adolescents to receive health care for sensitive matters under the same confidential terms as are afforded to adults. The primary care physician who looks

upon pregnancy prevention as being as much his responsibility as all other facets of preventative medicine—and acts on this responsibility—will be welcomed by many of his adolescent patients as meeting an essential need.

Physicians—especially pediatricians—can be the prime-movers in the attempt to decrease teenage pregnancy. But first they must be willing to re-educate themselves about adolescent gynecology and performing pelvic exams (Magee, 1975; Adler, 1983) and accept the fact that sizeable numbers of teenagers are at risk of pregnancy or sexually transmitted disease (Blum, 1987).

Parents

Sex education begins at home, although it does not necessarily need to be confined there. Several studies demonstrate that parental sex education may have some protective effect (i.e., delay onset of intercourse or increase use of contraception) (Strasburger, 1985b,c), while school-based sex education programs probably do no more than make teenagers more knowledgeable about sexual matters and their own and others' sexual attitudes. The need for joint parent-school ventures into this area is clear: such cooperation might enable increased numbers of parents to communicate effectively with their children and feel less apprehensive about material presented in school. But if society, in general, wants to diminish the toll of teenage pregnancy, then the need is clear—no more retreats! (Gordon, 1982; Kirby, 1984; Selverstone, 1985).

Society

While the concept of postponing adolescent sexual involvement is ideal, such an idea may not be practical. Certainly, the notion of "just say no" is far too superficial (and insulting to the intelligence of most adolescents) to offer much practical help (Strasburger, 1986). Giving teenagers the reasons *why* they should say "no" and the communication skills and assertiveness training they need to be able to resist sexual pressures may prove more fruitful, but such programs are still being field-tested (Howard, 1985). Acknowledging that teenagers are capable of saying "yes"—and that the decision is theirs alone—but trying to convince them that it is ultimately in their own best interests to say "no" may prove to be the wisest course to follow.

The evolution of teenage pregnancy programs (Weatherley et al., 1986) and school-based health clinics (Kenney, 1986) has contributed much to the efforts to lower the number of teenage pregnancies, but such efforts still need to be amplified. The prototypical clinic in St. Paul, Minnesota lowered pregnancy rates by more than 50% and showed contraceptive continuance rates of 93% at 12 months, for example (Kenney, 1986), but such clinics do not reach street youth, teenagers in elementary or middle schools, or even high school teens in communities that are opposed to such a concept. Wider dissemination of information and wider availability of contraceptives and counseling are still needed.

A noted child psychiatrist has observed: "The ambivalence of Western society toward sexuality—manifested by the conflicts between official attitudes and private behavior, and the pervasive emphasis on sex side by side with sanctions against its expression—accounts for the difficulty, so common in adolescence, of attaining the basis for a sense of competence, freedom, and pleasure as a sexually functioning adult" (Eisenberg, 1965). The proof of this pudding lies in the portrayal of sex on American television: until writers and producers show sex responsibly—sex within committed relationships, sex with bad consequences, sex accompanied by birth control—American children and adolescents will continue to receive large doses of sex education from a highly stimulating but inaccurate and misleading source (Strasburger, 1989a,b). The American Academy of Pediatrics and many other organizations have called for the airing of contraceptive advertising on national television (Committee on Adolescence, 1986). Such a step would represent "one small step" towards redressing an imbalance that has become increasingly worse in the past two decades.

References

Abrahamse AF, Morrison PA, Waite LJ: Teenagers willing to consider single parenthood: Who is at greatest risk? *Fam Plann Perspect* 20:13–18, 1988.

Adler J: Pelvic examination of the adolescent. *Res Staff Phys* 29:43–58, 1983.

Akpom AC, Akpom KL, Davis M: Prior sexual behavior of teenagers attending rap sessions for the first time. *Fam Plann Perspect* 8:203–206, 1976.

Alan Guttmacher Institute: *Teenage Pregnancy: The Problem that Hasn't Gone Away.* Yale University Press, New Haven, 1981.

Alan Guttmacher Institute: *Teenage Pregnancy in Developed Countries.* Yale University Press, New Haven, 1986.

Alan Guttmacher Institute: *Risk and Responsibility: Teaching Sex Education in America's Schools Today.* Alan Guttmacher Institute, New York, 1989.

Associated Press: Court Overturns 'Squeal Rule.' New Haven Journal-Courier, December 1, 1983.

Associated Press: Supreme Court Voids Florida Consent Law. Albuquerque Journal, May 19, 1989.

Baldwin W: Trends in adolescent contraception, pregnancy, and childbearing. In McAnarney ER (Ed): *Premature Adolescent Pregnancy and Parenthood.* Grune & Stratton, New York, 1983.

Blake J: The teenage birth control dilemma and public opinion. *Science* 180:708–712, 1973.

Blum RW: Contemporary threats to adolescent health in the United States. *JAMA* 257: 3390–3395, 1987.

Blum RW: *The State of Adolescent Health in Minnesota.* Univ. of Minnesota, Minneapolis, 1989.

Blum RW, Resnick MD, Stark TA: The impact of a parental notification law on adolescent abortion decision-making. *Am J Public Health* 77:619–620, 1987.

Bodine N: Minors and contraceptives: A constitutional issue. *Ecology Law Q* 859:860, 1973.

Braverman PK, Strasburger VC: Why adolescent gynecology?—Pediatricians and pelvic exams. *Pediatr Clin North Am* 36(3):471–488, 1989.

Broering J, Moscicki B, Millstein S: Sexual practices among adolescents. Paper presented at Society for Adolescent Medicine Annual Meeting. San Francisco, March 19–22, 1989.

Carlson M: The battle over abortion. *Time*, July 17, 1989, pp. 32–33.

Cartoof V, Klerman L: Parental consent for abortion: Impact of the Massachusetts law. *Am J Public Health* 76:397–400, 1986.

Cassidy J: US abortion ruling divides a nation. *The Sunday Times* (London), July 9, 1989, p. C4.

Center for Population Options: *Fact Sheet: Adolescent Sexuality and the Media.* Center for Population Options, Washington, DC, 1987.

Chamie M, Eisman S, Forrest JD: Factors affecting adolescents' use of family planning clinics. *Fam Plann Perspect* 14:126–139, 1982.

Coles R, Stokes G: *Sex and the American Teenager.* Harper & Row, New York, 1985.

Comerci G: Adolescent medicine and the pediatrician: Changes and controversies. Presented at American Academy of Pediatrics Annual Meeting. San Francisco, October 24, 1983.

Committee on Adolescence: Sexuality, contraception, and the media. *Pediatrics* 78:535–536, 1986.

Davis S: Pregnancy in adolescents. *Pediatr Clin North Am* 36(3):665–680, 1989.

Dawson DA: The effects of sex education on adolescent behavior. *Fam Plann Perspect* 18:162–170, 1986.

Demetriou E, Emans SJ, Masland RP: Dysuria in adolescent girls: Urinary tract infection or vaginitis? *Pediatrics* 70:299–301, 1982.

Dryfoos J: What the United States can learn about prevention of teenage pregnancy from other developed countries. *SIECUS Rep* XIV:1–7, 1985.

Dryfoos JG, Klerman LV: School-based clinics: Their role in helping students meet the 1990 objectives. *Health Educ Q* 15:71–80, 1988.

Edwards LE, Steinman ME, Hakanson EY: An experimental comprehensive high school clinic. *Am J Public Health* 67:765–766, 1977.

Eisenberg L: A developmental approach to adolescence. *Children* 12:131–135, 1965.

Elkind D: Understanding the young adolescent. *Adolescence* 13:127–134, 1978.

Elkind D: Teenage thinking: Implications for health care. *Pediatr Nurs* 2:383–385, 1984.

Ellerbee L: *"And So It Goes"—Adventures in Television.* G. P. Putnam's Sons, New York, 1986, p. 34.

Fine JS, Jacobson MS: Physician assessment of adolescent sexual activity. *Fam Plann Perspect* 18:233–237, 1986.

Fisher M, Marks A, Trieller K, et al: Are adolescents able and willing to pay the fee for confidential health care? *J Pediatr* 107:480–483, 1985.

Forrest JD, Silverman J: What public school teachers teach about preventing pregnancy, AIDS and sexually transmitted diseases. *Fam Plann Perspect* 21:65–72, 1989.

Fox GL: The family's influence on adolescent sexual behavior. *Child Today* 8:21–36, 1979.

Furstenberg FF, Moore KA, Peterson JL: Sex education and sexual experience among adolescents. *Am J Public Health* 75:1331–1332, 1985.

Gordon S: Sexuality education in the 1980s—No more retreats. *J Sex Ed Ther* 8:6–8, 1982.

Gordon S, Scales P, Everly K: *The Sexual Adolescent*, 2nd ed. Duxbury Press, North Scituate, MA, 1979.

Greenberg BS, Abelman R, Neuendorf K: Sex on the soap operas: Afternoon delight. *J Commun* 31:83–89, 1981.

Hardy JB, King TM, Repke JT: The Johns Hopkins' adolescent pregnancy program: An evaluation. *Obstet Gynecol* 69:300–306, 1987.

Harris L and Associates: *American Teens Speak: Sex, Myths, TV, and Birth Control.* Louis Harris and Associates, New York, 1986.

Harris L and Associates: Sexual Material on American Network Television During the 1987–88 Season. Planned Parenthood Association, New York, 1988.

Henshaw SK, Van Vort J: Teenage abortion, birth, and pregnancy statistics: An update. *Fam Plann Perspect* 21:85–88, 1989.

Herold ES, Goodwin MS: Why adolescents go to birth-control clinics rather than to their family physicians. *Can J Public Health* 70:317–320, 1979.

Hofferth SL, Kahn JR, Baldwin W: Premarital sexual activity among U.S. teenage women over the past three decades. *Fam Plann Perspect* 19:46–53, 1987.

Hofmann A: Identifying and counseling the sexually active adolescent is every physician's responsibility. *Clin Pediatr (Phila)* 11:625–629, 1972.

Hogan D, Astone N, Kitagawa E: The impact of social status, family structure, and neighborhood on the fertility of black adolescents. *Am J Sociol* 90:825–855, 1985.

Hoggart S: Abortion judgment creates States of war. *Sunday Observer* (London), July 9, 1989, p. 29.

Holder AR: *Legal Issues in Pediatrics and Adolescent Medicine*, 2nd ed. Yale University Press, New Haven, 1985.

Howard M: Postponing sexual involvement among adolescents. *J Adolesc Health Care* 6:271–277, 1985.

Hunt AD, Litt IF: Obtaining a sexual history and diagnostic labeling: The influence of ethnicity and age (abstr). *J Adolesc Health Care* 3:139, 1982.

Jaffe LR, Seehaus M, Wagner C, et al: Anal intercourse and knowledge of acquired immunodeficiency syndrome among minority-group female adolescents. *J Pediatr* 112:1005–1007, 1988.

Jessor SL, Jessor R: Transition from virginity to nonvirginity among youth: A social-psychological study over time. *Dev Psychol* 11:473–484, 1975.

Kenney AM: School-based clinics: A national conference. *Fam Plann Perspect* 18:44–46, 1986.

Kenney AM, Guardado S, Brown L: Sex education and AIDS education in the schools: What states and large school districts are doing. *Fam Plann Perspect* 21:56–64, 1989.

Kirby D: The effects of school sex education programs: A review of the literature. *J Sch Health* 50:559–563, 1980.

Kirby D: *Sexuality Education: An Evaluation of Programs and Their Effects, An Executive Summary*. Mathech, Inc., Bethesda, MD, 1984.

Lovick SR: What about school-based health clinics? *PTA Today* February, 1988, pp. 21–23.

Lovick SR, Wesson WF: *School-Based Clinics: An Update*. Center for Population Options, Washington, DC, 1986.

Magee J: The pelvic exam: A view from the other end of the table. *Ann Intern Med* 83:563–564, 1975.

Marsiglio W, Mott FL: The impact of sex education on sexual activity, contraceptive use and premarital pregnancy among American teenagers. *Fam Plann Perspect* 18:151–161, 1986.

Meyrowitz J: *No Sense of Place: The Impact of Electronic Media on Social Behavior*. Oxford University Press, New York, 1985.

Mosher WD, Bachrach CA: First premarital contraceptive use: United States, 1960–1982. *Stud Fam Plann* 18:83–95, 1987.

Mott FL, Haurin RJ: Linkages between sexual activity and alcohol and drug use among American adolescents. *Fam Plann Perspect* 20(3):128–136, 1988.

National Institute of Mental Health: *Television and Behavior: Ten Years of Scientific Progress and Implications for the Eighties*: Summary Report, vol. 1. National Institute of Mental Health, Bethesda, MD, 1982.

Nielson AC Company: *Report on Television*. A. C. Nielson Co., New York, 1984.

Orr MT: Private physicians and the provision of contraceptives to adolescents. *Fam Plann Perspect* 16:83–86, 1984.

Panel on Adolescent Pregnancy and Childbearing: Risking the future: A symposium on the National Academy of Sciences report on teenage pregnancy. *Fam Plann Perspect* 19:119–125, 1987.

Panel on Adolescent Pregnancy and Childbearing, National Research Council: *Risking the Future: Adolescent Sexuality, Pregnancy, and Childbearing*. National Academy Press, Washington, DC, 1987.

Piaget J: The intellectual development of the adolescent. In Caplan G, Lebovici E (eds): *Adolescence—Psychosocial Perspectives*. Basic Books, New York, 1969.

Reichelt PA: Changes in sexual behavior among unmarried teenage women utilizing oral contraception. *J Pop Behav Soc Environ Issues* 1:57–68, 1978.

Reichelt PA: Coital and contraceptive behavior of female adolescents. *Arch Sex Behav* 8:159–172, 1979.

The Roper Organization: *The 1985 Virginia Slims American Women's Opinion Poll*. The Roper Organization, New York, 1985.

Selverstone R: Sex education and the adolescent: Perspectives from a sex educator. *Semin Adolesc Med* 1:145–151, 1985.

Shakespeare W: *The Winter's Tale*, Act III, scene 3, lines 58–62. New American Library, New York, 1963, p. 90.

Sprafkin J, Silverman LT: Sex on prime time. In Schwarz M (ed): *TV and Teens*. Addison-Wesley, Reading, MA, 1982.

Sprafkin JN, Silverman LT: Update: Physically intimate and sexual behavior on prime-time television. *J Commun* 31:34–40, 1981.

Stout JW, Rivara FP: Schools and sex education: Does it work? *Pediatrics* 83:375–379, 1989.

Strasburger V: Sex, drugs, rock 'n' roll: An introduction. *Pediatrics* 76(Suppl):659–663, 1985a.

Strasburger VC: Sex, drugs, rock 'n' roll: Are solutions possible?—a commentary. *Pediatrics* (Suppl) 76:704–712, 1985b.

Strasburger VC: Normal adolescent sexuality: A physician's perspective. *Semin Adolesc Med* 1:101–115, 1985c.

Strasburger VC: When parents ask about the influence of TV on their kids. *Contemp Pediatr* 1:18–30, 1985d.

Strasburger VC: Teenagers and television. *Pediatr Ann* 14:814–820, 1985e.

Strasburger VC: Telling teens to say no is not enough. *Hartford Courant*, September 28, 1986.

Strasburger VC: Children, adolescents, and television 1989—II. The role of pediatricians. *Pediatrics* 83:446–448, 1989a.

Strasburger VC: Adolescent sexuality and the media. *Pediatr Clin North Am* 36(3):747–774, 1989b.

Strasburger VC, Eisner JM: Teenagers, physicians, and the law in Connecticut, 1982. *Conn Med* 46:80–84, 1982.

Strasburger VC, Eisner JM, Tilson JQ, et al: Teenagers, physicians, and the law in New England. *J Adolesc Health Care* 6:377–382, 1985.

Thornton A, Camburn D: The influence of the family on premarital sexual attitudes and behavior. *Demography* 24:323–330, 1987.

Trussell J: Teenage pregnancy in the United States. *Fam Plann Perspect* 20(6):262–272, 1988.

Update: Kids will be kids. *Fam Plann Perspect* 20(5):204, 1988.

Washington AE, Sweet RL, Shafer MB: Pelvic inflammatory disease and its sequelae in adolescents. *J Adolesc Health Care* 6:298–310, 1985.

Weatherley RA, Perlman SB, Levine MH, et al: Comprehensive programs for pregnant teenagers and teenage parents: How successful have they been? *Fam Plann Perspect* 18:73–78, 1986.

Young M: Self-esteem and sexual behavior among early adolescents. *Fam Life Educ* 7(4):16–19, 1989.

Zabin LS, Hirsch MB, Smith EA, et al: Adolescent pregnancy-prevention program: A model for research and evaluation. *J Adolesc Health Care* 7:77–87, 1986.

Zabin LS, Kantner JF, Zelnik M: The risk of adolescent pregnancy in the first months of intercourse. *Fam Plann Perspect* 11:215–222, 1979.

Zelnik M: Sexual activity among adolescents: Perspective of a decade. In McAnarney ER (ed): *Premature Adolescent Pregnancy and Parenthood.* Grune & Stratton, New York, 1983.

Zelnik M, Kantner JF: Reasons for nonuse of contraception by sexually active women aged 15–19. *Fam Plann Perspect* 11:289–296, 1979.

Zelnik M, Kantner JF: Sexual activity, contraceptive use and pregnancy among metropolitan-area teenagers: 1971–1979. *Fam Plann Perspect* 12:230–237, 1980.

Zelnik M, Kim YJ: Sex education and its association with teenage sexual activity, pregnancy, and contraceptive use. *Fam Plann Perspect* 14:117–126, 1982.

2

Prescribing
Oral Contraceptives

Victor C. Strasburger

Oral contraceptives (OCs) are currently the most popular, effective, and logical contraceptive method for the majority of sexually active teenage women. With careful patient selection and follow-up, providing OCs for teenagers can be a safe and rewarding endeavor for pediatricians. For teenagers, delaying a pregnancy until the young woman is older and married can be economically, educationally, and even physically "life-saving," at times. Pediatricians overburdened with well-baby physicals and toddlers with otitis media may experience a new sense of pride and accomplishment after a few of their teenaged patients come back from college (or invite them to their weddings) and tell them how that one intervention made a crucial difference in their lives. Information regarding the safety of oral contraceptives has all too frequently been misinterpreted or sensationalized in the media, leading to misperceptions and unwarranted concerns about OC use (Jones et al., 1980; Grubb, 1987). In addition, pediatricians who fear they may encourage promiscuity are sometimes reluctant to provide OCs to sexually active teenagers (Orr, 1984). Unfortunately, these two facts have combined to limit OC use in the teenage population; and teenage pregnancies, which could have been prevented, continue to exact a high socioeconomic toll.

An ideal contraceptive for adolescents would be easy to use and obtain, inexpensive, completely protective and reversible, separate from the coital act, and involve no health risks (Hofmann, 1984). While no contraceptive fills this bill completely, OCs and condoms come the closest. OCs have the advantages that they are dissociated from the sexual act and are the most effective contraceptive method available (Table 2–1). On the other hand, condoms offer protection against sexually transmitted diseases and may be more attractive from a public health point of view (Bergman, 1980). Both suffer from the significant disadvantage of requiring a high degree of motivation and advanced planning for use—which many teenagers may lack (Table 2–2) (Kreutner, 1987). Some adolescent programs are now recommending that their female patients use OCs *and* condoms for optimal pregnancy and disease prevention (Hatcher et al., 1988; Mishell, 1989), although this recommendation may be overly idealistic and impractical for most younger teens.

Two reports have touted diaphragms for teenage women: In the largest sample to date, 8% of a New York cohort of over 2,000 diaphragm users were teenagers, and 65% were still using their diaphragms a year later (Lane et al., 1976). In another, a study of a middle-class population, 27% of teenagers selected the diaphragm, and 72% continued their use of it for a year (Marks and Mueller, 1979). The diaphragm is an attractive choice for contraception because it offers some protection against symp-

Table 2-1   Theoretical and Actual Effectiveness of Various Contraceptive Methods

Method	Theoretical (%)	Practical (%)
Combination oral contraceptives	99.9	90–99
Progesterone-only contraceptives	98	90
IUD	98	96
Diaphragm	97	70–97
Condom	97	64–97
Spermicide	97	61–97
Condom + spermicide	99	95
Withdrawal	91	75

Adapted from Hofmann, 1984.

Table 2-2   Adolescent Contraception

	Pill	IUD	Diaphragm	Condoms
Motivation required	+ + +	0	+ + + +	+ +
Episodic sex	0	+	+	+
Frequent sex	+ + + +	+ + +	+ / −	+
Systemic side effects	+ +	+ + +	0	0
Messy	0	0	+ + + +	+ +
Male cooperation required	0	0	+ / −	+ + + +
Secrecy possible	Difficult	Easy	Difficult	Possible

Adapted from Kreutner, 1987.

tomatic gonorrheal infection (Stone et al, 1986), tubal damage (Cramer et al., 1987), cervical neoplasia (Wright et al., 1978), and human *Papillomavirus* infection (Celentano et al., 1987). Nevertheless, the amount of self-manipulation necessary for insertion and the messiness of the contraceptive cream or jelly make this an option for only the most motivated patients—usually, college students. Even then, the diaphragm may carry too high a risk of pregnancy for nulliparous young women who engage in frequent intercourse (Table 2-3) (Klitsch, 1988).

The cervical cap is a close cousin to the diaphragm and was recently approved for use in the United States (McIntyre, 1986), but it suffers from unacceptably high pregnancy rates: 17% at the end of 1 year and 38% at the end of 2 years, according to the most recent study (Powell et al, 1986). Likewise, the vaginal sponge requires self-insertion, planning, and carries a high failure rate (17% in the 1st year) (North and Vorhauer, 1985). Spermicides are readily available but also require planning, self-insertion, tolerance for messiness, and must be combined with use of condoms for maximum effectiveness. Currently, there are two intrauterine devices on the market: the Progestasert (Alza Corporation, Palo Alto, CA) and the Paraguard T380 (GynoPharma, Inc., Somerville, NJ) (Lewin, 1986). IUDs have an unacceptably high risk of infection, expulsion, and toxic sequelae, making them an inappropriate method of birth control for most adolescents or any nulliparous woman who plans to conceive in the future (Grimes, 1986; Lee et al., 1988; Mishell, 1989).

Most recently, the U.S. Food and Drug Administration has approved the use of Norplant, a progesterone that is implanted under the skin in the form of six matchstick-sized silicone capsules that are effective for 5 years. However, in European studies, Norplant was discontinued before 5 years by nearly 25% of women because of irregular menstrual bleeding (*Washington Post*, 1989).

Table 2–3   Intercourse Frequency and Failure of Barrier Contraceptives

Study group	N	Pregnancies/100 women during first 12 months of use
Nulliparous diaphragm users		
Intercourse <4×/wk	399	9.9
Intercourse >4×/wk	161	20.7
Nulliparous sponge users		
Intercourse <4×/wk	358	12.7
Intercourse >4×/wk	161	16.6

Data from McIntyre, 1986. Adapted from Hatcher, 1988.

Oral Contraceptives

Formulation

In the 1990 Physicians' Desk Reference (PDR) there are 63 different name-brand OCs listed (Table 2–4). The number and variety of different OCs can be confusing to the nongynecologist; but, in fact, a little experience with just a few different types of OCs is all that is required (Table 2–5).

All combination OCs contain estrogen and progestin components. The estrogen may be either mestranol or ethinyl estradiol, which are virtually identical after being metabolized in the liver (Hale, 1986), although ethinyl estradiol is thought to be 1.2–1.4 times more potent on a microgram-for-microgram basis (Hatcher et al., 1988). The progestin component may be any one of six: norethinedrone, norethindrone acetate, norethynodrel, ethynodiol diacetate, norgestrel, or levonorgestrel, which are each metabolized in different ways. In addition to their progestational effects, progestins may also exhibit estrogenic and antiestrogenic or androgenic effects (Table 2–6). The balance between the estrogenic and progestational factors determines an OC's effect on the endometrium (Blatzer, 1986; Gorrill and Marshall, 1986; Stubblefield, 1986).

The estrogen component was originally incriminated as the cause of major side effects. Since 1960, when the Federal Drug Administration (FDA) approved Enovid, the first oral contraceptive, the dose of estrogen has been reduced to 50 µg or less to minimize risks and side effects. Newer studies have shown that progestational components are also associated with certain risks (Meade et al., 1980; Kay, 1982), and, therefore, progestin doses have been decreased as well.

Multiphasic OCs, introduced in 1984, can now be recommended as agents of initial choice because they contain lower doses of both hormones, and the net effect is a reduction in the risk of thromboembolic events and fewer alterations in the lipid profile (Mishell, 1989).

Current multiphasic pills that contain levonorgestrel (e.g., Triphasil and Tri-Levlen) contain only about 10% as much progestin as those multiphasic pills with norethindrone (e.g., Ortho-Novum 7/7/7) (Mishell, 1989). However, highly androgenic progestins (levonorgestrel, norgestrel) appear to have an adverse effect on the lipid profile, while those that are estrogen-dominant (norethindrone, norethindrone acetate, ethynodiol diacetate) do not. (See Table 2–7 for the relative potencies of progestins in OCs.) While recent studies of low-dose pills, including multiphasic preparations, found no adverse changes in HDL or LDL cholesterol (Kloosterboer et

Table 2–4   Choosing a Low-Dose Oral Contraceptive

Group	Pill	Estrogen dose	Biological activity
Good initial choice (fixed dose)	Ortho 1/35 Ovcon 35	35 μg ethinyl estradiol 35 μg ethinyl estradiol	Progestational: Low Androgenic: Low Endometrial: Low
Good initial choice (multiphasic)	Ortho 7/7/7 Tri-Norinyl Tri-Levlen Triphasil	35 μg ethinyl estradiol 35 μg ethinyl estradiol 32 μg ethinyl estradiol (average)	Progestational: Low Androgenic: Moderate Endometrial: Moderate
Good back-ups	Levlen Lo-Ovral Nordette Norinyl 1/35 Ortho 1/35 Norinyl 1/50 Norlestrin 1/50 Ortho 1/50 Ovcon 1/50	30 μg ethinyl estradiol 30 μg ethinyl estradiol 30 μg ethinyl estradiol 35 μg ethinyl estradiol 35 μg ethinyl estradiol 50 μg mestranol 50 μg ethinyl estradiol 50 μg mestranol 50 μg ethinyl estradiol	Progestational: Moderate Androgenic: Moderate Endometrial: Moderate
Good for acne (estrogenic)	Ovcon 35 Ovcon 50 Demulen 1/35 Demulen 1/50 Ortho 1/50 Triphasil	35 μg ethinyl estradiol 50 μg ethinyl estradiol 35 μg ethinyl estradiol 50 μg ethinyl estradiol 50 μg ethinyl estradiol 32μg ethinyl estradiol (32 μg average)	Progestational: High Androgenic: Low Endometrial: Low/ Moderate
Rarely used	Loestrin 1/20	20 μg ethinyl estradiol	Progestational: Moderate Androgenic: Moderate Endometrial: Low
	Loestrin 1.5/30	30 μg ethinyl estradiol	Progestational: High Androgenic: High Endometrial: Low
	Norlestrin 2.5	50 μg ethinyl estradiol	Progestational: High Androgenic: High
	Ovral	50 μg ethinyl estradiol	Endometrial: High
Mini-pills	Micronor Nor Q.D. Ovrette	No estrogen No estrogen No estrogen	Progestational: Low Androgenic: Low Endometrial: Low

Adapted from Dickey, 1987.

Table 2–5   One Physician's Armamentarium: Six Oral Contraceptives

Starting pills: Ortho-Novum 1/35
                   Ovcon 35
                   Ortho-Novum 7/7/7
                   Triphasil
Acne: Demulen 1/35
Pill amenorrhea: Lo-Ovral

Table 2–6   OCs, Estrogen Effect, and Androgenicity: Implications for Acne

Progestin	Estrogenic effect
Norgestrel (Triphasil, Tri-Levlen, Lo-Ovral)	0.00
Norethindrone 1 mg (Norinyl, Ortho-Novum)	1.00
Ethynodiol diacetate 1 mg (Demulen)	3.44

Pill	Progestin	Relative androgen effect
Ovcon 35	0.4 mg norethindrone	0.14
Demulen 1/35	1 mg ethynodiol diacetate	0.21
Ortho 7/7/7	0.5, 0.75, 1 mg norethindrone	0.26
Triphasil/Tri-Levlen	0.05, 0.075, 0.12 mg levonorgestrel	0.29
Norinyl/Ortho 1/35	1 mg norethindrone	0.34
Lo-Ovral	0.30 mg norgestrel	0.47
Loestrin 1.5/30	1.5 mg norethindrone acetate	0.79

Adapted from Hatcher, 1988.

Table 2–7   Relative Potencies of Progestins in Oral Contraceptives

Class Compound	Progestational	Estrogenic	Androgenic
Gonane			
Levonorgestrel	10–20	0.00	9.4
Norgestrel	5–10	0.00	4.7
Estrane			
Norethindrone	1	1.0	1.0
Norethindrone acetate	1	1.52	1.6
Ethynodiol diacetate	1	3.44	0.63

Adapted from Mans ML: *A Manual for the House Staff on Obstetrics and Gynecology*, p. 148.

al., 1986), the triphasic pills with norgestrel—but not those with norethindrone—still significantly lowered the HDL_2 subfraction that is thought to be the "good" protective cholesterol (Percival-Smith et al., 1987; Crook et al., 1988; Knopp, 1988; LaRosa, 1988). Physicians should be aware of these differences and, based on the individual patient profile, select the formulation that provides the safest components in the lowest effective dosage.

Current research is aimed at combining low doses of estrogen with newer progestins, such as desogestrel (which has no effect on lipids), gestodene, and norgestimate (Hoppe and Gestoden, 1988; Mishell, 1989).

Mechanism of Action

Combination OCs are thought to work at several different levels of the reproductive system (Blatzer, 1984):

1. At the pituitary level, OCs inhibit gonadotropin-releasing hormone (GnRH), thereby blocking the mid-cycle surge of luteinizing-hormone (LH) that is responsible for ovulation.
2. At the ovarian level, OCs inhibit follicular maturation beyond the primary follicle stage.

3. At the endometrial level, OCs cause thinning of the endometrium, creating a less hospitable environment for implantation.
4. At the cervical level, OCs transform cervical mucus into a thicker, scantier, more impermeable substance.

Contraindications

The FDA has delineated five absolute contraindications to OC use (Shearin and Boelhke, 1989). Significantly, few of them are relevant to the adolescent population:

1. Thrombophlebitis, thromboembolic disease, cerebrovascular accidents, or past history of any of these
2. Impaired liver function
3. Known or suspected breast cancer or estrogen-dependent neoplasia
4. Undiagnosed abnormal vaginal bleeding
5. Known or suspected pregnancy

Relative contraindications are considerably more controversial, and here the risks and benefits of OCs must carefully be weighed, along with potential alternative forms of contraception. Common sense dictates that true migraine headaches and preexisting hypertension probably belong on the above list as well. OCs cause an increased tendency towards clotting and a decreased hemovascular ability to dissolve clots by producing changes in viscosity, platelet adhesiveness, and levels of clotting factors VII, fibrinogen, and antithrombin III (Table 2–8) (Meade, 1982; Corson, 1986). In adult women, the relationship between migraines and strokes remains unclear despite several studies, but since migraine consists of a vasoconstrictive phase in cerebral vessels, putting an additional coagulation booster into such a system seems unwise (Collaborative Group for the Study of Stroke in Young Women, 1978; Greydanus, 1981; Meade, 1988). Likewise, the incidence of thrombotic stroke could probably be decreased if hypertensive patients were not given OCs (Kulig, 1985). Certainly, patients with either migraine headaches or borderline hypertension are much better candidates for the progestin-only Mini-pill (Hatcher et al., 1988).

Other *relative* contraindications include (Neinstein and Katz, 1986):

1. Diabetes mellitus
2. Epilepsy
3. Sickle cell anemia
4. Systemic lupus erythematosus
5. Hyperlipidemia
6. Gallbladder disease or renal disease

OCs should be discontinued within 2–4 weeks of elective surgery because of their clotting propensity. In addition, the efficacy of OCs may be affected by other medications being taken simultaneously (Table 2–9). Finally, teenagers who smoke should be strongly cautioned that their risks of serious complications are probably increased, although the confirmatory data all deal with adult women, usually over the age of 35 (Rosenfield, 1978).

Risks

Adolescents are the ideal age-group to be taking OCs because all of the known associated risks increase with age. In addition, to put the risk of taking OCs in proper

Table 2–8   Laboratory Changes in Patients Taking OCs

	Increased	Decreased
Plasma proteins	Prealbumin Immunoglobulins Transferrin Thyroid-binding globulin Plasminogen Fibrinogen Angiotensinogen	Albumin Haptoglobin Renin
Hormones	Thyroxine Cortisol	T3 resin uptake Urinary 17-OH steroids
Other	Platelets Iron, TIBC Factors II, VII, IX Triglycerides Cholesterol	HDL level

Adapted from Neinstein, 1986.

Table 2–9   Drugs That May Interfere with OCs

Drug	Mechanism of action	Solution
Anticonvulsants Phenobarbital Phenytoin	Induction of microsomal liver enzymes; more rapid estrogen metabolism	Use another method, drug, or higher dose OC (50 μg)
Antibiotics Penicillin Ampicillin Metronidazole Tetracycline	Enterohepatic circulation disturbance; induction of microsomal enzymes	Use another drug or back- up method
Sedatives Benzodiazepines Chloral hydrate Antimigraines	Increased microsomal liver enzymes	Use another drug or back- up method
Antacids	Decreased intestinal absorption of progestins	Use back-up method

Adapted from Dickey, 1987.

perspective, it must be compared with ordinary day-to-day risks (Table 2–10) and the risk of pregnancy or abortion (Table 2–11) (Dinman, 1980; Petitti, 1986). Considering all women of childbearing age, for example, the risk of pregnancy and childbirth is 25 times greater than the risk of induced abortion and eight times greater than the risk of contraceptive-induced mortality (Rosenberg and Rosenthal, 1987). With adolescents, these figures may be even more dramatic; yet exact data that are confined to adolescent populations are unavailable.

Although one reads mortality figures for the 15- to 19-year-old age group of 1.2/100,000 users/year for nonsmokers and 1.4/100,000 users/year for smokers (Tietze, 1977), in fact *in the world's medical literature there is only a single report of a birth control pill-related death of an adolescent*—a 17-year-old in Sweden who died in 1968 from a thrombotic stroke (preceded by a long history of headaches) (Ask-Upmark

Table 2–10   Voluntary and Involuntary Risks in Everyday Life

Risks	Deaths/person/yr, odds
Voluntary	
Smoking, 20 cigarettes/day	1 in 200
Drinking, 1 bottle wine/day	1 in 13,300
Playing football	1 in 25,000
Automobile racing	1 in 10,000
Motorcycling	1 in 50
Professional boxing	1 in 14,300
Skiing	1 in 1,430,000
Involuntary	
Hit by automobile	1 in 20,000
Earthquake (California)	1 in 588,000
Tornados (Midwest)	1 in 455,000
Lightning	1 in 10 million
Falling aircraft	1 in 10 million
Leukemia	1 in 12,500
Influenza	1 in 5,000
Meteorite	1 in 100 billion

Adapted from Dinman, 1980.

Table 2–11   Risks of Contraception and Pregnancy

Risks	Deaths/person/yr, odds
Contraception	
Oral contraception (*all* women)	
Smoker	1 in 16,000
Nonsmoker	1 in 63,000
IUD user	1 in 100,000
Barrier methods	None
Laparoscopic tubal ligation	None
Pregnancy	
Full-term pregnancy	1 in 10,000
Illegal abortion	1 in 3,000
Legal abortion	
Before 9 wks	1 in 400,000
Between 9–12 wks	1 in 100,000
Between 13–16 wks	1 in 25,000
After 16 wks	1 in 10,000

Adapted from Hatcher, 1988.

et al., 1969). In addition, since newer low-dose formulations of the pill have only become available and widely used within the last 10 years, many of the risk studies are now out-of-date. For example, a recent study of healthy oral contraceptive users and comparable nonusers at Group Health Cooperative in Seattle from 1977–1981 encompassed 54,971 woman-years of OC use and demonstrated only a slight excess mortality for OC-users (1.3 times). There were no deaths from cardiovascular illness or stroke, and only one death from liver cancer in the contraceptive group (Porter et al., 1987). Clearly, with the use of low-dose formulations and careful patient selection, the risk of mortality associated with OCs in adolescents is an important but primarily theoretical consideration. According to the most recent studies (which are much more likely to include large numbers of women older than 20 years of age, rather than teenagers), the following vascular risks of OCs have been found:

Venous thromboembolism: 3–11 times increased risk (Connell, 1984; Helmrich et al., 1987)

Thrombotic stroke: 2–5 times increased risk (Vessey et al., 1984; Helmrich et al., 1987)

Hypertension: 3 times increased risk (Kols et al., 1982; Helmrich et al., 1987; Woods, 1988). This is probably due to an increase in angiotensinogen levels, even on the 35-μg pills (Khaw and Peart, 1982). However, a recent large study of black women showed no increase in mean arterial blood pressure (Blumenstein et al., 1980).

Myocardial infarction: 2–4 times increased risk in studies done in the late 1970s, involving pills which contained 50 μg or more of estrogen (Dalen and Hickler, 1981). More recently, studies have failed to show an increased risk in either users of low-dose pills (Mant et al., 1987; Porter et al., 1987; Hatcher et al., 1988) or previous users (Stampfer et al., 1988). Among women who use OCs and smoke, most myocardial infarctions are attributable solely to smoking (Goldbaum et al., 1987).

Subarachnoid hemorrhage: 5 times increased risk (Petitti et al., 1979).

All of these risks are far more common in women over the age of 35 and older women who smoke. Teenagers are probably at *much* lower risk, although exact data are unavailable. In addition, the venous problems are now thought to be estrogen-associated, while arterial problems are thought to be caused by progestin-induced increases in atherogenic lipids (Knopp, 1986; Meade, 1988).

OCs and the Risk of Cancer

According to a 1985 Gallup Poll, 76% of women and 62% of men think that use of oral contraceptives involves "substantial risks" (Digest, 1985). Of these risks, those surveyed cited cancer more than any other problem (31% women, 27% men). In fact, OCs *lower* the risk of ovarian (Centers for Disease Control, 1987a; Vessey et al, 1987) and endometrial cancer (Centers for Disease Control, 1987b); the risk of breast and cervical cancer remains unsettled, and there is no known association with either pituitary adenomas (Pituitary Adenoma Study Group, 1983) or malignant melanomas (Holly, 1986). The only known association with cancer results from increases in three very rare types of tumors—prolactinomas, benign liver tumors, and hepatocellular carcinomas (Amtrup et al., 1980; Helling and Wood, 1982; Shy et al., 1983; Hennekens et al., 1984; Rosenberg et al., 1984; Stadel et al., 1985; Forman et al., 1986; Fortney et al., 1986; Neuberger et al., 1986; Webster, 1986; Centers for Disease Control, 1987a,b). All of these tumors are known to occur in adult women only. There have been a few cases of hepatocellular adenomas occurring in women aged 20–25 years; and although these are benign tumors, 10%–15% of cases progress to rupture and hemorrhage, with a high mortality rate (Hofmann, 1984).

At least 4 large cohort studies and 10 case-control studies in the past decade have found no association between OCs and breast cancer (Centers for Disease Control, 1983; Centers for Disease Control, 1986; Holly, 1986; Hatcher et al., 1988). An FDA advisory panel recently reviewed these studies and three others—two of which had found an increased risk of breast cancer in some former OC users (Kay and Hannaford, 1988; Stadel et al., 1988; Miller et al., 1989). Because of the preponderance of data showing no effect and the conflicting nature of the data showing that certain subgroups of former users might be at increased risk, the FDA decided that no change in the way OCs are used or prescribed is currently warranted (Golin, 1989; Johnson, 1989).

The possibility of a link between OCs and cervical cancer has concerned researchers for many years, but only recently have studies controlled for number of sexual partners and age at first intercourse—known high-risk factors. Within the past five years, several studies have documented an increased risk of 1.3–1.8 times for women who use OCs, with the higher figure applying to those who used birth control pills longer (Vessey et al., 1983; WHO Collaborative Study, 1985; Brinton et al., 1986; Beral et al., 1988). One possible mechanism to explain this phenomenon is that the pill could act as a cocarcinogen with other agents (e.g., cigarettes, herpes virus, human *Papillomavirus*) (Lincoln, 1984). Another possibility is a bias of ascertainment: pill users are followed more closely with annual PAP smears; therefore, cervical cancers would be more readily detected in that group. Overall, the association between OCs and cervical cancer remains to be elucidated, and there are still several recent studies which show no increased risk (Clarke et al., 1985; Hellberg et al., 1985; Irwin et al., 1988; Reeves et al., 1989). Furthermore, since few sexually active teenagers use OCs for any extended length of time (thereby minimizing their estrogen exposure), it would seem unlikely that an association with dysplasia is highly significant in this age group (Hofmann, 1984).

OCs and Pelvic Inflammatory Disease (PID)

OCs may be both protective against and hospitable to different organisms causing PID. One Swedish study documented PID occurring half as frequently among OC-users as nonusers and suggested that this protection may apply to both gonococcal and chlamydial salpingitis (Wolner-Hanssen et al., 1985). However, 15 of 17 published reports describe a positive association between OCs and *lower* genital tract chlamydial cervicitis (Washington et al., 1985a), and theoretically this *may* predispose to higher rates of chlamydial PID. And one recent study found a 70% increase in gonococcal cervical infections as well (Louv et al., 1989). Despite this, some researchers have reasoned that while OCs may increase the colonization of the lower genital tract, the thicker cervical mucus may actually decrease dissemination of the gonococcus or chlamydia into the adnexae (Washington et al., 1985b).

Other Risk Factors

A number of problems have been posed about OCs that have not withstood scientific scrutiny. OCs do *not* inhibit skeletal growth in adolescents: the doses used are too small, and teenage females have already attained 97% of their height potential by the time of their menarche (Hofmann, 1984). Menstruation usually resumes within 1–3 months of discontinuing OCs, and 98% of women are ovulatory by the third cycle (Tyrer, 1984). In the latest study, OCs did not have any adverse effects on glucose metabolism after use for 6 months when only low-dose formulations were tested (Van Der Vange et al., 1987).

Recently, a report from the 1988 World Congress on HIV in Stockholm found that African prostitutes using OCs were two to three times more likely to become infected with HIV than other prostitutes. The mechanism by which OCs might facilitate passage of the virus into the bloodstream is unknown, and this study represents a preliminary report only (Associated Press, 1988).

Beneficial Effects of Oral Contraceptives

Aside from their high degree of effectiveness in preventing pregnancy, OCs are probably life-saving in preventing tubal pregnancies, lowering the risk of PID, and decreasing the incidence of endometrial and ovarian cancer—the most common and the most fatal of gynecologic malignancies, respectively (Derman, 1986). In addition, OCs are the treatment of choice for sexually active teenagers who suffer from dysmenorrhea, may help to alleviate symptoms of premenstrual syndrome, decrease the incidence of benign breast disease, and have other significant beneficial side effects as well (Table 2–12) (Derman, 1986). In assessing overall risk-benefit ratios for adolescents using OCs, the benefits far outweigh the risks for the large majority of potential users.

How to Prescribe Birth Control Pills for Adolescents

Teenagers desiring oral contraceptives must be able to understand the risks and benefits of such treatment, i.e., be able to give an informed consent. Ordinarily, this means that they will be near the age of majority and qualify as a "mature minor." Since the age of majority is 18 years in all states, age 15 or above is usually considered to be "near" the age of majority. However, courts have given wide latitude to health professionals to decide exactly who is or is not "mature," and no physician has ever been successfully sued for prescribing OCs to a minor (nor has any suit been filed in the past 30 years) (Strasburger et al., 1985). Obviously, how the risks and benefits are explained will greatly influence the adolescent's thinking on the issue. Explaining that there is a theoretical risk of mortality due to taking the pill without explaining that this risk of mortality is 10–25 times greater for a pregnancy or abortion is unintentionally deceptive. Most teenagers have received inaccurate information about OCs (Table 2–13) (Herold and Goodwin, 1980), and it is important for physicians to be aware of some of the more common misconceptions (e.g., the pill "causes" cancer, pregnancy, heart attacks, etc.) An appropriate medical and sexual history needs to be taken (Table 2–14), and a thorough physical examination and pelvic examination should be done. In the rare instance of a teenager seeking OCs before initiating sexual intercourse and having a high level of anxiety about her first pelvic exam, the exam can be delayed

Table 2–12   Noncontraceptive Benefits of OCs

Benefit	Relative risk
Iron deficiency anemia	0.57
Menorrhagia	0.52
Endometrial cancer	0.50
Ovarian cancer	0.60
Breast cancer	0.96
Breast fibroadenoma	0.50
Fibrocystic breast disease	0.40
Functional ovarian cysts	0.07
Rheumatoid arthritis	0.49
Pelvic inflammatory disease	0.50
Ectopic pregnancy	0.01
Dysmenorrhea	0.37
Premenstrual syndrome	0.71
Acne	0.84

Adapted from Kulig, 1985.

Table 2–13   Where Do Teenage Girls Obtain Information on Side-Effects of the Pill?

Source	% Mentioning this source
Mass media	51
Girlfriends	49
Sex education class	25
Mother	15
Boyfriend	4
Sister	3
Physician	3

Adapted from Herold, 1980.

Table 2–14   Screening History for Oral Contraceptives

Please circle the appropriate answer or fill in the blank.

1. Have you ever been hospitalized? .... Yes   No

Have you ever had:

2. Surgery .... Yes   No
3. High blood pressure .... Yes   No
4. Frequent headaches .... Yes   No
5. Jaundice or hepatitis .... Yes   No
6. Gall bladder disease .... Yes   No
7. Diabetes .... Yes   No
8. Phlebitis or blood clots .... Yes   No
9. Heart murmur .... Yes   No
10. Epilepsy or seizures .... Yes   No
11. Any sexually transmitted disease:
     Syphilis, gonorrhea, chlamydia, warts, or pelvic inflammatory disease ... Yes   No
12. Family history of:
     Heart trouble .... Yes   No
     Diabetes .... Yes   No
     Cancer .... Yes   No

Please answer:

13. Do you wear contact lenses? .... Yes   No
14. Please list any medicines taken regularly and what they are for:

15. Age of onset of first period .... _____
16. How often do your periods come? .... _____
17. How long do they last? .... _____
18. Any discomfort with periods? .... _____
19. Any bleeding between periods? .... _____
20. What day did your last menstrual period start? .... _____
21. Age at time of your first intercourse .... _____
22. Current frequency of intercourse .... _____
23. Have you ever been pregnant? .... _____
24. What type of contraception have you used? .... _____
25. Date of your last pelvic exam? .... _____
26. Do you smoke cigarettes? How many? .... _____

intercourse has occurred (Turetsky and Strasburger, 1983). A screening exam should also include measurement of blood pressure, Tanner staging, a PAP smear, culture for gonorrhea, culture or test for chlamydia (if available), a complete blood count (CBC), test for syphilis (VDRL), and a urinalysis. If the patient's family fits a high cardiac risk profile, tests for cholesterol, triglycerides, and lipoprotein panels may also be appropriate. Teenagers who smoke should be *strongly discouraged* from continuing to smoke.

Since the average cost of a package of OCs is between $10 and $15, the physician can encourage compliance by giving the teenager a sample package or two along with her 6-month prescription, and by scheduling a 6-week visit to check blood pressure and side effects.

It is important to note that breakthrough bleeding for the first 1–3 months is not unusual in patients on low-dose oral contraceptives. Physicians who counsel their patients that such bleeding is usually temporary will probably obtain the best compliance. This management of breakthrough bleeding helps ensure that patients are not stepped up to higher dose OCs unnecessarily.

Giving teenagers periodic "rests" from oral contraceptives achieves nothing more than increasing their risk of pregnancy. In most patients, discontinuing use of birth control pills will result in resumption of their normal pre-pill menstrual pattern, regardless of how long they have taken oral contraceptives.

Recent studies have shown compliance rates ranging from 48%–84% (3 months) and from 34%–55% (12 months) for teenage girls taking OCs (Litt et al., 1980; Sher et al., 1982; Emans et al., 1987). Good compliers were older, suburban, had a single partner, had intercourse more than once a week, made their own appointments, "set the agenda" for the health visit, and displayed satisfaction with the pill at the initial visit (Litt et al., 1980; Sher et al., 1982). Poor compliers were younger, urban, had no college plans, were dissatisfied with the health visit, had side effects from the pill, and had no parental involvement with the visit (Sher et al., 1982; Emans et al., 1987). Pediatricians should be cognizant that confidentiality may be a key issue for many adolescents. Only 32% of pediatricians in one study said that they would be willing to prescribe OCs for a 15-year-old patient, and many would insist on parental consent, despite no legal requirement to do so (Orr, 1984).

Which Pill to Choose

With 63 birth control pills available and with the hormonal properties of each preparation not immediately apparent from reading the PDR or the package, choosing a pill can be a difficult decision. Physicians should always begin with a 28-day pill that contains less than 50 µg of estrogen (Ortho-Novum 1/35, Norinyl 1/35, Ovcon 35, Ortho-Novum 7/7/7, Tri-Norinyl, Triphasil, or Tri-Levlen). In fact, in January 1988 the FDA's Fertility and Maternal Health Drugs Advisory Committee recommended that all OCs containing more than 50 µg of estrogen be eliminated from the market, and pharmaceutical companies agreed to voluntarily withdraw them by October 1988 (Update, 1988). Type and amount of progestin may also be an important consideration. For example, the multiphasic Ortho-Novum 7/7/7 and Tri-Norinyl contain a weaker progestin (norethindrone) than Tri-Levlen and Triphasil (levonorgestrel).

Other factors may determine the initial choice of pill. For instance, a teenager with acne will benefit from a pill with high estrogenic activity and low androgenic activity (e.g., Ovcon 35, Demulen 1/35, or Ortho-Novum 1/50), whereas a high androgenic pill will exacerbate her problem (e.g., Ovral, Lo-Ovral). As discussed previously, intermenstrual spotting or breakthrough bleeding usually diminishes after two to three months. But if a teenager will not tolerate this problem, even after counseling, a change in OC may be necessary. If started on a multiphasic OC, the patient can be put on a constant dose pill. A pill with high progestational and endometrial effects (e.g., Lo-Ovral, Nordette, Ovral) can be useful for some patients.

For good patient management, the physician should become familiar with the advantages and disadvantages of each formulation. Certain side effects can be overcome, while others require cessation of OCs altogether (Table 2–15). For example, nausea or vomiting can usually be relieved by taking the pill at bedtime or trying to diminish the estrogen content. Pill amenorrhea (i.e., failure to have withdrawal bleeding) occurs in approximately 5% of pill users and may be associated with either norethindrone as the progestational agent or low-dose OCs in general. A change to a stronger progestin (e.g., norgestrel as in Lo-Ovral) or to a pill with a higher estrogen content (though not exceeding 50 μg) is usually sufficient to alleviate this problem. If amenorrhea persists despite switching pills or if symptoms are present, a pregnancy test may be necessary. Fortunately, recent research demonstrates that there is little risk of taking low-dose OCs during the first trimester of pregnancy (Stewart et al., 1987).

Physicians should be aware that often it is not the risk of *severe* side effects that results in discontinuation of OCs but rather the nuisance of minor side effects. For this reason, pills with less than 30 μg of estrogen (e.g., Loestrin 1/20) should probably be avoided because of the risk of spotting. In addition to breakthrough bleeding (5%–10% of patients), weight gain is perceived to be a major drawback of taking OCs, even though some recent studies dispute the notion that even 10% of patients will gain weight on the pill (Carpenter and Neinstein, 1986). The relationship between depression and OCs remains controversial, but pyridoxine hydrochloride (20 mg twice daily) can be tried before OCs are discontinued (Slap, 1981; Kreutner, 1987). OCs should also be discontinued with any evidence of hypertension, unexplained chest pain, increased frequency or severity of headaches, severe unexplained right upper quadrant pain, or development of galactorrhea. It is important for patients to understand that probably 90% of teenagers can take OCs without any side effects whatsoever.

Table 2–15   Management of Problems with Oral Contraceptives

Problems	Management
Acne	Low-androgenic pill
Nausea	Take pill at bedtime or with meals
	Use 30–35 μg pill
Fluid retention	Low-estrogenic pill
Increased appetite	Low-androgenic pill
Hypertension	D/C pill
	Try Mini-pill
Headaches	Consider d/c pill
Breakthrough bleeding	Wait 2–3 cycles, then switch from a multiphasic to a constant dose OC, a moderate progestational pill, or a 50-μg pill
Depression	Try 20 mg pyridoxine twice daily; try 30-μg pill or Mini-pill
Dry eyes	Try progestin-dominant pill

Starting the Pill

Because the newer birth control pills are such low-dose formulations, they must be taken at the same time every day to minimize the chances of failure or of breakthrough bleeding. Linking the taking of the pill to some other routine behavior (e.g., brushing teeth at night) is useful. The pill can be started on the first Sunday after the period begins, on day 5 of the menstrual cycle, or on day 1 of the menstrual cycle—whichever system the physician prefers. There is nothing sacred about doing this, however, other than maximizing the pill's effectiveness during the first cycle (estimated to be 95%–97%). The question of using a back-up method for the first cycle is often academic, since most teenagers are using no contraceptive method before beginning OCs. They are therefore far better protected in the first cycle than they have been. Nevertheless, patients should be informed that the pill is probably 2%–5% less effective in the first cycle, and a back-up method for the first month is advisable.

Patients will ordinarily begin withdrawal bleeding while taking the placebo pills in the package. If they miss one pill, they should take it as soon as they remember it and use a back-up method for that cycle, although they are probably well protected. Missing two or more pills will probably be signaled by breakthrough bleeding. In this case, the patient should continue taking her pills but use another method of contraception as well for the remainder of the cycle. It is often useful to display a sample package to the adolescent while giving these kinds of instructions.

Patients should be told not to discontinue the pill for any reason without checking with the physician first. They will need to call immediately if they develop severe headaches, chest pains, abdominal pains, or leg pains. Other medications—particularly antibiotics—may hamper the pill's effectiveness, and teenagers should be cautioned about this and reminded that the pill is a drug and should be mentioned any time the patient seeks medical attention.

Follow-up is important, particularly the 6-week visit to check blood pressure and side effects. After that, visits can be scheduled as needed but probably should be every 2–6 months, depending on the patient. An annual pelvic exam with PAP smear, VDRL, GC culture, and chlamydial test should be performed. Although the pill decreases plasma levels of certain vitamins and minerals (e.g., vitamins B1, B2, B6, B12; folate, zinc), there is no evidence that this is clinically significant, and no additional supplementation is required (Dickey, 1987).

Multiphasic Oral Contraceptives

The newest development in contraceptive technology has been the development of biphasic and triphasic pills. These are an attempt to keep levels of hormones administered to the lowest possible dosages, while still imitating the normal menstrual sequence and preventing pregnancy. Since they are as effective as the low-dose monophasic pills and contain lower overall dosages of both estrogen and progesterone, multiphasic pills are a logical and attractive choice as an initial pill or as a "step-down" pill for patients on higher-dose formulations (Policar, 1986). The physician should review the multiphasic regimen with the patient, explaining how the colors relate to the sequence in which the pills must be taken. The patient should be warned that missing even one pill can diminish effectiveness.

Before multiphasics were introduced, the numbers in the name of an oral contraceptive usually referred to the dosage. Ortho-Novum 1/35, for example, means that the pill contains 1 mg of progestin and 35 μg of estrogen throughout the cycle. With multiphasics, however, numbers refer not to dosage but to sequence. Ortho-Novum 7/7/7, for example, means that the concentration of progestin varies for each of the first 3 weeks, while the estrogen content remains the same.

Ortho-Novum 7/7/7 is one type of multiphasic. In another type, represented by Triphasil and Tri-Levlen, both the estrogen and the progestin concentrations vary (The Medical Letter, 1985).

The primary advantage of using a multiphasic compound that contains an estrane or low-potency progestin is its neutral effect on the lipid profile. Unlike compounds containing gonane progestins, the estranes do not elevate levels of low density lipoproteins (LDL) or depress levels of high density lipoproteins (HDL) (Ellsworth, 1986). (See previous discussion under "Formulation.") Since certain cardiovascular complications—stroke and ischemic heart disease, in particular—seem to be related more to the type of progestin used rather than to the estrogen content (Ellis, 1987), this point is important to remember.

Progesterone-only Pill (Mini-pill)

Progesterone-only oral contraceptives are difficult to use with adolescents. Since such pills have higher failure rates, including the risk of ectopic pregnancy, and a higher incidence of irregular bleeding, they are infrequently used and account for only 1% of all OCs sold (Grimes, 1986). The pregnancy rate is 2.5 to 3.7/100 woman-years because ovulation is not completely inhibited (Van Der Vange et al., 1987). In fact, the Mini-pill prevents ovulation in only 15%–40% of cycles (Hatcher et al., 1988). Rather, its contraceptive action is accomplished by thickening cervical mucus, making the mucus more impermeable to penetration by sperm, and possibly by altering tubal motility. The Mini-pill is taken daily, without interruption, and bleeding can be unpredictable. Therefore, its use with adolescent patients—where compliance is a major factor and pregnancy must always be suspected—is problematical. Nevertheless, when combination pills are contraindicated in certain patients (e.g., migraine headaches, hypertension, sickle cell disease, congenital heart disease), the Mini-pill may be worth trying (Graham and Fraser, 1982; Shearin and Boelhke, 1989).

Postcoital Contraception

The risk of pregnancy from a single episode of sexual intercourse at mid-cycle is estimated to be around 14% (Hatcher et al., 1988). Adolescent women who are raped are subject to this risk and may elect to take preventive medication if it is offered. In addition, college students occasionally request emergency contraception after unprotected intercourse.

For many years, diethylstilbestrol (DES) was the only "morning-after" pill available. In a dosage of 25 mg twice daily for 5 days, it frequently made patients extremely nauseous and exposed them to a 10% risk of ectopic pregnancy (Kreutner, 1987). More recently, insertion of copper IUDs (Kulig et al, 1980), use of oral ethinyl estradiol or conjugated estrogens (Lippes et al., 1976; Dixon et al., 1980, Schilling, 1984), and combination BCPs (Yuzpe and Lancee, 1977) have been employed, with far better results. Yuzpe pioneered the use of Ovral as a postcoital oral contraceptive, employing two tablets taken within 72 hours of intercourse, followed by two additional tablets 12 hours later (Yuzpe and Lancee, 1977; Smith and Ross, 1978; Yuzpe, 1979;

Editorial, 1983; Johnson, 1984; Percival-Smith and Abercrombie, 1987). The pregnancy rate was only 1.6%, and the number of side effects was minimal. In a recent study of 867 college women, this technique averted 70% of potential pregnancies, although the side effects were more significant (30% nausea, 20% nausea and vomiting, 49% no side effects) (Percival-Smith and Abercrombie, 1987). While the FDA has not specifically approved Ovral for this use, this technique represents a doubling-up of OCs, which is commonly done when a pill is missed, for example, and would therefore seem both effective and safe.

Conclusion

Birth control pills have undergone an evolutionary transformation in the past 10 years, making them far safer and easier to use than previously thought. Sexually active adolescents have always comprised the ideal group for taking OCs, both because of their unique psychology (i.e., the need to dissociate contraception from the sexual act) and because they are subject to few of the thromboembolic risks of older women. The toll of teenage pregnancy is sufficiently high that the benefits of OCs far outweigh the risks in the adolescent age group. Pediatricians who choose to familiarize themselves with the principles of adolescent gynecology and contraception will find this a rewarding and important endeavor.

References

Amtrup F, Slottved J, Svanholm H: Liver cell carcinoma in young women possibly induced by oral contraceptives. *Acta Obstet Gynecol Scand* 59:567–569, 1980.

Ask-Upmark E, Glas J, Stenram U: Oral contraceptives and cerebral arterial thrombosis. *Acta Med Scand* 185:479–481, 1969.

Associated Press: Pill use raises AIDS risk, *Albuquerque Journal*, June 17, 1988.

Beral V, Hannaford P, Kay C: Oral contraceptive use and malignancies of the genital tract. *Lancet* 2:1331–1334, 1988.

Bergman AB: Condoms for sexually active teenagers. *Am J Dis Child* 134:247–249, 1980.

Blatzer FR: Formulation and noncontraceptive uses of the new, low-dose oral contraceptive. *J Reprod Med* 29(Suppl):503–510, 1984.

Blatzer FR: Measurements of androgenicity—the spectrum of progestogen activity. *J Reprod Med* 31(Suppl):864, 1986.

Blumenstein BA, Douglas MB, Hall WD: Blood pressure changes and oral contraceptive use: A study of 2,676 black women in the southeastern United States. *Am J Epidemiol* 112:539–552, 1980.

Brinton LA, Huggins GR, Lehman H, et al: Long-term use of oral contraceptives and risk of invasive cervical cancer. *Int J Cancer* 38:339–344, 1986.

Carpenter S, Neinstein LS: Weight gain in adolescent and young adult oral contraceptive users. *J Adolesc Health Care* 7:342–344, 1986.

Celentano DD, Klassen AC, Weisman CS, et al: The role of contraceptive use in cervical cancer: The Maryland cervical cancer case-control study. *Am J Epidemiol* 126:592–604, 1987.

Centers for Disease Control: Long-term oral contraceptive use and the risk of breast cancer. *JAMA* 249:1591–1595, 1983.

Centers for Disease Control (Cancer and Steroid Hormone Study) and the National Institute of Child Health and Human Development (the CASH Study): Oral contraceptive use and the risk of breast cancer. *N Engl J Med* 315:405–411, 1986.

Centers for Disease Control (Cancer and Steroid Hormone Study): The reduction in risk of ovarian cancer associated with oral-contraceptive use. *N Engl J Med* 316:650–655, 1987a.

Centers for Disease Control (Cancer and Steroid Hormone Study): Combination oral contraceptive use and risk of endometrial cancer. *JAMA* 257:796–800, 1987b.

Clarke EA, Hatcher J, McKeown-Eyssen GE, et al: Cervical dysplasia: Association with sexual behavior, smoking, and oral contraceptive use. *Am J Obstet Gynecol* 151:612–616, 1985.

Collaborative Group for the Study of Stroke in Young Women: Oral contraception and increased risk of cerebral ischemia or thrombosis. *N Engl J Med* 288:871–878, 1978.

Connell EB: Oral contraceptives: The current risk-benefit ratio. *J Reprod Med* 29(Suppl):513–523, 1984.

Corson SL: Contraceptive steroid effects on nonreproductive organ systems. *J Reprod Med* 31(Suppl):865–878, 1986.

Cramer DW, Goldman MB, Schiff I, et al: The relationship of tubal infertility to barrier method and oral contraceptive use. *JAMA* 257:2446–2450, 1987.

Crook D, Godsland IF, Wynn V: Oral contraceptives and coronary heart disease: Modulation of glucose tolerance and plasma lipid risk factors by progestins. *Am J Obstet Gynecol* 158:1612–1620, 1988.

Dalen JE, Hickler RB: Oral contraceptives and cardiovascular disease. *Am Heart J* 101:626–639, 1981.

Derman R: Oral contraceptives: Assessment of benefits. *J Reprod Med* 31(Suppl):879–886, 1986.

Dickey RP: *Managing Contraceptive Pill Patients*, 5th ed. Creative Infomatics, Durant, OK, 1987.

Digest: Americans exaggerate health risks of the pill, underestimate effectiveness of all contraceptives. *Fam Plann Perspect* 17:128–129, 1985.

Dinman BD: The reality and acceptance of risk. *JAMA* 244:1226–1228, 1980.

Dixon GW, Schlesselman JJ, Ory HW, et al: Ethinyl estradiol and conjugated estrogens as postcoital contraceptives. *JAMA* 244:1336–1339, 1980.

Editorial: Postcoital contraception. *Lancet* 1:855–856, 1983.

Ellis JW: Multiphasic oral contraceptives: Efficacy and metabolic impact. *J Reprod Med* 32:28–36, 1987.

Ellsworth H: Focus on Triphasil. *J Reprod Med* 31(Suppl):559–564, 1986.

Emans SJ, Grace E, Woods ER, et al: Adolescents' compliance with the use of oral contraceptives. *JAMA* 257:3377–3381, 1987.

Forman D, Vincent TJ, Doll R: Cancer of the liver and the use of oral contraceptives. *Br Med J* 292:1357–1361, 1986.

Fortney JA, Bonhomme M, Grubb GS, et al: Oral contraceptives and hepatocellular carcinoma. *Br Med J* 292:1392–1393, 1986.

Goldbaum G, Kendrick JS, Hogelin GC, et al: The relative impact of smoking and oral contraceptive use on women in the United States. *JAMA* 258:1339–1342, 1987.

Golin M: O.C. pill/cancer decision 'on hold' awaiting new, longterm research. *Adolesc Med Newsletter* 16(1):2, 1989.

Gorrill MJ, Marshall JR: Pharmacology of estrogens and estrogen-induced effects on nonreproductive organs and systems. *J Reprod Med* 31(Suppl):842–847, 1986.

Graham S, Fraser IS: The progestogen-only mini-pill. *Contraception* 26:373–388, 1982.

Greydanus DE: Alternatives to adolescent pregnancy: A discussion of the contraceptive literature from 1960 to 1980. *Semin Perinatol* 5:53–90, 1981.

Grimes DA: Reversible contraception for the 1980s. *JAMA* 255:69–75, 1986.

Grubb GS: Women's perceptions of the safety of the pill: A survey in eight developing countries. *J Biosoc Sci* 19:313–321, 1987.

Hale R: Currently available formulations. *J Reprod Med* 31(Suppl):557–558, 1986.

Hatcher RA, Guest F, Stewart F, et al: *Contraceptive Technology 1988–1989*, 14th ed. Irvington Publishers, New York, 1988.

Hellberg D, Valentin J, Nilsson S: Long-term use of oral contraceptives and cervical neoplasia: An association confounded by other risk factors. *Contraception* 32:337–346, 1985.

Helling TS, Wood WG: Oral contraceptives and cancer of the liver: A review with two additional cases. *Am J Gastroenterol* 77:504–508, 1982.

Helmrich SP, Rosenberg L, Kaufman DW, et al: Venous thromboembolism in relation to oral contraceptive use. *Obstet Gynecol* 69:91–95, 1987.

Hennekens CJ, Speizer FE, Lipnick RJ, et al: A case-control study of oral contraceptive use and breast cancer. *J Natl Cancer Inst* 72:39–42, 1984.

Herold ES, Goodwin MS: Perceived side effects of oral contraceptives among adolescent girls. *Can Med Assoc J* 123:1022–1026, 1980.

Hofmann AD: Contraception in adolescence: A review. *Bull WHO* 62:151–162, 331–344, 1984.

Holly EA: Cutaneous melanoma and oral contraceptives: A review of case-control and cohort studies. *Recent Results Cancer Res* 102:108–117, 1986.

Hoppe G: Gestoden: An innovative progestogen. *Contraception* 37:493–501, 1988.

Irwin KL, Rosero-Bixby L, Oberle MW, et al: Oral contraceptives and cervical cancer risk in Costa Rica. *JAMA* 259:59–64, 1988.

Johnson JH: Contraception: The morning after. *Fam Plann Perspect* 16:266–270, 1984.

Johnson JH: Weighing the evidence on the pill and breast cancer. *Fam Plann Perspect* 21:89–92, 1989.

Jones EF, Beniger JR, Westoff CF: Pill and IUD discontinuation in the United States, 1970–1975: The influence of the media. *Fam Plann Perspect* 12:293–300, 1980.

Kay C: Progestogens and arterial disease: Evidence from the Royal College of General Practitioners' Study. *Am J Obstet Gynecol* 142:762–765, 1982.

Kay CR, Hannaford PC: Breast cancer and the pill—a further report from the Royal College of General Practitioners' oral contraception study. *Br J Cancer* 58:675–680, 1988.

Khaw K-T, Peart WS: Blood pressure and contraceptive use. *Br Med J* 285:403–407, 1982.

Klitsch M: FDA approval ends cervical cap's marathon. *Fam Plann Perspect* 20:137–138, 1988.

Kloosterboer HJ, van Wayjen RG, van den Ende A: Comparative effects of monophasic desogestrel plus ethinyloestradiol and triphasic levonorgestrel plus ethinyloestradiol in lipid metabolism. *Contraception* 34:135–144, 1986.

Knopp RH: Arteriosclerosis risk: The roles of oral contraceptives and postmenopausal estrogens. *J Reprod Med* 31(Suppl):913–921, 1986.

Knopp RH: Cardiovascular effects of endogenous and exogenous sex hormones over a woman's lifetime. *Am J Obstet Gynecol* 158:1630–1643, 1988.

Kols A, Rinehart W, Piotrow P, et al: Oral contraceptives in the 1980's. *Popul Rep[A]* No. 6, 1982.

Kreutner AK: Adolescent contraception. *Primary Care* 14:121–138, 1987.

Kulig JQ, Rauh JL, Burket RL, et al: Experience with the copper-7 intrauterine device in an adolescent population. *J Pediatr* 96:746–750, 1980.

Kulig JW: Adolescent contraception: An update. *Pediatrics* 76(Suppl):675–680, 1985.

Lane ME, Arceo R, Sobrero AJ: Successful use of the diaphragm and jelly by a young population: Report of a clinical study. *Fam Plann Perspect* 8:81–86, 1976.

LaRosa JC: The varying effects of progestins on lipid levels and cardiovascular disease. *Am J Obstet Gynecol* 158:1621–1629, 1988.

Lee NC, Rubin GL, Borucki R: The intrauterine device and pelvic inflammatory disease revisited: New results from the Women's Health Study. *Obstet Gynecol* 72:1–8, 1988.

Lewin T: "Searle, Assailing Lawsuits, Halts U.S. Sale of Intrauterine Devices." *New York Times*, Feb. 1, 1986, p. 1.

Lincoln R: The pill, breast and cervical cancer, and the role of progestogen in arterial disease. *Fam Plann Perspect* 16:55–63, 1984.

Lippes J, Malik T, Tatum HJ: The post-coital copper T. *Adv Plann Parent* 11:24–29, 1976.

Litt IF, Cuskey WR, Rudd S: Identifying adolescents at risk for non-compliance with contraceptive therapy. *J Pediatr* 96:742–745, 1980.

Louv WC, Austin H, Perlman J, et al: Oral contraceptive use and the risk of chlamydial and gonococcal infections. *Am J Obstet Gynecol* 160:396–402, 1989.

Mant D, Villard-MacKintosh L, Vessey MP, et al: Myocardial infarction and angina pectoris in young women. *J Epidemiol Community Health* 41:215–219, 1987.

Marks A, Mueller M: The diaphragm: An appealing and effective contraceptive for many teenagers. *Pediatr Res* 13:328, 1979.

McIntyre SL, Higgins, JE: Parity and use-effectiveness with the contraceptive sponge. *Am J Obstet Gynecol* 155:796–801, 1986.

Meade TW: Oral contraceptives, clotting factors, and thrombosis. *Am J Obstet Gynecol* 142:758–761, 1982.

Meade TW: Risks and mechanisms of cardiovascular events in users of oral contraceptives. *Am J Obstet Gynecol* 158:1646–1652, 1988.

Meade TW, Greenberg G, Thompson SG: Progestogens and cardiovascular reactions associated with oral contraceptives and a comparison of the 50 and 30 mcg estrogen preparations. *Br Med J* 280:1157–1161, 1980.

The Medical Letter: Triphasil—a new triphasic oral contraceptive. *Med Lett Drugs Ther* 27(688):48, 1985.

Miller DR, Rosenberg L, Kaufman DW, et al: Breast cancer before age 45 and oral contraceptive use: New findings. *Am J Epidemiol* 129:269–280, 1989.

Mishell DR Jr: Contraception. *N Engl J Med* 320:777–787, 1989.

Neinstein LS, Katz B: Contraceptive use in the chronically ill adolescent female. *J Adolesc Health Care* 7:123–133, 350–360, 1986.

Neuberger J, Forman D, Doll R, et al: Oral contraceptives and hepatocellular carcinoma. *Br Med J* 292:1355–1357, 1986.

North BB, Vorhauer BW: Use of the Today contraceptive sponge in the United States. *Int J Fertil* 30:81–84, 1985.

Orr MT: Private physicians and the provision of contraceptives to adolescents. *Fam Plann Perspect* 16:83–86, 1984.

Percival-Smith RKL, Abercrombie B: Post-coital contraception with DL-Norgestrel/ethinyl estradiol combination: Six years experience in a student medical clinic. *Contraception* 36:287–290, 1987.

Percival-Smith RK, Morrison BJ, Sizto R, et al: The effect of triphasic and biphasic oral contraceptive preparations. *Contraception* 35:179–187, 1987.

Petitti DB: Epidemiologic assessment of the risk of oral contraception. *J Reprod Med* 31(Suppl):887–891, 1986.

Petitti DB, Wingerd MA, Pellegrin F: Risk of vascular disease in women. *JAMA* 242: 1150–1154, 1979.

Pituitary Adenoma Study Group: Pituitary adenomas and oral contraceptives: A multicenter case-control study. *Fertil Steril* 39:753–760, 1983.

Policar M: Clinical experience with multiphasic oral contraceptives. *J Reprod Med* 31(Suppl):939–945, 1986.

Porter JB, Jick H, Walker AM: Mortality among oral contraceptive users. *Obstet Gynecol* 70:29–32, 1987.

Powell MG, Mears BJ, Deber RB, et al: Contraception with the cervical cap: Effectiveness, safety, continuity of use, and user satisfaction. *Contraception* 33:215–232, 1986.

Reeves WC, Brinton LA, Garcia M, et al: Human papillomavirus infection and cervical cancer in Latin America. *N Engl J Med* 320:1437–1441, 1989.

Rosenberg L, Miller DR, Kaufman DW, et al: Breast cancer and oral contraceptive use. *Am J Epidemiol* 119:167–176, 1984.

Rosenberg MJ, Rosenthal SM: Reproduction mortality in the United States: Recent trends and methodological considerations. *Am J Public Health* 77:833–836, 1987.

Rosenfield A: Oral and intrauterine contraception: A 1978 risk assessment. *Am J Obstet Gynecol* 132:92–106, 1978.

Schilling LH: Postcoital contraception: Student choices and effectiveness. *J Am Coll Health* 32:239–243, 1984.

Shearin RB, Boelhke JR: Hormonal contraception. *Pediatr Clin North Am* 36(3):697–716, 1989.

Sher PW, Emans SJ, Grace EA: Factors associated with compliance to oral contraceptive use in an adolescent population. *J Adolesc Health Care* 3:120–123, 1982.

Shy KK, McTiernan AM, Daling JR, et al: Oral contraceptive use and the occurrence of pituitary prolactinoma. *JAMA* 249:2204–2207, 1983.

Slap G: Oral contraceptives and depression—impact, prevalence and cause. *J Adolesc Health Care* 2:53–64, 1981.

Smith RP, Ross A: Post-coital contraception using dl-norgestrel/ethinyl estradiol combination. *Contraception* 17:247–252, 1978.

Stadel BV, Lai S-H, Schlesselman JJ, et al: Oral contraceptives and premenopausal breast cancer in nulliparous women. *Contraception* 38:287–299, 1988.

Stadel BV, Rubin GL, Webster LA, et al: Oral contraceptives and breast cancer in young women. *Lancet* 2:970–973, 1985.

Stampfer MJ, Willett WC, Colditz GA, et al: A prospective study of past use of oral contraceptive agents and risk of cardiovascular disease. *N Engl J Med* 319:1313–1317, 1988.

Stewart FH, Guest F, Stewart G, et al: *Understanding Your Body*. New York, Bantum, 1987.

Stone KM, Grimes DA, Magder LS: Personal protection against sexually transmitted diseases. *Am J Obstet Gynecol* 155:180–188, 1986.

Strasburger VC, Eisner JM, Tilson JQ, et al: Teenagers, physicians, and the law in New England. *J Adolesc Health Care* 6:377–382, 1985.

Stubblefield PG: Selection of steroid combinations for oral contraceptives of maximum benefit. *J Reprod Med* 31(Suppl):922–928, 1986.

Tietze C: New estimates of mortality associated with fertility control. *Fam Plann Perspect* 9:74–76, 1977.

Turetsky RA, Strasburger VC: Adolescent contraception: Review and recommendations. *Clin Pediatr* 22:337–341, 1983.

Tyrer LB: Oral contraception for the adolescent. *J Reprod Med* 29(Suppl):551–559, 1984.

Update: Thumbs down on high-dose pills. *Fam Plann Perspect* 20(3):110–111, 1988.

Van Der Vange N, Kloosterboer HJ, Haspels AA: Effect of seven low-dose combined oral contraceptive preparations on carbohydrate metabolism. *Am J Obstet Gynecol* 156:918–922, 1987.

Vessey M, Metcalfe A, Wells C, et al: Ovarian neoplasms, functional ovarian cysts, and oral contraceptives. *Br Med J* 294:1518–1520, 1987.

Vessey MP, Lawless M, McPherson K, et al: Neoplasia of the cervix uteri and contraception: A possible adverse affect of the pill. *Lancet* 2:930–934, 1983.

Vessey MP, Lawless M, Yeates D: Oral contraceptives and stroke: Findings in a large prospective study. *Br Med J* 289:530–531, 1984.

Washington AE, Gove S, Schachter J, et al: Oral contraceptives, *Chlamydia trachomatis* infection and pelvic inflammatory disease: A word of caution about protection. *JAMA* 253:2246–2250, 1985a.

Washington AE, Sweet RL, Shafer MB: Pelvic inflammatory disease and its sequelae in adolescents. *J Adolesc Health Care* 6:298–310, 1985b.

Washington Post: FDA panel backs five-year implants for birth control. April 28, 1989.

Webster L: Epidemiology of oral contraceptives and the risk of breast cancer. *J Reprod Med* 6(Suppl):540–545, 1986.

WHO Collaborative Study of Neoplasia and Steroid Contraceptives: Invasive cervical cancer and combined oral contraceptives. *Br Med J* 290:961–965, 1985.

Wolner-Hanssen P, Svensson L, Mardh P-A, et al: Laparoscopic findings and contraceptive use in women with signs and symptoms suggestive of acute salpingitis. *Obstet Gynecol* 66:233–238, 1985.

Woods JW: Oral contraceptives and hypertension. *Hypertension* (Suppl. II) II(3):11–15, 1988.

Wright NJ, Vesey MP, Kenward B, et al: Neoplasia and dysplasia of the cervix uteri and contraception: A possible protective effect of the diaphragm. *Br J Cancer* 38:273–279, 1978.

Yuzpe AA: Postcoital contraception. *Int J Gynaecol Obstet* 16:497–501, 1979.

Yuzpe AA, Lancee WJ: Ethinylestradiol and dl-norgestrel as a postcoital contraceptive. *Fertil Steril* 28:932–936, 1977.

Recommended Reading

Dickey RP: *Managing Contraceptive Pill Patients*, 5th ed. Durant, Oklahoma: Creative Infomatics, 1987. Available from Irvington Publishers, Broadway, New York, NY 10003.

Hatcher RA, Guest F, Stewart F, et al: *Contraceptive Technology 1988–1989*, 14th ed. New York: Irvington Publishers, 1988–89. Available from publisher.

3

Barrier Contraception

Samuel K. Parrish, Jr.

Barrier methods of contraception include the condom, diaphragm, cervical cap, vaginal sponge, and vaginal spermicidal inserts. All barrier methods of contraception function by preventing sperm from gaining entrance to the cervical canal. Some methods that function as barrier contraceptives also have spermicidal activity (e.g., vaginal sponge, vaginal spermicidal inserts, and diaphragms when used with spermicidal gels) and are discussed in this chapter.

Barrier methods of contraception have been used for centuries and are described in literature dating as early as the 19th Century B.C. Vaginal tampons coated with oil, honey, and other materials are described in Egyptian papyri. Egyptian and Chinese art shows characters prominently wearing penile sheaths or condoms. The forerunners of diaphragms and cervical caps were likely halves of fruit which were placed into the vagina, covering the cervix in much the same way as diaphragms are presently used.

In the scientific literature, the condom was advocated as early as 1560 by Gabriello Fallopio, who recommended the use of treated linen sheaths for the prevention of syphilis. Barrier methods of contraception were the only effective means of contraception available for use until the development and distribution of oral contraceptives and intrauterine devices in the 1960s. With the availability of these two means of contraception, the use of barrier methods decreased significantly. Concerns about the safety of intrauterine devices and oral contraceptives combined with a public health awareness of an increase in sexually transmitted disease, particularly infection with the human immunodeficiency virus, have led to a resurgence in the popularity of many barrier methods of contraception. The pregnancy rates of the barrier methods are given in Table 3–1.

The Condom

Commonly known as rubbers, Trojans, prophylactics, jimmie hats, protection, and hoods, condoms are thin sheaths made of latex rubber or lamb cecum membrane that fit over the erect penis, acting as a mechanical barrier to prevent semen from entering the vagina. Condoms are available in either plain, contoured, or ribbed styles and have either a flat or reservoir-tipped receptacle to receive semen on ejaculation. Condoms may be unlubricated or lubricated with dry or "wet" materials, usually silicon or glycerine compounds. Condoms are available in two sizes, the regular (2 inches in flat width and 7.1 inches in length) and the smaller "Hugger" condom (1.93 inches in flat width and 6.3 inches in length). Since 1975 condoms have been available with spermicidal lubricants, the most common being nonoxynol-9. Condoms are most often

Table 3–1   Pregnancy Rates of Various Barrier Methods of Contraception

Method	Pregnancies per 100 woman years use
Condom	10
Diaphragm	13
Cervical cap	17.4–20
Vaginal sponge	15.8
Vaginal inserts	18

used alone but may be used in combination with spermicidal foams and gels for contraception.

Availability

Condoms may be purchased at drug stores and pharmacies and are distributed in vending machines in locations such as public restrooms and college dormitories. Condoms are also available at no cost at many family planning agencies, community clinics, or sexually transmitted disease programs. The cost of condoms ranges from 20 cents to $2.50, and they may be purchased in single or multiple packs.

Effectiveness

The consistent and proper use of condoms provides the sexually active adolescent with an effective and inexpensive means of contraception. The theoretical effectiveness of condoms is 95% when used alone and 99% when used with spermicidal foams. However, in actual use, the effectiveness is cited at 90% when used alone and 95% when used in combination with spermicides. A 1973 U.S. National Study of Family Growth cited 6.6% of couples experienced condom failure within one year of condom use.

Common Sources of Condom Failure

Unprotected foreplay is the most commonly cited source of condom failure. Careless removal of the condom or failure to remove the penis from the vagina following ejaculation resulting in semen spillage is also frequently reported. Condom tearing is rarely reported with appropriate use. Condom tearing may be reported when an oil-based lubricant, such as Vaseline, is used (Table 3–2).

Protection Against Sexually Transmitted Diseases

The effectiveness of condoms in preventing sexually transmitted disease relies on proper use of the condom and the elimination of unprotected foreplay prior to insertion of the penis into the vagina. Both latex and membrane condoms provide protection from illnesses commonly spread by contact with semen. Infections spread through contact with skin lesions are less effectively prevented by condom use. In vivo and in vitro protection against *Neisseria gonorrhoeae*, *Chlamydia trachomatis*, syphilis, and moniliasis is provided by both latex and lamb membrane condoms. In laboratory studies, latex condoms offer protection against cytomegalovirus, hepatitis B, and human immunodeficiency virus (Feldblum and Fortney, 1988; MMWR, 1988; Reitmeijer et al., 1988).

Table 3–2   Sources of Condom Failure

Unprotected foreplay
Incomplete application of condom covering only tip of penis
Careless removal of the condom resulting in semen spillage
Failure to remove the penis from the vagina immediately following intercourse resulting in
    semen spillage
Tearing of the condom during intercourse
Use of oil-based lubricant resulting in weakening or tearing of the condom during use

Specific Concerns, Complications, and Comments About Condoms

Condoms Might Break.   Condom breakage is reported in 1.5%–10% of all condoms used (*Consumer Reports*, 1989). Condom breakage occurs most often when condoms are stored improperly in warm or moist areas (such as a wallet or in the glove compartment of an automobile). Condom breakage is also reported when condoms are used after their expiration date (which is printed on the package). Tearing of the condom is reported when condoms are used with oil-based lubricants, such as Vaseline or hand lotions. Only water-based lubricants, such as glycerine, K-Y, or surgical jellies, should be used with condoms.

Condoms Interrupt the Sexual Act.   In order for the condom to be an effective means of contraception and protection against sexually transmitted disease, it must be applied after the male has achieved erection, but before *any* sexual contact has occurred. The application of the condom can be made a part of the foreplay for adolescents who are motivated to use condoms properly.

Condoms May Cause Skin Rashes or Allergies.   Condom dermatitis has been reported, but remains extremely rare. Patients who are sensitive to condoms may be allergic to either the latex or chemical substances used in the manufacture of the condom, such as antioxidants or dithiocarbamates. Some users may be sensitive to chemical lubricants used in condom preparation. For such patients, the lamb "skin" condoms may be tolerated. Also condoms manufactured with silicon or "dry" lubricant substances or nonlubricated condoms may be tolerated (Fisher, 1987).

The Condom Might Fall Off During Intercourse or After Ejaculation.   Users of condoms should be advised to withdraw the penis from the vagina immediately following ejaculation before the penis becomes flaccid to avoid the condom falling off and leakage of semen into the vagina. The penis should be held tightly around the base of the condom to prevent its slipping off, the condom removed, and the penis washed before any activity continues. For individuals who complain that condoms slip off during intercourse, the smaller "hugger" style condoms or Mentor brand condoms (Mentor Corp., Minneapolis, MN) are recommended. Hugger condoms offer a tighter fit, and Mentor condoms are prepared with an inner adhesive band approximately 3 cm from the tip which prevents the condom from slipping during intercourse.

Condoms Decrease Sensation During Intercourse.   In some instances men will report a decrease in sensitivity during intercourse when wearing condoms. However, almost 50% of men using condoms reported that decreased sensation allowed for prolonged sexual activity (*Consumer Reports*, 1989) and judged this as an actual advantage of using condoms. The adolescent male who experiences premature ejaculation may find that the decrease in sensitivity may allow for more satisfactory sexual experiences. For some adolescent females, the use of lubricated condoms may decrease vaginal irritation due to excessive friction during the sexual act.

Asking My Partner to Use a Condom Is Embarrassing.   For many adolescents asking a sexual partner to use a condom at the moment at which sexual excitement is at its peak is quite difficult and embarrassing. Youngsters should be encouraged and counseled to discuss the use of condoms prior to sexual activity of any sort. It must be stressed that contraception should always be used and that "just this time" is enough to cause an unintended pregnancy that will certainly be as embarrassing as asking a partner to use condoms.

Condoms Are Messy to Use.   Using lubricated condoms may be distasteful for the inexperienced, but with practice they become less messy. In addition, the use of the condom eliminates the discharge of semen from the vagina following intercourse that many adolescents find unpleasant.

Condoms and the Adolescent Patient

Condoms provide an effective, low-cost means of contraception and are appropriate for most adolescent patients. The practitioner may choose to recommend condoms to adolescents who are motivated to avoid pregnancy and sexually transmitted diseases. The use of the condom has the benefit of allowing the male partner to be involved and share in contraceptive responsibility. The availability of condoms without the involvement of medical personnel, through drug stores, vending machines, or free clinics, should make the condom accessible to all who desire to use them.

For adolescents with multiple or new sexual partners, the condom offers some degree of protection against sexually transmitted diseases, including infection with human immunodeficiency virus. Adolescents engaging in infrequent sexual activity who do not desire to take oral contraceptives daily may find the condom an appropriate means of contraception. Condoms are also appropriate for the adolescent who is unable to use other barrier methods of contraception, such as diaphragms and cervical caps or vaginal sponges and inserts.

In order for condoms to be an effective means of both contraception and protection against sexually transmitted disease they must be on hand and used. This necessitates that the adolescent anticipate sexual activity or at least recognize the possibility for sexual activity during an encounter. For the adolescent who finds anticipating sexual activity to be a source of guilt or discomfort because he feels that planning to have sex is inappropriate, the condom is not the best method of contraception to use.

Instructions to Patients on Proper Use of Condoms

1. Hold the tip of the condom, and squeeze out the air. This leaves some room for semen when you come (ejaculate). Put the condom on the end of your penis.
2. Keep holding the tip of the condom. Unroll it onto your erect penis. Unroll the condom all the way down to the hair.
3. Put the condom on *before* you enter your partner.
4. You can use a lubricant like "K-Y" or a contraceptive gel. Lubricants like Vaseline or grease *should not* be used.
5. After you come (ejaculate): hold onto the condom and pull out while your penis is still hard.
6. Use a *new* condom *every time* you have sex. Use a condom *only once* and then throw it away.

7. Don't store condoms for a long time in your wallet or near heat.
8. All condoms sold in the United States meet the same standards for strength and quality.

(Adapted from *How to Use a Condom*, Family Planning Council Southeastern Pennsylvania.)

The Cervical Cap

The cervical cap was first developed in the 1800s. This small rubber dome-shaped apparatus fits tightly across the cervix, preventing the entrance of semen into the uterus. The cervical cap is intended to be used in combination with a spermicidal gel which is placed inside the cap prior to its insertion. The cervical cap has not been widely used in the United States. The Food and Drug Administration approved the cervical cap for use in 1988, although it presently remains under investigation (Klitsch, 1988).

Availability

The cervical cap must be fitted by personnel trained in its use and may not be available in all locations.

Effectiveness

The cervical cap has a pregnancy rate of 17.4–20 pregnancies per 100 woman years (8.0–48 in studies reviewed) (Smith and Lee, 1984; Powell et al., 1986).

Protection Against Sexually Transmitted Disease

No data are available to document the effectiveness of the cervical cap in the prevention of sexually transmitted disease. It is felt that the cervical cap offers minimal protection against infection in the same manner as the diaphragm.

Fitting the Cervical Cap

1. The candidate for a cervical cap first undergoes a routine speculum examination and Pap smear with special attention noting cervical lesions or signs of cervicitis which contraindicate the use of the cap.
2. The size and shape of the cervix is estimated. An average sized and round cervix is best suited for cervical cap use.
3. A bimanual examination is performed in order to determine cervical and uterine placement. A severely anteverted uterus will make fitting the cap difficult and increase the likelihood of displacement during intercourse. A midplane or retroverted uterus is most appropriate for fitting and proper use.
4. With one hand the practitioner spreads the patient's labia, and using the other hand the cap is compressed and inserted into the end of the vagina and onto the cervix.
5. Stability of the cap is determined by pushing on the cap, simulating movement likely encountered during intercourse.

6. Gaps between the cap rim and cervix should be checked. The entire cervix should be covered by the cap.
7. The seal of the cap should be evaluated by indenting the cap and observing for 30 seconds. If the indentation disappears immediately, the seal may be inadequate.

After the appropriate cap size has been determined and fitted, the patient should be taught to observe her cervix with the use of a hand mirror. She should then be taught to insert the cap correctly. The patient should also be taught to remove the cervical cap. Some caps are manufactured with a small string to aid in removal.

The patient should be instructed to return from home with the cap inserted in order to assess proper placement. The patient should feel no discomfort with the cap in place. The patient should be instructed to remove the cap within 24–48 hours after placement (Brokaw et al., 1988).

Special Concerns, Complications, and Comments About the Cervical Cap

Difficulty in Insertion   Although cap insertion may be complicated and cumbersome, most individuals motivated to use the cervical cap for contraception are able to be instructed properly in its use.

Displacement During Use   Between 10% and 40% of all women using the cervical cap have reported at least one episode of displacement of the cap during normal use. This is the most frequently reported complication and cause of unintended pregnancy associated with the use of cervical caps (Powell et al., 1986).

Odor Associated with Cervical Cap Use   Between 5% and 17% of women using the cervical cap report an unpleasant vaginal odor associated with use. The odor is most often noted following intercourse and is associated with the presence of semen (Klitsch, 1988).

Length of Time the Cervical Cap May Be Left in Place   The patient is instructed to leave the cervical cap in place for 24–48 hours. For many patients this allows for more spontaneous sexual activity. However, the patient must be instructed to remove the cap within 48 hours and to clean the cap appropriately in order to prevent premature deterioration of the cervical cap (Eichhorst, 1988).

Abnormal Pap Smears Associated with the Cervical Cap   It is not recommended that individuals with abnormal Pap smears use the cervical cap as a means of contraception.

The Cervical Cap and the Adolescent Patient

At present, no studies are available documenting the use of the cervical cap in adolescent patients. One study of women attending a University of California-Berkeley family planning project found that approximately 50% of users experienced unplanned pregnancies while using the cervical cap as a means of contraception. In adolescents who are highly motivated, the cervical cap may serve as an effective means of contraception. However, the cervical cap should be reserved for use in women who are unable or unwilling to use oral contraceptives or condoms, and for whom a comfortable fit is impossible with a diaphragm.

The cervical cap is more difficult to insert than the diaphragm, and for individuals who are uncomfortable manipulating their labia and inserting the device, the cap should not be used.

The Diaphragm

The diaphragm is a latex dome which is mounted on a circular rim containing a metal spring. Commonly manufactured diaphragms range in size from 45–105 mm in diameter. Proper use calls for the diaphragm to fit comfortably behind the symphysis pubis and snugly against the vaginal wall.

The diaphragm is intended for use in combination with spermicidal gels which are placed inside the cap, thus providing a physical barrier and chemical means of contraception to the user.

Availability

Diaphragms are available by prescription through pharmacies and at most family planning programs. Diaphragms range in size from 45–105 mm in diameter. Styles differ depending upon the type of spring mechanism mounted in the rim, with an arcing spring the most commonly used.

Effectiveness

The accepted pregnancy rate associated with diaphragm use is 13 pregnancies per 100 woman years or 87% effectiveness. Higher pregnancy rates are found among "new" users and also among younger patients. A high failure rate of the diaphragm is generally attributed to motivational and behavioral factors (Porter et al., 1983).

The most commonly cited reasons for failure of the diaphragm include the lack of consistent use, inappropriate fit, and breakage from improper storage and care of the diaphragm.

Protection Against Sexually Transmitted Disease

The diaphragm, when used alone, does not offer protection against the major sexually transmitted diseases. When used in combination with spermicidal gels or foams containing nonoxynol-9, some protection is provided against *N. gonorrhoeae*, *Trichomonas*, herpes, and candidal infections. However, the diaphragm must not be considered an appropriate means of protection against these or other sexually transmitted diseases.

Fitting the Diaphragm

The diaphragm requires proper fitting by a trained practitioner. Diaphragms vary both in size and in the type of spring enclosed in the ring. Springs may be coiled, flat, or arcing. The arcing spring is the most easily inserted and most widely used type of diaphragm.

The visit for fitting the diaphragm is an important one, and the patient must be given an appropriate amount of time during which questions and concerns regarding the diaphragm may be discussed.

1. A speculum examination is performed for routine cultures and Pap smear. Special note is taken of the presence of cystocele or rectocele which will contraindicate the use of a diaphragm.
2. The distance from the posterior fornix to the pubic bone is measured. This is performed by placing the second finger into the vagina and feeling downward to

locate the posterior fornix with the finger tip. The point at which the proximal portion of the second finger touches the symphysis pubis is noted. This distance is used to estimate the length of the vagina.

3. A sizing ring or fitting diaphragm is chosen which most closely matches the length of the vagina as previously determined. The diaphragm is folded and inserted into the vagina, pushing downward towards the posterior fornix until it is located at a point behind the pubic bone. The diaphragm is then tilted into place, with the ring located behind the pubic bone.

4. The diaphragm should be checked to determine proper fit. A finger tip should be able to be placed between the diaphragm rim and the lateral vaginal wall. The patient may be aware of the presence of the diaphragm, but should not experience discomfort.

5. The diaphragm should cover the cervix entirely, and should not be easily dislodged. The patient may be asked to bear down or Valsalva which may dislocate the diaphragm if the fit is too tight.

6. A finger should be placed between the rim of the diaphragm and the vaginal wall, and the diaphragm should be removed. The patient should then be instructed to place the diaphragm properly. The patient should be instructed in locating the pubic symphysis, as well as in feeling to determine that the diaphragm covers the cervix completely.

7. After the patient has inserted the diaphragm herself, the examiner should again perform a manual examination to ensure proper fit.

8. The patient should be instructed to attempt placement of the diaphragm at home and return to be examined with the diaphragm in place. At this visit, the patient should be asked about discomfort while wearing the diaphragm as well as difficulties encountered in placement. Patients may place the diaphragm while standing with one leg elevated (often standing with one foot on a small stool or on the toilet) or lying on their side.

9. The patient should be instructed always to use a spermicidal gel when using the diaphragm. The spermicidal gel should be placed inside the diaphragm cap prior to its insertion.

Specific Concerns, Complications, and Comments Regarding the Diaphragm

Timing of Use   The diaphragm may be inserted up to 2 hours prior to intercourse and should be left in place for at least 6 hours following intercourse. This requires the patient to acknowledge that a sexual act is likely to occur. For the youngster who is unable to anticipate sexual activity, this is a difficult requirement to fulfill and may make the diaphragm an inappropriate means of contraception to use.

Embarrassment with Insertion   Some adolescents may be uncomfortable with the self-manipulation necessary to insert the diaphragm properly. This is often noted at the visit for fitting the diaphragm. Some of these youngsters may be taught to insert a diaphragm properly, but individuals who remain uncomfortable should be counseled in the use of other means of contraception.

Refitting and Readjustment   Individuals using the diaphragm should be reexamined in 6 months after first use in order to be refitted. Vaginal stretching is often noted within the first 6 months of diaphragm use. Also in youngsters who are experiencing growth, the need for readjustment may be noted.

Medical Conditions That are Contraindications for Diaphragm Use   Uterine prolapse, cystocele, rectocele, poor vaginal tone, and an inability to feel the cervix are all
contraindications of diaphragm use in the adolescent patient.

Urinary Tract Infection Associated with Diaphragm Use   Vaginal colonization with
Escherichia coli and subsequent urinary tract infection are reported to be associated
with diaphragm use. In individuals with a history of recurrent urinary tract infection,
the diaphragm is contraindicated as a means of contraception (Fihn et al., 1985).

Allergy to the Diaphragm   Allergies to the latex diaphragm are quite rare. Individuals
who report rashes or discomfort secondary to diaphragm use may be sensitive to the
spermicidal gel used or sensitive to the diaphragm. Some individuals may require
discontinuance of diaphragm use due to discomfort.

The Diaphragm and the Adolescent Patient

The diaphragm is an effective means of contraception for the motivated adolescent who
is unwilling or unable to use oral contraceptives, condoms or other barrier methods.
The youngster who is comfortable with her body and is able to manipulate her genitalia
in order to achieve proper insertion is an appropriate candidate for diaphragm use. The
diaphragm requires placement prior to use, which necessitates some degree of planning
sexual activity. For individuals who are unable to anticipate intercourse, the diaphragm
will present considerable difficulty for proper use.

In many instances, the younger adolescent patient is unable to properly use the
diaphragm due to embarrassment at insertion or to an inability to anticipate or delay
sexual activity in order for the diaphragm to remain in place for an appropriate amount
of time prior to use. Therefore, the diaphragm may be more suitable for use in the older
adolescent patient.

The Vaginal Contraceptive Sponge

Available in the United States since 1983, the vaginal contraceptive sponge is a cup-
shaped device measuring 5–6 cm in diameter and 1.5 cm thick. The contraceptive
sponge is manufactured from a polyurethane polymer and is impregnated with nonox-
ynol-9 spermicide. The sponge is available under the tradename Today Contraceptive
sponge™ (Lemberg, 1984).

Availability

The vaginal contraceptive sponge is widely available and may be purchased in pack-
ages of three sponges for approximately $1.00 per sponge. No prescription or physician
visit is necessary in order to use the contraceptive sponge. The contraceptive sponge
may be available at some family planning agencies within local communities.

Effectiveness

In studies of effectiveness using the vaginal contraceptive sponge, 15.8 pregnancies
per 100 woman years of use were reported. This rate is somewhat less than protection
provided by appropriate diaphragm use (Lemberg, 1984).

The vaginal contraceptive sponge provides protection against unintended pregnancy in three ways: 1) Spermicidal activity of nonoxynol-9 is the primary means of contraception provided by the vaginal sponge. The Today sponge contains 30% by weight of nonoxynol-9 as manufactured. This spermicide is activated by moisture and is slowly released. The sponge is felt to provide adequate spermicidal protection for a period of 24–48 hours. 2) Mechanical protection by absorption of semen by the polyurethane sponge. This is felt to decrease the number of sperm available for fertilization and to provide contraceptive function. 3) Mechanical blockage—the sponge, when properly applied, covers the cervix, thereby blocking semen from entering the cervical os.

Protection Against Sexually Transmitted Disease

The vaginal contraceptive sponge offers some protection against *N. gonorrhoeae* and *C. trachomatis*. Although potentially important, the vaginal contraceptive sponge should not be used as a primary means of protection against sexually transmitted disease (Rosenberg et al., 1987a, 1987b).

Specific Concerns, Complications, and Comments Regarding the Vaginal Sponge

Toxic Shock Syndrome   Although individual cases of toxic shock syndrome have been reported associated with use of the vaginal contraceptive sponge, toxic shock syndrome remains exceedingly rare. Studies to evaluate the effect of contraceptive sponges on the growth and toxin production of *Staphylococcus aureus* suggest that the contraceptive sponge inhibits the production of toxin associated with toxic shock syndrome (Dart and Levitt, 1985; Remington et al., 1987).

Although toxic shock syndrome is not considered a major problem associated with the use of vaginal contraceptive sponges, women using the vaginal sponge are advised not to leave the sponge in place for more than 24 hours when experiencing their menstrual periods (Edelman et al., 1984).

Sponge Tearing and Retention   When the contraceptive sponge was initially introduced, problems were noted with tearing of the sponge upon removal. Sponges presently available are reinforced with polyester at the site of the retrieval loop in order to address this concern. Tearing of the contraceptive sponge is most often associated with the use of the contraceptive sponge for a period of time greater than 48 hours. If a patient experiences tearing of the contraceptive sponge, she should be told to seek appropriate medical attention for removal.

Allergic Reaction   Allergic reaction to the polyurethane contraceptive sponge was reported in 4.3% of patients studied in one series (Lemberg, 1984). The most commonly reported symptom of allergic reaction was vaginal itching. Patients reporting persistent vaginal itching with sponge use should be counseled to choose another method of contraceptive protection.

Discomfort with Intercourse   Awareness of the contraceptive sponge and discomfort on intercourse due to vaginal dryness has been reported in association with vaginal contraceptive sponge use. Vaginal dryness is reportedly due to the ability of the contraceptive sponge to absorb vaginal fluid during intercourse. Patients reporting this as a persistent complaint with sponge use may need to be counseled to seek another form of contraception.

Odor with Vaginal Sponge Use   If the vaginal sponge is left in place for greater than 24 hours after use, vaginal odor may be experienced due to retention of vaginal fluid and semen within the polyurethane sponge. Patients should be counseled to remove the sponge within 24 hours in order to avoid an offensive odor (Chvapil et al., 1985).

The Contraceptive Sponge and the Adolescent Patient

The vaginal contraceptive sponge presents a low-cost, relatively effective means of contraception for the adolescent who is able to use this method properly. The use of the vaginal contraceptive sponge requires appropriate placement, within the vagina and covering the cervix. For the adolescent who is unable or unwilling to insert the sponge, this method is inappropriate. The sponge offers the adolescent the advantage of increased spontaneity for sexual contact as well as protection for multiple sexual acts with a single application of the contraceptive sponge. The sponge also offers some degree of protection against the most commonly encountered sexually transmitted diseases.

The rate of effectiveness of the contraceptive sponge is relatively low in comparison with the condom and diaphragm when properly used. It should, therefore, not be recommended as a "first line" method of protection against unintended pregnancy for the adolescent.

Vaginal Insert Spermicides

Vaginal inserts have been used as a means of contraception for over 5,000 years. Spermicidal agents are available in numerous forms and dosages and include foams, gels, creams, suppositories, tablets, and films. Currently, nonoxynol-9 and octoxynol-9 are the most widely used chemical substances for spermicidal activity. Both nonoxynol-9 and octoxynol-9 are surface-active agents which coat and break down the cell membrane of sperm cells, thereby preventing conception.

Availability

Vaginal spermicides are widely available without prescription through commercial sources and at many family planning agencies. The average cost to consumers varies depending upon the preparation desired.

Effectiveness

The effectiveness of vaginal insert contraceptive preparations varies considerably from 1.55–29 pregnancies per 100 women per year. Commonly cited is a pregnancy rate of 18 per 100 women per year.

Protection Against Sexually Transmitted Disease

Laboratory and clinical studies have suggested some protection against essentially all organisms causing sexually transmitted diseases. While not completely protective, vaginal spermicidal agents when combined with barrier methods such as condoms, offer significant protection against sexually transmitted disease (North, 1988).

Concerns, Complications, and Comments About Vaginal Insert Spermicides

Difficulty with Insertion   All vaginal spermicides require insertion into the vagina as near the cervix as possible. For some individuals, this may initially be difficult. Most patients can be taught a proper method of insertion.

Discomfort During Use   Although allergic reaction to spermicidal agents has been reported, it remains quite rare. Individuals who are allergic to either the spermicide or carrier compound should utilize an alternative method of contraception.

Risk to Pregnancy When Contraception Occurs While Using Spermicides   There is no association between the use of vaginal spermicides and birth defects (Kowal, 1981).

Need for Repeated Use   Vaginal spermicides must be inserted into the vagina each time intercourse is to occur. The spermicide must be in place for 15–20 minutes before beginning intercourse. Individuals who are strongly motivated to use vaginal insert spermicides are able to exercise such timing accordingly.

Vaginal Insert Spermicides and the Adolescent Patient

Because of the high failure rate and necessity for insertion into the vagina, many adolescent patients may be unwilling or unable to use this method properly. As with most contraceptive methods, timing and consistency of use is essential for optimal function of this method of contraception. The vaginal insert methods are not a first line method of contraception for adolescents.

For the adolescent who is unable to use oral contraceptives but who desires a highly effective means of contraception as well as increased protection against sexually transmitted disease, the combination of condoms and vaginal spermicidal preparations offers such protection. It is recommended that the vaginal contraceptives be used in conjunction with condoms for adolescents who choose either method for protection against unintended pregnancy.

References

Brokaw AK, Baker NNM, Haney SL: Fitting the cervical cap. *Nurse Pract* 7:49–55, 1988.

Chvapil M, Droegemueller W, Heine MW, MacGregor JC, Dotters D: Collagen sponge as vaginal contraceptive barrier: critical summary of seven years of research. *Am J Obstet Gynecol* 3:325–329, 1985.

Consumer Reports: Can you rely on condoms? *Consumer Rep*, March 1989, pp 135–142.

Dart RC, Levitt MA: Toxic shock syndrome associated with the use of the vaginal contraceptive sponge (letter). *JAMA* 13:1877, 1985.

Edelman DA, Harper J, McIntyre SL: A comparative trial of the Today contraceptive sponge and diaphragm. *Am J Obstet Gynecol* 7:869–876, 1984.

Eichhorst BC: Contraception. *Primary Care* 3:437–456, 1988.

Feldblum PJ, Fortney JA: Condoms, spermicides, and the transmission of human immunodeficiency virus: a review of the literature. *Am J Public Health* 1:52–54, 1988.

Fihn SD, Latham RH, Roberts P, Running K, Stamm WE: Association between diaphragm use and urinary tract infection. *JAMA* 2:240–245, 1985.

Fisher A: Condom dermatitis in either partner. *Cutis* 4:281–285, 1987.

Klitsch M: FDA approval ends cervical cap's marathon. *Fam Plann Perspect* 3:137–138, 1988.

Kowal D: Study raises questions of spermicide safety. *Contracept Technol Update* 1:49–51 1981.

Lemberg E: The vaginal contraceptive sponge: a new non-prescription barrier contraceptive. *Nurse Pract* 10:24–37, 1984.

MMWR: Leads from the MMWR. *JAMA* 13:1925–1927, 1988.

North BB: Vaginal contraceptives, effective protection from sexually transmitted diseases for women? *J Reprod Med* 3:307–311, 1988.

Porter CW, Waife RS, Holtrop HR: *Contraception: The Health Provider's Guide*, ed 1. Grune & Stratton, New York, 1983.

Powell MG, Means BJ, Deber R, Fergusen D: Contraception with the cervical cap: effectiveness, safety, continuity of use and user satisfaction. *Contraception* 3:215–232, 1986.

Reitmeijer CAM, Krebs JW, Feorino PM, Judson FN: Condoms as physical and chemical barriers against human immunodeficiency virus. *JAMA* 12:1851–1853, 1988.

Remington KM, Butler RS, Kelly JR: Effect of the Today contraceptive sponge on growth and toxic shock syndrome toxin-1 production by Staphylococcus aureus. *Obstet Gynecol* 4:563–569, 1987.

Rosenberg MJ, Feldblum PJ, Rojanapithayakorn W, Sawasdivorn W: The contraceptive sponge's protection against Chlamydia trachomatis and Neisseria gonorrhea. *Sex Transm Dis* 3:147–152, 1987a.

Rosenberg MJ, Rojanapithayakorn W, Feldblum PJ, Higgins JE: Effect of the contraceptive sponge on chlamydial infection, gonorrhea, and candidiasis. *JAMA* 17:2308–2312, 1987b.

Smith GG, Lee RJ: The use of cervical caps at the University of California, Berkeley: a survey. *Contraception* 2:115–123, 1984.

4

Consent and Confidentiality
Critical Issues in Providing Contraceptive Care

Adele D. Hofmann

Confidentiality is an important factor in the delivery of adolescent health care (Hofmann, 1989; Johnson and Tanner, 1989; Irwin, 1986). The American Academy of Pediatrics, the American Academy of Family Physicians, and the American College of Obstetricians and Gynecologists, among others, recently issued a joint policy position stating that all adolescents should "have an opportunity for examination and counseling apart from parents and the same confidentiality [should] be preserved as between the . . . adult and the provider* (American Academy of Pediatrics, 1989).

The Confidentiality Option—Pragmatic Need

The requirement of adolescents for confidentiality is based, in part, on developmental truisms and pragmatic need and, in part, upon a new legal concept of the mature minor and a constitutional entitlement to privacy in health care. From the pragmatic perspective, the developmental pursuit of emancipation and autonomy finds many young people secretly involved in various health risk behaviors. Sexual intimacy and substance use are prime examples. Many of these risk-takers will not advise parents of their behavior, even if in need of medical attention, and would rather delay care or put it off altogether rather than have their families know.

  The reason for this silence is not only the fear of parental retribution for forbidden acts but also the more subtle but no less constraining fear of hurting their families with the consequent loss of parental esteem and diminished parental love. Although these fears often are more a matter of fantasy than fact, with most parents willing to be much more supportive than their adolescent believes, fear still inhibits teen-to-parent communication.

  A further reason for noncommunication rests in the nature of emancipation itself, not just the type of behavior involved. The purpose of emancipation is for the adolescent to separate from earlier childhood dependency ties and develop a sense of independence and autonomy in preparation for adulthood. If teenagers were to tell

---

*This policy position also recommends that adolescents should be firmly encouraged to involve their parents and states that confidentiality can not be preserved in life-threatening situations.

parents everything that happened in their lives this would make matters much less their own and unacceptably threaten a return to dependency. Teenagers need to put temporary emotional distance between them and their parents until their sense of independence is secured.

As a consequence of all these factors, necessary medical care may not be obtained until symptoms progress to a point where they can no longer be hidden or worries about health overcome fears of parental wrath. Yet avoidance only acts to increase the adolescent's likelihood of health harm.

Physicians who assume the role of a nonjudgmental "extraparental adult" do not suffer from this developmentally based distancing process and problems in intergenerational communication. Accordingly, adolescents welcome the opportunity to share confidences with the physician even if they are unable to share them with parents.

Nor can confidentiality be breached and parents notified without the minor's permission. Should a physician do so, he or she will totally lose the patient's trust and any ability to help.* This not only applies to the particular patient at hand but also to adolescents in the community as the word soon spreads and the physician becomes known as one who tells. At the same time, simply knowing rarely improves the parents' ability to control an emancipating offspring. Most parents are well aware of this dilemma and welcome the physician's intervention.

Confidentiality and Contraception

Nowhere is the confidentiality option more critical than in providing preventive care to sexually active teens if the epidemic of unintended teen pregnancies is to be checked. In a recent survey, one of every four teenagers visiting a Planned Parenthood clinic stated that parental notification would be an unacceptable condition for their attendance. If notification were mandatory, 98% of these young women would continue to be sexually active but use a less effective, nonprescription contraceptive method or no method at all. Only 2% would consider being abstinent† (Torres, 1980). Similar results have been found in other polls as summarized in Table 4-1.

The need of adolescents for confidential contraceptive services also enjoys broad societal support. This was amply illustrated by the events that followed the 1982 attempt of the Department of Health and Human Services (DHHS) to promulgate regulations *mandating* parental notification for minors receiving contraceptive services from Title X-funded family planning programs, rather than simply *encouraging* it, as was specified in the congressional appropriations legislation. As soon as the proposed regulations became known, some 75 national organizations united together with more than 40 states and the District of Columbia in firm opposition to what rapidly became known as the DHHS "squeal rule." Included in this formidable array of opponents were the American Academy of Pediatrics, the American College of Physicians, the American Medical Association, the Children's Defense Fund, Girls' Clubs of America, the National Education Association, the Salvation Army, the Society for Adoles-

---

*Exception should be made to this rule for adolescents in imminent danger of serious harm. The cardinal example is a youth with suicidal ideation. Parents must be informed of the problem so that appropriate protective steps can be taken.

†The data also show that two out of every three adolescents in family planning programs report that their parents already know of their attendance or that they would not have any objection to parental notification.

Table 4–1　Published Reports of Surveys of Adolescents on the Perceived Impact That Mandatory Parental Notification Would Have on Family Planning Clinic Use

Author	Date	Population	Results
Torres	1980	1,170 females <18 yr attending a family planning clinic	44% of parents did not know of adolescent's clinic attendance; 23% would not attend if parents had to know; 21% would continue having sex using a less effective method or none at all; only 2% would stop sex.
Zabin & Clark	1981	1,200 females <18 yr at 1st family planning clinic visit	31% had delayed obtaining contraceptives due to fear of parental discovery.
Zabin & Clark	1983	Teens attending a family planning clinic	44% would not have attended if their parents had to know.
Herceg-Baron & Furstenberg	1982	200 females <18 yr at 1st visit to a family planning clinic	58% said their parents did not know of their clinic attendance.
Kenney et al.	1982	Teen females attending 3 different family planning clinics	Clinic attendance fell by 10%–50% following news reports of the DHHS proposal for mandatory parental notification (see text).
Planned Parenthood Federation of America	1986	National opinion poll of 1,000 12–17-year-olds	32% believed teenagers less likely to use birth control if parental permission were required.

cent Medicine, and the Young Women's Christian Association, among many others. It was the common opinion that the "squeal rule" could only mean more pregnant teens. Subsequent court challenges sought and successfully obtained a permanent injunction. Federal judges in both New York and Washington, D.C. ruled that the regulations were invalid and could not be enforced because they unacceptably exceeded congressional intent and the scope of authorizing legislation (Alan Guttmacher Institute, 1983). The Reagan administration elected to let the matter drop without seeking Supreme Court review and the "squeal rule" was put to rest (Center for Population Options, 1984).

Other efforts to legally restrain adolescent sexual behavior have met with a similar lack of success. A few states have attempted to require the reporting of voluntarily sexually active girls to appropriate authorities under the provisions of statutory rape laws and child abuse/molestation laws. One recent enactment in California, for example, required the reporting of any sexually active minor under age 14 as a case of child abuse, even if she was sexually active by choice and legally obtaining medical care on her own consent, as for a sexually transmitted disease. The statute was permanently enjoined by the California courts on the grounds that consensual sexual behavior by a minor adolescent, even if under the age of 14, did not comprise sexual abuse, and mandatory reporting impermissibly invaded the minor's state constitutional privacy rights (English, 1986). To the author's knowledge, no such laws are now operative in any state, and voluntary sexual intercourse is not sufficient cause for the mandatory reporting of adolescent girls or their partners for either statutory rape or sexual abuse.*

The Confidentiality Option—A New Constitutional Entitlement

The right of *mature* minors to consent to health care on their own also has emerged as a new constitutional entitlement, particularly in relation to reproductive services. Rulings of the U.S. Supreme Court over the past two decades have defined a new relationship between adolescents, their parents, and the State, a relationship in which, for the first time, at least some minors have independent standing of their own without the need for adult representation.

How this came about is a particularly interesting tale. Prior to the 1960s, the law primarily viewed minors in paternalistic and protective terms. Adults (usually parents, but sometimes the state) made all decisions for minors on their behalf in what was believed to be their best interests. Young people had no independent standing and no voice or representation of their own until majority which, at that time, was age 21.

Change first began in 1967 with the landmark case of *In re Gault (387 U.S. 1, 1967)*. Gerald Gault, a 15-year-old Arizona schoolboy of dubious reputation, had made an obscene phone call to one of his high school teachers who then filed charges against him. Following a brief hearing, the Arizona juvenile authorities packed Gerald off to a state training farm for an indefinite term which could be as long as six years (or until age 21). The U.S. Supreme Court reversed the juvenile court's decision on the basis that Gerald had not been given any of the due process protections of the Bill of Rights, as was generally true of the entire juvenile justice system. For example, Gerald had been denied the right to know the charges being levied against him at the time he was accused; he was not given any opportunity to question his accuser in court, and he was not given a transcript of the proceedings following his hearing. The Court, however, stopped short of extending *all* the Bill of Rights to minors and specifically withheld the right to a jury trial and the right to bail as being inconsistent with the rehabilitative ideals of the juvenile justice system in having prompt, secret hearings which would not label youths as criminals. Later cases continued to address the question of due process in the juvenile justice system and also extended this to students in matters of school suspensions (Hofmann, 1980).

In 1969 the landmark case of *Tinker v. the Des Moines Independent School District* (393 U.S. 503) established the right of minors to free speech. John and Mary Tinker and Christopher Eckhart, three young adolescents, had joined their parents' protest of the Vietnam war by wearing black armbands. The principal of the children's school, however, did not approve of protest in the classroom and stated that any students wearing armbands on the school premises would be immediately suspended. John, Mary, and Christopher did go to school with the bands and were sent home. The Supreme Court found for the young people, declaring that freedom of speech is not for adults alone and that "state operated schools cannot be enclaves of totalitarianism."

The Court, however, has not yet gone so far as to endow all minors with all civil rights by a long shot and, as often as not, continues to view young people as subject to

---

*It should be noted that statutory rape laws continue to apply to male partners and they may b. criminally charged should anyone desire to do so, such as the girl's parents. The only point being made here is that health care providers and other professionals are not *required* to report the case to the authorities and may continue to give the girl confidential care.

adult dominion and control. In *Tinker*, for example, although the right of minors to free speech was established, the Court went on to say that schools could limit free speech if it posed a threat to the maintenance of school order. In *Ingraham v. Wright* the Court refused to support the contention that corporal punishment in schools constituted cruel and unusual punishment, stating instead that it was an appropriate and time-honored method of discipline (Mlyniec, 1978). Nor would the Court even take up the question of whether stripping and physically searching students or searching their lockers and desks without warrants comprised unfair search and seizure. But the concept of seeing some minors in some circumstances as entitled to adult constitutional rights had been introduced. This was a very new perspective.

At about the same time as the Supreme Court was looking at civil rights for minor youth, it also was examining the rights of women to control their own fertility without state regulation. Initially, laws prohibiting the prescription and sale of contraceptives to married women were declared unconstitutional. Later this was extended to unmarried women as well (Paul and Pilpel, 1979). Then, in 1973 in *Roe v. Wade* (410 U.S. 113) and *Doe v. Bolton* (410 U.S. 179) the Court ruled that states could not prohibit women from voluntarily terminating their pregnancies before fetal viability. The sum effect of these cases was to establish a new right to privacy in matters of reproductive health care, a right by which a woman's decisions about her fertility are hers alone to make in consultation with her physician. No other entity, whether the state or an individual, may be given a third party veto power (Hofmann and Pilpel, 1973; Hofmann, 1980; Paul and Pilpel, 1979).

In the mid 1970s, minors' constitutional rights and women's reproductive rights were joined in a series of cases that asked whether minor adolescents had the same privacy rights in reproductive health care as did adults. In *Carey v. Population Services International* (431 U.S. 678, 1977) the Supreme Court ruled that states could not prohibit drugstores from selling contraceptives to minors regardless of age in the interests of legislating morality. And in *Planned Parenthood of Central Missouri v. Danforth* (428 U.S. 52, 1976) the U.S. Supreme Court said that minors who were mature enough to become pregnant also were mature enough to be entitled to privacy in the abortion decision and that states could not require parental consent.

Later, in *Baird v. Bellotti* (U.S. No. 78-329, 78-330, 1979) the Court modified *Danforth* by saying that states could require parental consent or notification before a minor's abortion, provided there also was a bypass mechanism for those who did not want to involve their parents. A constitutionally permissible procedure was suggested in which the girl could request a judicial hearing to determine whether she was mature enough to give an informed consent. If deemed mature, she then would be entitled to make her own abortion decision as if an adult. Only if deemed immature could the judge decide what course was in the girl's best interest; this could be either parental involvement or termination without parental knowledge. The "Bellotti" provision has now been enacted in a number of states.

How future decisions of the Court will affect adolescent reproductive health care remains to be seen. The recent decision in *Webster v. Reproductive Health Services* (U.S.L.W. 5023 (U.S. July 3, 1989) (No. 88-605)) does not affect adolescents any more than adults and Bellotti provisions still apply. There are, however, two cases currently before the Court which do have bearing. Both *Hodgeson v. Minnesota* (853 F.2D 1452 (1988)) and *Slaby v. Akron Center for Reproductive Health* (U.S.L.W. 2106 (U.S. Aug. 12, 1988) (No. 86-3664)) address abortions and parental notification issues. At this point in time, one cannot say whether the outcome of these cases will substantively change minors' access to pregnancy termination.

The Supreme Court's rulings on minors and reproductive care, however, almost exclusively deal with the abortion issue. Only in *Carey* was contraception addressed in a limited manner (drugstore sales, not physician prescription). Prescriptive contraception is a lesser form of reproductive care than abortion, and, if anything, less rigorous standards would apply. Certainly the standards would not be more restrictive.

One of the most important outcomes of these cases was the emergence of the mature minor doctrine. This doctrine states that any minor who is sufficiently mature as to be able to understand the benefits and risks of the proposed therapies and make a reasoned choice from among them is competent to give an informed consent and should be entitled to do so. Indeed, the ability of a minor to give an informed consent has been a pivotal question throughout the evolution of minors' consent law, whether statutory, case, or constitutional.

In summary, mature minors are legally entitled to consent to contraceptive services and to enjoy the associated confidentiality on a wide variety of grounds. This includes the following:

- Supreme Court rulings on minors and abortions as translated to apply to contraception
- The resounding defeat of DHHS's "Squeal Rule" and mandated parental notification
- The widespread support of free access to contraceptive services for teens by professional organizations and agencies advocating for children and youth
- The rejection of child abuse and statutory rape laws as legitimate causes for the mandatory reporting of voluntarily sexually active girls
- The fact that while there have been several temporary injunctions against providing minors contraception without parental consent over the years, none of them have ever become permanent
- No case has yet been found in which damages were awarded against a physician for providing contraceptive services to a minor of any age on her own consent

State Law

Despite the evolution of the mature minor doctrine as a fundamental legal principle, most health care providers still look for statutory and regulatory direction within their particular state in determining precisely when a minor may consent on her own. The longstanding tradition of requiring parents to consent for their minor offspring's health care, excepting in an emergency, is well entrenched. Most health professionals understandably desire very specific legal permission to do otherwise.

It is of historical interest to note that the requirement of parental consent for the treatment of a minor was never statutorily addressed. Rather, the rule derives from an interpretation of old English common law on contracts and torts in which consenting to health care is seen as a contract between a physician and patient. Minors, however, are not considered competent to enter into a contract. Only a parent or legal guardian can do this on the minor's behalf. If a physician touches or treats a minor without a valid contract (consent), then the physician is technically committing an unauthorized touching, or assault and battery. Negligence is a separate issue relating to an alleged harm resulting from treatment.

These old common law precepts, however, have never been absolutely applied. First, the courts have always granted wide latitude to physicians in treating minors without parental consent in emergencies. Second, no one has yet been able to find a case where damages were awarded against a physician for treating a minor on the minor's own consent for any condition, including surgery, as long as the minor was 16 years of age or older. Nor have damages been awarded against any physician for prescribing contraceptives to a sexually active minor of *any* age on her own consent (Paul and Pilpel, 1979).

It would be very difficult, today, to pursue a case of assault and battery successfully through the courts for treating a mature minor on his or her own consent when the patient was obviously benefitted and the physician had appropriately documented both the minor's ability to give an informed consent and the reason for not involving parents (Morrissey et al., 1986).

These general principles, however, have not been sufficient in and of themselves to open the health care doors to all youths in need of confidential care, and virtually every state has enacted one or more statutes permitting some minors to consent to some forms of health care under some circumstances. These laws are of two general types. The first is based on the minor's status, such as being emancipated, married, or mature, and the second is based on the minor's medical need, such as care-related to sexual activity and substance abuse. In some instances a minimum age of eligibility applies; this usually is at age 12 years but may be as high as age 15. Table 4–2 categorizes these laws, but it is beyond the scope of this paper to define each state's permissions, and the reader is referred to Morrissey et al., 1986, for a detailed state-by-state analysis.

The Law and Contraception

It is safe to say that minor adolescents may be provided confidential birth control services on their own consent in any jurisdiction in the United States. About half of the states have statutes specifically permitting minors to consent to contraceptive care. None specifically prohibit it without exception. Others have statutes and/or state agency policies mandating that state-funded family planning services be provided to all people without regard to sex, age, race, income, number of children, marital status, citizenship, or motive.

In states without specific statutory enablements or funding policies, support can be found in federal regulations governing programs receiving funds under Title XIX and XX of the Social Security Act and/or Title X of the Family Planning Services Act; these regulations also require that recipients provide services to any minor desiring them without regard to marital status, age, or parenthood. Even were a state to require parental consent for contraceptive services to minors, this is most likely to be unconstitutional in light of recent Supreme Court rulings as previously discussed. A case in point is Florida where parental consent is required for contraceptive care unless the physician deems that the minor would suffer a health hazard if services were not provided. In actuality, most Florida teenagers are being provided confidential contraceptive care without any litigational problems (Morrissey et al., 1986).

Parental Notification

There is no state in which health providers are *required* to tell parents about prescribing birth control for a minor. Most statutes, however, permit this if considered necessary

Table 4–2   Categories of Minors Who May Consent to their Own Health Care by Statute, Policy, and Common Law Exception in at Least Some Jurisdictions

By minor's status

Emancipated minors

1.   Living away from home with parental permission and earning one's living by bona fide employment (traditional definition; limited to minors over 16 as compulsory school laws apply to younger teens and limit earning power).
2.   Living away from home and managing one's own financial affairs; parental permission and source of income not relevant; a minimum age may or may not apply. Primarily intended to meet needs of alienated youth and runaways.
3.   By court decree of emancipation; eligibility requirements similar to #2 above plus having lived away from home for a reasonable period of time (6 months) and indication that the separation is permanent.
4.   Minors who are living at home but employed and contributing to their own support.

Mature minors (see text)

Minors who are or have been married

Minors who are parents (usually for both self and child)

High school graduates

By nature of medical record

Sexuality related

1.   Sexually transmitted diseases; sometimes expanded to any reportable communicable disease or any infectious disease.
2.   Diagnosis and treatment of pregnancy (usually excludes abortion which is dealt with in a separate statute)
3.   Pregnancy prevention/contraception/family planning services
4.   Termination of pregnancy

Substance abuse

Mental health care (a minimum age of 14 or 16 usually applies)

1.   Admission to a mental hospital
2.   Ambulatory mental health services

Emergency; variable from life and limb saving to treatment for any health endangerment; consent of minor not required.

for the minor's health. Even here, however, the decision of a physician to notify parents without the minor's permission probably is in violation of the minor's constitutional privacy rights. This question has not yet been addressed by the courts, but there is very strong support for such an argument.

This does not mean that parental involvement should not be explored. Indeed, this is an appropriate management consideration quite apart from what the law does and does not allow. This issue should be discussed routinely and adolescents *encouraged* to let their parents know or to let the physician do this for them.

Implementing Confidentiality in the Health Care System

Confidentiality in adolescent health care is not simply what the law allows but also how effectively the law is put into practice. This begins with the patient's entry into the health care system, proceeds through the actual patient-provider encounter, and ends with the documentation of the encounter in the health record and health record privacy. Table 4–3 outlines these steps and potential barrier issues.

Table 4–3   Confidentiality Issues for Minor Adolescents Obtaining Contraception at Different Points in the Health Care System

Services' availability and accessibility:
  Location: Near school, home, or convenient bus line so can get to health facility on own
  Hours: Appointments available at times when not required to be in school or expected at home
  Entry/waiting room privacy: Can enter facility and wait in waiting room without significant risk of unintended discovery by friends, relatives, others
  Fees: Services and supplies are low cost

The patient-physician interaction:
  Given opportunity to see physician on own
  Can consent to own contraceptive care
  Physician assurance as to confidentiality

Health record privacy:
  Confidential information in the record separated from other information
  Provisions made to avoid parental access
  Release to third parties only with the minor's consent (except as mandated by law)

All the enabling laws in the world will be futile if privacy and confidentiality are not implemented in actual clinical practice. Privacy in regard to location and the type of health services being given is an example. Compare a primary care provider's private practice office with a family planning clinic. Being observed by a friend or relative in the private practitioner's office would not be particularly embarrassing, as the girl could be there for any one of a hundred different reasons, but discovery in a family planning program where the reason for the adolescent's presence is abundantly clear could be quite another matter. In the latter setting, the potential for embarrassment in simply being there can well act as a barrier to care. At the same time, without an advance arrangement with parents to pay unitemized bills, only a limited number of adolescents can afford to pay a private practitioner's fees, while most family planning programs are subsidized and low cost.

Other more subtle barriers also may be present, particularly in private practitioners' offices. In some cases, the cause is simply a lack of awareness due to limited training and experience in adolescent medicine. But in other cases, sidestepping confidentiality may be a more deliberate avoidance of what this author terms the "Pandora's Box syndrome." Adolescents have a reputation for being difficult to manage and posing complex problems. If the physician opens a confidential discussion of health risk behaviors, a myriad of thorny problems might well emerge. Not only could these problems be very time-consuming and totally wreck the schedule of a busy practitioner, but they also could be very hard to manage. Various ways in which this reluctance can be manifest include the following:

- Failure to see adolescents by themselves for part or all of each visit and continuation of the primary transactional alliance with parents
- Failure to include evaluation of sexual risk-taking as a part of routine adolescent health care
- Inadequate office equipment for performing pelvic examinations
- Inadequate training and/or skills in performing pelvic examinations
- Inadequate information about adolescent contraceptive counseling and prescription
- No plans for unitemized billing of parents or other appropriate financial arrangements

While it is beyond the scope of this paper to deal with each of these aspects in detail, we will discuss how to implement the law in clinical practice, how to establish the confidentiality option with parents, what to do about parental confrontation if it occurs, and the question of who pays the bills.

Implementing the Law in Clinical Practice

Know the Law

The first and most important point is to be familiar with the law in the state where the practice is located. In regards to contraceptive care, we again note that there is firm legal support for providing confidential services in every state. Specific regional information can be obtained from any of the following resources:

- Family law divisions of local bar associations
- State and county medical societies
- Family planning programs
- Adolescent medicine programs
- State and local health and social service agencies
- Hospital attorneys
- Malpractice carrier attorneys

It should be kept in mind that applicable statutes are not always crystal clear about legislative intent and that federal and state funding policies may also apply. In these instances, what the law permits is susceptible to variable interpretation, and each advisory resource may view the law somewhat differently from the other, depending on their representations. Family planning programs, for example, tend to be consumer-oriented and view the law as more enabling of minor's consent than would hospital or malpractice attorneys, whose primary objective is to protect the health provider from any litigational risks. Bar associations and county medical societies tend to be more balanced in their interpretation in not only representing the interests of the professional but also being consumer advocates in varying degrees. None of these resources, however, will make any recommendations that are not fully supportable.

Establish Policies and Practices about Confidential Care in Advance

There are a number of ways in which confidentiality can be comfortably and effectively introduced into the clinical setting. The following are some possibilities:

- Routinely see every adolescent alone for part or all of each visit. Establish this as a standard of care with all parents.
- Periodically assess health risk behaviors. Introduce ways in which this can be effectively and easily accomplished. Self-administered patient questionnaires can be useful and time-saving.
- Incorporate counseling on health risk prevention into anticipatory guidance for adolescents. In counseling on pregnancy prevention, include discussion of safe sex practices, contraception, and other aspects of responsible sexual behavior.
- Decide whether gynecologic care and pelvic exams will be done by the practitioner or by referral. If by referral, ensure that the confidentiality option exists in the referral resource as well.

- Routinely discuss confidential care with the adolescent and whether parental involvement is possible. If not possible, how does the adolescent plan on handling parental enquiries about doctor visits and/or discovery of contraceptives should either occur?
- Establish office procedures for adolescents to make their own appointments.
- Establish billing and payment options.
- Educate and train office personnel about adolescents, how to interact with them in a positive manner and avoid confrontation.
- Establish procedures to protect confidential information in the patient's record, including the possibility of dual records.
- Develop a list of low-cost referral resources including Planned Parenthood clinics, other local family planning clinics, adolescent medicine clinics, school-based adolescent clinics, department of health clinics for adolescents, community clinics, etc.

Establishing the Confidentiality Option with Parents

Establishing the confidentiality option with parents in advance and having their agreement to their teenagers being seen on her own and in confidence together with their willingness to pay blind or unitemized bills can go a long way toward preventing later confrontations and upset. If the adolescent has been cared for by the practitioner since childhood, a parent conference can be held when the patient reaches early puberty, or around 10–12 years of age. If the patient is adolescent at the time of entering care, confidentiality issues can be a part of the initial orientation.

The purpose of this conference is to inform parents of the need of adolescents for confidential care and to secure their agreement. Specifically, the discussion can cover adolescent developmental issues, health risk behaviors, and why confidentiality is important, as previously discussed. It may also be helpful to point out that seeing the adolescent alone serves as an educational experience in self-representation and independent utilization of the health care system.

In discussing confidentiality with the adolescent, it also is wise to plan how she intends on handling parental enquiries about what went on. At the very least, parents often ask what happened when they have accompanied the teen to the office and the physician has spent time with the patient alone. Even if the visit was by the patient alone, parents may ask the teenager about a received unitemized bill or, if contraceptive supplies are prescribed, these may be inadvertently discovered. Young people need to know that there are no absolute confidentiality guarantees and that for this and other reasons, it might be far easier for them to involve their parents from the beginning.

Awkward Situations

Any physician rendering adolescents confidential care sooner or later will either receive a telephone call from a calm but curious parent about what happened or from an angry parent outraged at the physician's audacity in seeing their adolescent without their permission. In dealing with any confrontational situation, counterdefensive measures need to be strictly avoided, as they only add fuel to the fire of parental wrath. Rather, the reason for the parents' distress needs to be recognized and acknowledged. This is much more easily accomplished when the confidentiality option has been established in advance and the physician and parents are in a partnership. In this situation, parents recognize their disability due to developmental exigencies and usually are comfortable in sharing the responsibility for their adolescent with another.

But this is not always the case. Two common situations occur. The first is when parents know of the visit and call the physician to enquire about what occurred. These parents are curious, not angry. They are concerned about their offspring but understand the physician's position. If confidentiality has already been discussed, a simple reminder may suffice. Alternatively, it can be suggested that they go right to the source and ask their daughter what happened. If revelation is insisted upon, a joint conference with the parent and adolescent to discuss the problem usually finds some sort of resolution. This will be considerably easier if the adolescent has already thought of how to handle parental enquiries as was suggested in the section on implementing confidentiality.

Far more difficult are the parents who call in anger, having just discovered the adolescent's visit or found her contraceptives. The distress of these parents is most understandable. They have been responsible for their offspring ever since he or she was born, and it is not easy to surrender the parenting role to another. Parents also are particularly vulnerable to upset if they have not been in very good control of their adolescents' behavior in the first place and may feel that whatever little control they do have is being further eroded. In turn, this leads to feelings of powerlessness and frustration, then the launching of a self-justifying attack on another in an effort to regain position and power.

The most effective way of handling the situation is to empathize with parents' anger over the phone and immediately set up an appointment with the family to discuss the problem the following day. This allows for an overnight cooling off period. Once the meeting is convened, the physician again empathizes with the parents and encourages them to express their concerns. Unless there are specific reasons to the contrary, the adolescent also should be present and given time to express his or her views. The true nature of the problem, which usually is intergenerational conflict, quickly emerges, and the physician can then easily switch gears and change the meeting from one of personal accusation to a family therapy session in which problems in intrafamily dynamics are defined and solutions explored.

While this strategy usually works well, it is true that every once in a while one encounters a parent who continues to threaten suit. But, as we have already noted, physicians who provide teenagers with confidential contraceptive services are acting well within the law. Unless it is alleged that the patient had somehow been harmed by the treatment and negligence also is involved, the likelihood of such a case even coming to litigation is all but nonexistent.

Other parents sometimes focus on punishing the adolescent by forced early marriage, filing criminal charges against her partner for statutory rape, persistent verbal assault, physical beatings, locking the youth out of the home, and permanently disowning her. Fortunately, these are very rare occurrences. When they do occur, management consists of mobilizing various social service resources.

Record Documentation

In the event of any legal action, record documentation is important. In validating the physician's decision to provide a minor with confidential care, notations should be made about the following:

- That the patient was mature and capable of giving an informed consent
- That an informed consent was obtained
- That parental involvement was encouraged and refused by the patient
- The nature and extent of risk to the patient if no treatment is given.

A second physician opinion sometimes is recommended to lend support to the first physician's decisions. In the matter of minors' consent law, however, this is not thought to be necessary (Morrissey et al., 1986).

Financial Responsibility

If a physician sees adolescents on their own consent, who is responsible for paying the bill? Legally, most minors' consent statutes specifically exempt parents from any financial liability. Even if there are no such provisions, there is the general presumption that they cannot be held responsible for services which they did not agree to, i.e., which they did not contract for.*

At the same time, few private physicians can absorb more than a limited number of teenagers when payment for services does not even meet office overhead costs. Some of the ways in which this dilemma has been handled include the following:

Payment by parents of periodic unitemized bills per advance agreement. This is probably the most practical option in private practices where adolescents may be seen for both confidential and nonconfidential care. Anticipatory planning for confidential adolescent care with parents has already been discussed in detail.

Full payment by the adolescent. Not all adolescents are wholly indigent. Many do work after school; others have substantial allowances. They may be capable of paying right away or on a time-payment basis if given the option. Like anything else in life, there is no free lunch. While payment issues should not be a barrier to contraceptive services for teens, it still is appropriate to review how much they can pay.

Partial payment by adolescent. Physicians need to decide whether they are willing to see some adolescents at cost or at a loss. Other options may not be available. While seeing teenagers should not be a chronic and continuing loss-leader, there will be times when providing contraceptive care to an adolescent and preventing an unintended pregnancy will be worth it.

Third-party payment options

Public assistance: Care providers who accept Medicaid generally can submit bills to the payor agency if they know the adolescent's Medicaid number; parental signatures are not needed for claim submission, and no notice of claim disposition is sent to the head of household. In some states, the girl also will have to produce an authorization sticker. These requirements may be insurmountable for some teens but not for others.

Unless generally emancipated (and not just for the purposes of health care), minors cannot obtain public assistance on their own and can only receive it upon their parent's application for AFDC. Independent Medicaid is not an option.

---

*This does not apply to emergency care of minors where parents generally are expected to pay even if they were not present and had not consented. This is based on the presumption that if the parents had known of their offspring's emergency they would have wanted the child treated and would have consented. Consequently, their agreement to emergency care is always implicit.

Private insurers: Few adolescents have their own private health insurance. This would happen only if they were employed and receiving insurance as a benefit. Otherwise, most adolescents who have private insurance are covered under family policies in which one or the other parent is the primary policy holder. The reason for making this distinction is that any claims filed with private insurers for the care of a minor generally must be signed by the parent (as both guardian and policy holder); this individual also receives notice of all claim dispositions.

HMO members: Probably the only situation where adolescents can receive completely confidential care under their parents' insurance plan is when this is an HMO, as it is a prepaid system and notice of services rendered is not sent to the policy holder.

Referral to a subsidized or low-cost resource. There are a number of community programs which receive various grants and other subsidies enabling them to provide low-cost or free care to adolescents. Such resources include family planning programs, hospital-based adolescent medical services, school-based adolescent health services, free clinics, community clinics, and department of health-sponsored teen clinics.

The Medical Record

None of the minors' consent to health care statutes addresses the question of health record privacy as well. Rules pertaining to the reporting of certain communicable diseases and of gunshot and stab wounds continue to apply. Third party payors also require the release of diagnostic information if they are to process a claim. In addition, an adolescent's confidential record may be subpoenaed in connection with court cases, just as anyone else's.

The greatest risk of breach of confidentiality, however, lies in the requests of parents, schools, and various social agencies for copies of the health record. This is particularly problematic when the record contains both information which the parent is aware of and information which is confidential to the adolescent alone. Patients now have the right to see their medical record and obtain a copy of it unless there is information which might be harmful to them. In the case of minors, this right of access devolves on parents. In fulfilling such requests, few record rooms consider the problem of dual entries, and the photocopy machine is an indiscriminate copier.

The same applies to information requested by schools and social agencies. For it is the parent who gives permission for information release, and once again the entire contents of the medical chart commonly is sent on. The adolescent is never even aware of such requests. Although there are no statutes on the subject, it would be consistent with other aspects of minors' consent law to state that information generated as a result of an adolescent's confidential visit should only be released by that adolescent.

Any physician recording confidential information in adolescents' charts needs to be aware of this dilemma and to take some sort of protective steps. This includes not putting any more information in the record than absolutely necessary, having a dual record with one portion reserved for confidential care, and establishing any other procedures that may be needed to monitor information requests and ensure that the adolescent's confidences are only released with the adolescent's permission.

There are a few instances where health record confidentiality for minors actually has been addressed in the law and where it is a violation to reveal information even to parents without the minor's express consent. Most of these laws apply to records held in federally funded health care programs, with the strictest rules applying to the records of minors receiving drug abuse treatment. These provisions are detailed in Morrissey et al. (1986).

Benefits of Minors' Consent Laws

Confidentiality is an essential element of adolescent health care, and the law addressing this issue provides many benefits:

- It establishes the ethical principle that health protection of minors has priority over other considerations.
- It allows minors to gain earlier access to needed health care and prevents unnecessary health harm.
- It encourages adolescents to assume self-responsibility in health care.
- It acknowledges that young people do have the capacity for independence in health care prior to an arbitrary age of majority through the mature minor rule.
- It endows minors with the constitutional right of privacy in reproductive health care.
- It recognizes that adolescents are neither children nor adults but are their own unique entities at a very special time in the life cycle.

References

Alan Guttmacher Institute: Federal judges reject DHHS parent notice rule. *Washington Memo*, February 3, 1983.

American Academy of Pediatrics: Policy statement: Confidentiality in Adolescent Health Care. *AAP News*, April 1989, p. 9.

Center for Population Options: Administration shelves squeal rule. *Issues and Action Update* 3(1):1, Winter 1984.

English A: Health and privacy rights of young adolescents upheld. *Youth Law News* 79(5):14–17, Sept-Oct, 1986.

Herceg-Baron IR, Furstenberg FF Jr: Adolescent contraceptive use: the impact of family support systems, in Fox GL (ed): *The Childbearing Decision: Fertility Attitudes and Behavior*. Sage Publications, Beverly Hills, CA, 1982.

Hofmann AD: A rational policy toward consent and confidentiality in adolescent health care. *J Adolesc Health Care* 1:9–17, 1980.

Hofmann AD: Legal issues in adolescent medicine, in Hofmann AD, Greydanus DE: *Adolescent Medicine*, 2nd ed. Appleton-Lange, Norwalk, CT, 1989.

Hofmann AD, Pilpel HP: The legal rights of minors. *Pediatr Clin North Am* 20(4):989–1004, 1973.

Irwin CE: Why adolescent medicine. *J Adolesc Health Care* 7:2S–12S, 1986.

Johnson RL, Tanner NM: Approaching the adolescent patient, in Hofmann AD, Greydanus DE (eds): *Adolescent Medicine*, 2nd ed. Appleton-Lange, Norwalk, CT, 1989.

Kenney AM, Forrest JD, Torres A: Storm over Washington: the parental notification proposal. *Fam Plann Perspect* 14(4):185–197, 1982.

Mlyniec WL: The impact of the *Ingraham* decision, in *Proceedings: Conference on Corporal Punishment in Schools: A National Debate (February 18–20, 1977)*, National Institute of Education, U.S. Department of Health, Education and Welfare, 1978.

Morrissey JM, Hofmann AD, Thrope JC: *Consent and Confidentiality in the Health Care of Children and Adolescents: A Legal Guide*. New York: The Free Press, 1986.

Paul EW, Pilpel HP: Teenagers and pregnancy: the law in 1979. *Fam Plann Perspect* 11(5):297–302, 1979.

Planned Parenthood Federation of America: *American Teens Speak: Sex, Myths, TV, and Birth Control*. Louis Harris and Associates, New York, 1986.

Torres A: Telling parents: clinic policies and adolescents' use of family planning and abortion services. *Fam Plann Perspect* 12(6):284–292, 1980.

Zabin LS, Clark SD Jr: Why they delay: a study of teenage family planning clinics. *Fam Plann Perspect* 13(5):205–217, 1981.

Zabin LS, Clark SD Jr: Institutional factors affecting teenagers' choice and reasons for delay in attending a family planning clinic. *Fam Plann Perspect* 15(1):25–9, 1983.

5

A Color Guide to Gynecologic Problems

Paula K. Braverman

The American Academy of Pediatrics' Task Force on Pediatric Education published recommendations in 1978 encouraging program directors to include more curriculum related to adolescent health care (Comerci et al., 1987). Gynecology was one of the areas that pediatricians felt to be particularly deficient in their training programs. Surveys have shown that interest in gynecology does exist (Neinstein and Shapiro, 1986). With education and experience that increase the level of comfort and expertise, basic medical gynecology can be performed by the primary care provider as part of the comprehensive health care of the adolescent. Referral to a gynecologist can be reserved for those conditions that require more sophisticated evaluation and treatment (Braverman and Strasburger, 1989).

Equipment

The basic equipment needed to perform a complete gynecology exam includes an examination table with stirrups; specula; supplies to perform the Papanicolaou smear (PAP); urine pregnancy test kits; culture media or antigen detection kits to identify various causes of vaginitis, including sexually transmitted diseases; and saline and 10% potassium hydroxide (KOH) for the office microscopic evaluation of vaginal and cervical secretions.

Specula come in various sizes including the Graves, Pederson, Huffman, and pediatric. The Graves is frequently too wide (1⅜ inches) for most nulliparous adolescents while the pediatric is too short (3 inches) for the length of the adolescent vaginal canal. The Pederson (1 × 4½ inches) is excellent for the sexually active female, and the Huffman is usually ideal for the virginal adolescent because of its small width (½ inch) along with a sufficient length (4½ inches) (Huffman et al., 1981; Emans and Goldstein, 1982).

PAP Smears

PAP smears are useful to assess the estrogen response of vaginal epithelium as well as screen for malignancy of the vagina, cervix, or uterus. They should be performed on all sexually active females as well as those with a history of exposure to diethylstilbestrol (DES). Several studies have shown a significant number of abnormal PAP smears in the sexually active adolescent population. This is especially relevant in view of the current concern about human *Papillomavirus* and its association with cervical carcinoma (Emans and Goldstein, 1982; Russo and Jones, 1984; Moscicki, 1989).

Vaginal specimens can be obtained by scraping the vaginal walls with a wooden spatula. For the cervical specimen, one scrapes the cervix using a rotating motion such that the spatula samples the entire circumference of the cervix. A cotton swab may be inserted into the endocervical canal to obtain columnar endocervical cells. A cytobrush may also increase the yield of endocervical cells. The specimen is not considered adequate if the squamocolumnar junction is not sampled. The slide(s) are fixed and sent to the laboratory for cytological evaluation (Huffman et al., 1981; Emans and Goldstein, 1982).

A maturation index may also be obtained by the PAP method. The maturation index is a measure of the vaginal estrogen response that assesses the proportion of superficial, intermediate, and parabasal cells. Parabasal cells, which predominate in a poor estrogen environment, are small round cells with large nuclei. With an estrogen response, intermediate and superficial cells appear that are larger and have progressively smaller nuclei, respectively (Huffman et al., 1981; Emans and Goldstein, 1982).

Other Common Tests

Currently, urine pregnancy tests are available that are extremely sensitive and specific without interference from other substances present in urine. They can detect human chorionic gonadotropin (HCG) in amounts as low as 50 mIU and may be rapidly performed. The results may be available in five minutes (Hatcher et al., 1988).

Saline preparation of vaginal/cervical secretions may reveal the presence of white and red blood cells, *Trichomonas vaginalis*, bacterial vaginosis (clue cells), or yeast forms. Ten percent KOH preparation destroys most cellular elements while leaving yeast forms intact, thus making them more apparent (Emans and Goldstein, 1982; Gilchrist and Rauh, 1985).

Culture or transport media are available for *Neisseria gonorrhoeae*, *Chlamydia trachomatis*, *Trichomonas vaginalis*, *Candida* species, and viruses (*Herpes simplex*). Direct fluorescent antibody (DFA) tests are also available for some microbes such as *N. gonorrhoeae*, *C. trachomatis*, and *T. vaginalis*. Enzyme immunoassay (EIA), which objectively measures an antigen-antibody reaction by spectrophotometry, is available for *C. trachomatis* (Emans and Goldstein, 1982; Holmes et al., 1984; Morbidity and Mortality Weekly Report, 1985).

Pelvic ultrasound is a noninvasive imaging technique that allows one to view pelvic anatomy. Fluid, pelvic masses (solid or cystic), and uterine characteristics (size, content, and configuration) can be viewed without radiation or surgical intervention.

Basic Pelvic Examination

The pelvic examination begins with inspection of the external genitalia to evaluate for the presence of nonambiguous genitalia, clitoral size, distribution and character of pubic hair, signs of mucosal estrogenization, patency of the hymen, normal morphology of the urethra, and presence of any lesions, masses, or discharge. The clitoris is usually 2–4 mm, and a width greater than 5 mm is suggestive of an endocrinologic or genetic abnormality. A well estrogenized mucosa is dull and pink, while poorly estrogenized mucosa is red and thinner. An imperforate hymen presents as a bulging of the perineal area without an apparent opening to the vaginal canal between the labia minora. Vaginal agenesis appears as a dimple in the vaginal area surrounded by a ruffled ridge of tissue representing the hymen. The urethra is found just anterior to the hymenal ring below the clitoris and should be assessed for eversion, discharge, or growths (Huffman et al., 1981; Emans and Goldstein, 1982).

Two common nonvenereal abnormalities can be seen during examination of the external genitalia. One is folliculitis, which represents infection of the follicles causing small inflammatory papules. The other condition is hidradenitis suppurativa. This is a chronic condition that usually begins after puberty and is caused by plugging of the apocrine glands with keratin followed by bacterial invasion. The glands can rupture with resultant painful abscesses, which can drain purulent material and cause significant scarring (Hurwitz, 1981).

After insertion of the speculum, the vagina and cervix can be visualized. The vaginal mucosa in an estrogenized individual appears pink and dull with rugae. The presence of discharge does not always indicate infection. A normal white mucous discharge may be present. This is called leukorrhea and represents the desquamation of vaginal epithelium. DES can cause vaginal abnormalities, including red granular areas called vaginal adenosis. This drug also placed individuals at risk for clear cell adenocarcinoma (Huffman et al., 1981; Emans and Goldstein, 1982).

The normal cervix is round and protrudes from the vaginal walls. The cervix also has a dull pink appearance because it is covered with stratified squamous epithelium. The cervical os of a nulliparous female is small and round, while that of a parous female is transverse in configuration. Cervical cyanosis can be seen in pregnancy. One normal developmental finding in adolescents is the ectropion, which is a red, rough area surrounding the os and represents the endocervical columnar cells extending onto the exocervix. This is completely normal and is only of concern if it is very large or extends onto the lateral vaginal walls. Such individuals may have been exposed to DES. Individuals exposed to DES may have other cervical abnormalities, including a peak in the anterior border (cockscomb), hypoplasia, a hood, and pseudopolyps (Huffman et al., 1981; Emans and Goldstein, 1982).

Sexually Transmitted Diseases (STDs)

There are various sexually transmitted diseases that can be seen in sexually active adolescents. The first is *Neisseria gonorrhoeae*—a gram-negative diplococcus found on mucosal surfaces, including the cervix, urethra, rectum, and pharynx. Physical exam may reveal a purulent greenish-yellow cervical or urethral discharge and/or a rectal discharge that may contain blood. It is important to remember that this infection may be totally asymptomatic. A cervical gram stain may show gram-negative diplococci. However, in the female this is only suggestive of gonococcal infection— not pathognomonic—since other *Neisseria* species that are nonpathogenic may be found in the female vagina. Direct inoculation of a *warmed* Thayer Martin plate, which is immediately transported to the laboratory and placed in a CO_2-rich environment, is the ideal method for isolating this organism. Transport media which contain a CO_2 pellet are available and facilitate transportation of the specimen. Direct fluorescent antibody methods have also been introduced to the market (Emans and Goldstein, 1982; Holmes et al., 1984).

In addition to pelvic inflammatory disease, Bartholin's gland abscess and disseminated gonorrhea infection are major complications of *N. gonorrhoeae* infection in women. In the former condition, the infected major vestibular gland in the labia minora becomes swollen and extremely tender. Gonorrhea disseminates in 1% of the cases, causing fever, migratory polyarthralgias, tenosynovitis, and skin lesions. The skin lesions begin as erythematous papules and progress to pustules or hemorrhagic necrotic lesions. These lesions are most common on the hands and feet (Emans and Goldstein, 1982; Holmes et al., 1984).

Chlamydia trachomatis is the most common sexually transmitted disease in the United States. It causes mucopurulent cervicitis, urethritis, conjunctivitis, and pelvic inflammatory disease. As with gonorrhea, it is frequently asymptomatic. This organism is an obligate intracellular parasite, with one strain infecting columnar epithelial cells. *Chlamydia* culture is considered the "gold standard" for detection but is expensive and not readily available. Results are not usually available for 5–7 days. Direct fluorescent antibody (DFA) is a rapid method, which has been shown to have excellent sensitivity and specificity. It also has the advantage of allowing one to assess the adequacy of the sample. However, the accuracy of this method is dependent upon the ability of the technician performing the test. Enzyme immunoassay (EIA) is another rapid test that objectively measures an antigen-antibody response by spectrophotometric analysis. It is less sensitive than the other methods and does not allow for assessment of the adequacy of the sample (Holmes et al., 1984; Morbidity and Mortality Weekly Report, 1985).

Pelvic inflammatory disease is a complication of both gonorrhea and chlamydia. It is a polymicrobial disease with ascent of the organisms into the uterus, fallopian tubes, and contiguous pelvic areas. Sequelae include: infertility, ectopic pregnancy, chronic pain, and tuboovarian abscess. Laparoscopy reveals swollen fallopian tubes which may have exudate extruding from the fimbriated ends (Emans and Goldstein, 1982; Holmes et al., 1984; Washington et al., 1985).

Trichomonas infection is caused by a flagellated protozoan called *Trichomonas vaginalis*. It classically causes a frothy, green, malodorous discharge that can be associated with itching, burning, and even intermenstrual bleeding. The vulva may appear extremely erythematous and swollen. The cervix may be friable and may have "strawberry spots," which represent areas of ecchymosis. As with other STDs, this infection can also remain asymptomatic. The organism may be cultured, and a direct fluorescent antibody method has also been released for identification. However, it may also be rapidly identified on a saline preparation of cervical/vaginal secretions. Unfortunately, wet preps will miss 25% of women with *Trichomonas* infection (Emans and Goldstein, 1982; Holmes et al., 1984).

Bacterial vaginosis, otherwise known as gardnerella vaginitis and nonspecific vaginitis, may be a sexually transmitted disease. However, it has also been found in individuals who are not sexually active. This infection is associated with the presence of the organism *Gardnerella vaginalis*. Women with this infection have also shown an increase in the number of vaginal anaerobic organisms. This has led to the theory that bacterial vaginosis may represent a disruption of normal flora. The typical discharge is malodorous, thin and gray-white, with a vaginal pH >4.5. There may be vaginal burning and itching but usually there is minimal vaginal inflammation. Saline preparation reveals clue cells and minimal numbers of white blood cells. Clue cells are epithelial cells that are covered with bacteria and have ragged borders. Gram stain reveals gram-variable coccobacilli. If the discharge is mixed with potassium hydroxide

Supplies for the Pelvic Examination

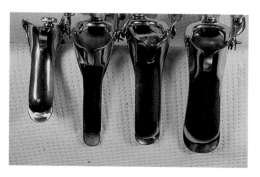

5-1 Specula (left to right): pediatric, Huffman, Pederson, Graves.

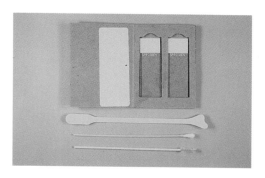

5-2 Two-slide PAP in cardboard transport container with spatula, cotton swab, and cytobrush.

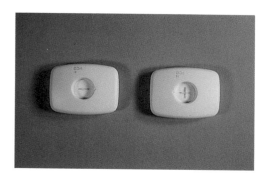

5-3 Example of urine pregnancy test with positive and negative results (Testpack[R]-Abbott).

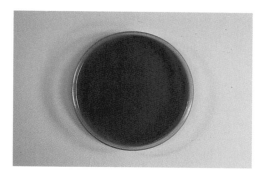

5-4 Thayer Martin plate for *Neisseria gonorrhoeae* culture.

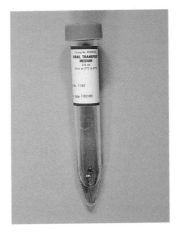

5-5 Viral culture transport tube.

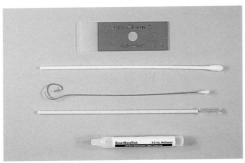

5-6 Supplies to perform direct fluorescent antibody for *Chlamydia trachomatis,* including slide, dacron culture swabs, cytobrush, and fixative (MicroTrak[R]-Syva).

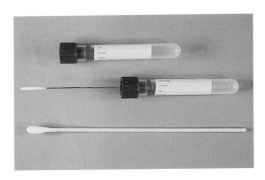

5-7 Supplies for enzyme immunoassay, including transport tube and swabs (Chlamydiazyme[R]-Abbott).

Pap Smears

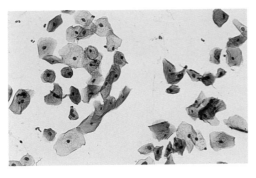

5-8 Normal PAP smear with superficial and intermediate epithelial cells.

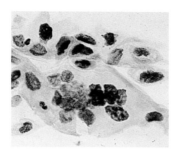

5-9   Severe dysplasia.

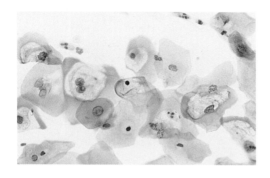

5-10   Koilocytes on PAP smear.

Saline Preparations

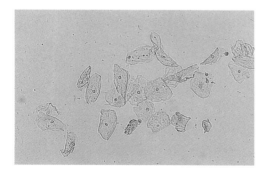

5-11   Normal well estrogenized epithelial cells in saline. Green dye has been added to provide contrast without affecting cellular morphology.

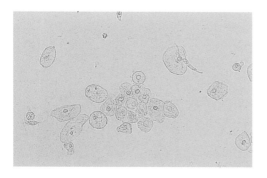

5-12   Saline preparation of vaginal secretions from prepubertal female. Note poorly estrogenized epithelial cells which are round and have a larger nucleus to cytoplasm ratio than those in figure 5-11.

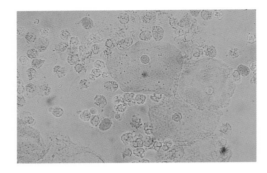

5-13   Saline preparation with white blood cells and epithelial cells.

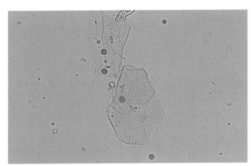

5-14   Saline preparation with epithelial cells and red blood cells.

Examination of the Genitalia

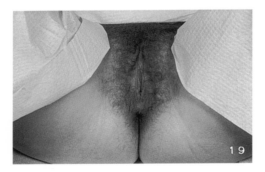

5-15   Normal Tanner 5 female: labia majora and pubic hair.

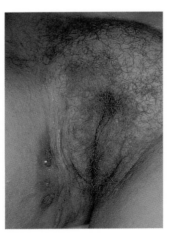

5-16   Hidradenitis suppurativa.

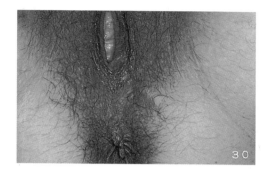

5-17 Normal labia minora—increased pigmentation.

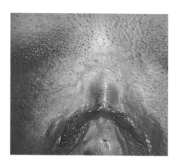

5-18 Normal urethra.

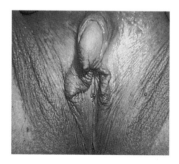

5-19 Clitoromegaly.

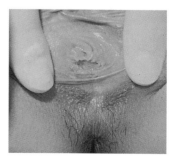

5-20 Vaginal agenesis with ruffled appearance in area of hymen and blind dimple.

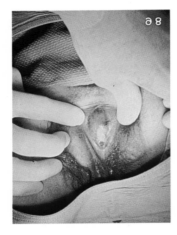

5-21 Imperforate hymen with bulging of perineum between labia minora.

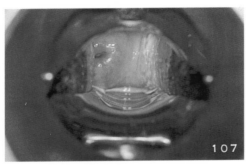

5-22 Normal vaginal rugae with pink dull epithelium.

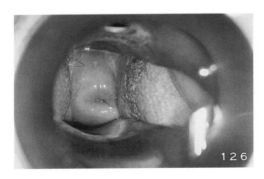

5-23 Normal nulliparous cervix with round cervical opening and pink dull squamous epithelium.

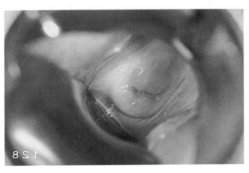

5-24 Parous cervix with transverse opening.

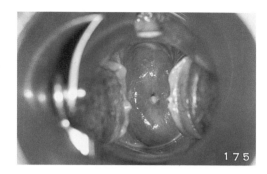

5-25   Cervical cyanosis of pregnancy.

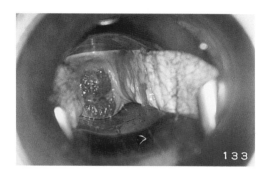

5-26   Ectropion.

Sexually Transmitted Diseases

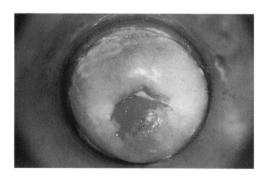

5-27   Gonococcal cervicitis with purulent discharge from the os.

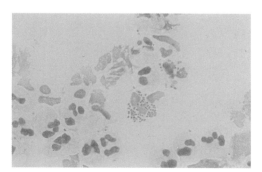

5-28   Gram stain of urethra with gram-negative diplococci.

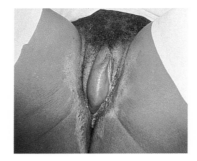

5-29 Bartholin's gland abscess.

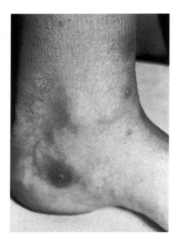

5-30 Skin lesion on foot of patient with disseminated gonorrhea infection.

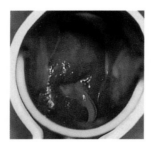

5-31 Chlamydia cervicitis with mucopurulent discharge.

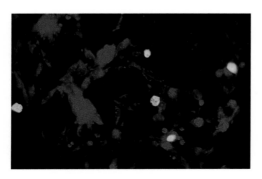

5-32 *Chlamydia trachomatis* culture confirmation using Syva MicroTrak®. Note fluorescent green bodies consistent with positive confirmation.

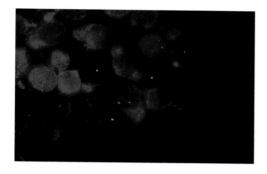

5-33 *Chlamydia trachomatis*—direct fluorescent antibody of cervical specimen using Syva MicroTrak®.

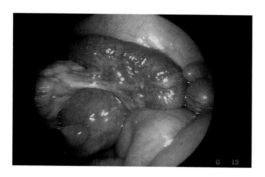

5-34 Laparascopic view of pelvic inflammatory disease.

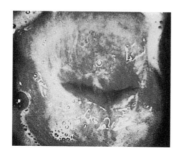

5-35 *Trichomonas vaginalis* with frothy discharge.

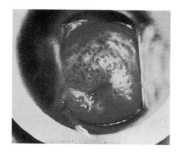

5-36 Strawberry cervix.

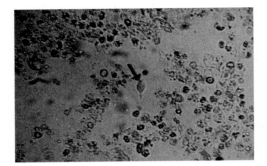

5-37 *Trichomonas vaginalis* on saline preparation (*arrow*). Note flagella and oval shape which is different than surrounding white blood cells. Movement of the flagella can frequently be seen on a fresh preparation.

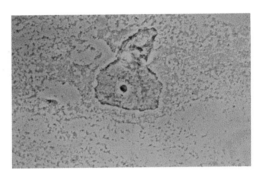

5-38 Clue cell from bacterial vaginosis. Note stippled appearance and ragged borders of epithelial cell.

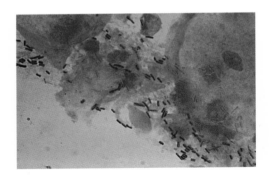

5-39 Gram stain of a vaginal smear with coccobacilli found in bacterial vaginosis.

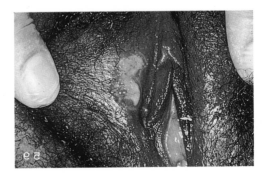

5-40 Chancre of primary syphilis located on mucosa between the labia minora and labia majora.

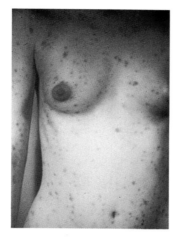

5-41 Rash of secondary syphilis on torso.

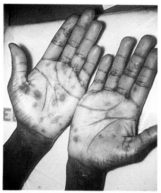

5-42 Rash of secondary syphilis on palms.

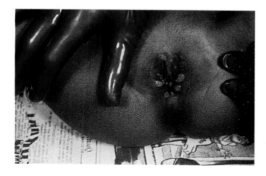

5-43 Condylomata lata—secondary syphilis.

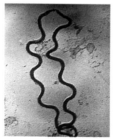

5-44 Darkfield examination demonstrating spirochete—*Treponema pallidum*.

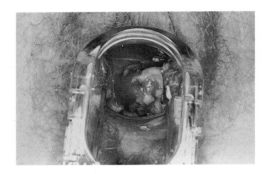

5-45 Thick white vaginal discharge from *Candida albicans*.

5-46 *Candida albicans* colonies ▶ growing on fungal media slant.

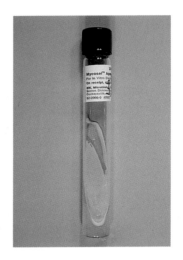

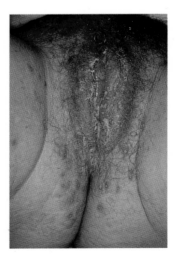

5-47 KOH preparation showing hyphae with budding.

5-48 Primary *Herpes simplex* with ulceration and labial edema.

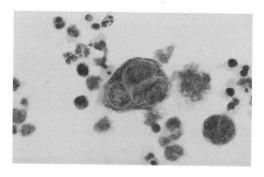

5-49 Tzanck prep—multinucleated giant cell.

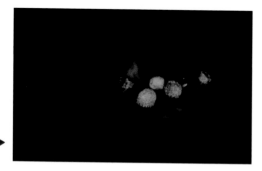

5-50 Fluorescent antibody confirmation for *Herpes simplex* virus II culture (Syva MicroTrak®). ▶

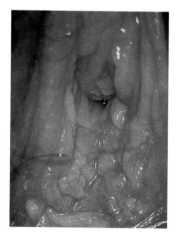

5-51 Condylomata acuminata on labia prior to application of acetic acid.

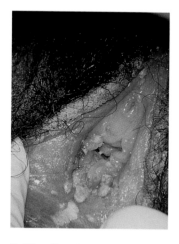

5-52 Condylomata acuminata on labia after application of acetic acid. Note white appearance to lesions (acetowhite reaction).

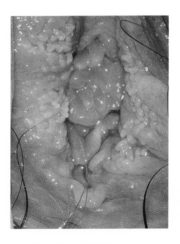

5-53 Acetowhite reaction on mucosa with small papular growths which are not as apparent to the naked eye prior to the application of acetic acid.

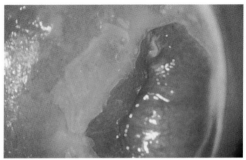

5-54 Condylomatous lesions on cervix after application of acetic acid.

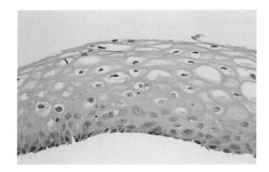

5-55 Biopsy of cervical condyloma showing koilocytes.

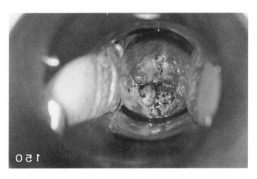

5-56 Cervical carcinoma.

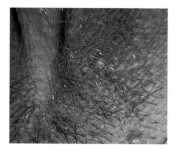

5-57   Molluscum contagiosum.

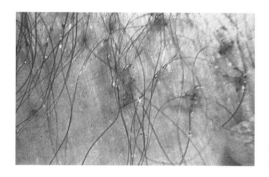

5-58   Pediculosis pubis with nits attached to hair shafts and lice.

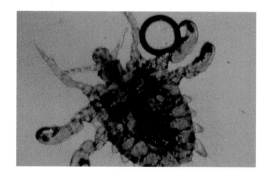

5-59   Crab louse—*Phthirus pubis*.

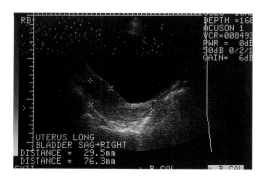

Pelvic Ultrasound

5-60   Normal long view of uterus outlined with markers.

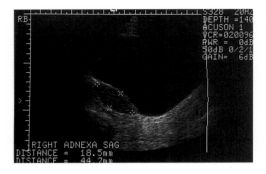

5-61 Normal adnexa outlined with markers.

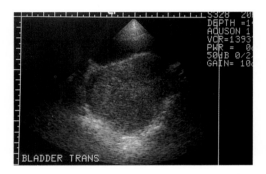

5-62 Adnexal mass-torsion of hemorrhagic ovarian cyst.

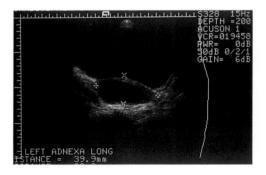

5-63 Ovarian cyst outlined with markers.

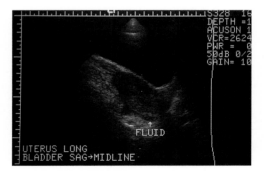

5-64 Fluid in cul-de-sac.

(KOH), an amine odor is produced. This is referred to as a positive whiff test (Emans and Goldstein, 1982; Holmes et al., 1984).

Syphilis is caused by a corkscrew-shaped spirochete—*Treponema pallidum*. The rates of this infection are increasing in some regions of the United States. Individuals with syphilis will classically progress through four stages if they remain un-treated. During the first stage, primary syphilis, there is a painless hard chancre at the site of inoculation that may be accompanied by inguinal adenopathy. Darkfield exam-ination of secretions from this lesion reveals the spirochete. This lesion heals on its own, regardless of treatment, and several weeks to months later secondary syphilis occurs. Lesions of secondary syphilis include a diffuse maculopapular rash, which may also be present on the palms and soles and pink-grey masses in the genital area known as condylomata lata. The latency stage may last for years and is followed by the tertiary stage, which is uncommon in the current age of antibiotics. Serological testing is usually used to confirm this diagnosis (Emans and Goldstein, 1982; Holmes et al., 1984).

Monilial vaginitis, otherwise known as a yeast infection, is caused by various fungi commonly including *Candida albicans*. Classically, the individual presents with an erythematous edematous vulva and a thick white clumped vaginal discharge. Diagnosis can be made by visualizing budding or branching hyphae on saline or 10% KOH preparation. The organisms can also be grown on a fungal culture media. It should be remembered that candida is a normal inhabitant of the vagina and a positive culture may not be clinically significant. Conditions that may predispose to this infection include diabetes, pregnancy, and the use of antibiotics (Emans and Goldstein, 1982; Holmes et al., 1984).

Herpes simplex is a DNA virus that causes painful blisters and ulcerations on mucosal membranes. Both types I and II can be found in the perineal area. The vulva may be extremely edematous with painful inguinal adenopathy and a profuse watery vaginal discharge. Various techniques may be utilized to confirm the diagnosis. Ideally, a fresh lesion should be cultured. Direct fluorescent antibodies may distinguish between types I and II. A Tzanck prep may also be obtained by scraping the base of a lesion and staining the specimen to show multinucleated giant cells (Emans and Gold-stein, 1982; Holmes et al., 1984).

Condylomata acuminata is caused by human *Papillomavirus* (HPV). This virus typically causes single or multiple papular growths with a white to reddish color. Al-though usually painless, pruritus may be present. It has become apparent that small papular growths on the vulva and vestibular area may represent *Papillomavirus* infection and that subclinical infection may exist on seemingly normal mucosa. The application of 3%–5% acetic acid causes a white reaction which, with the aid of a colpo-scope, makes abnormal tissue, including warts, more apparent. This acetowhite reaction represents coagulation of protein in the nuclei and cytoplasm of abnormal cells. Use of a colposcope helps to identify abnormal areas which may require biopsy (Moscicki, 1989).

The concern about HPV infection is related to the apparent association between this virus and cervical carcinoma. There have been an increasing number of abnormal PAP smears in the adolescent population. In some areas, HPV is more prevalent than *C. trachomatis*. Culture techniques are not available for this virus, and DNA hybridization is currently the only method for definitive diagnosis. PAP smears or biopsy may show koilocytes which are suggestive of *Papillomavirus* infection. Koilo-cytes are superficial or intermediate squamous cells with evidence of perinuclear cavitation, irregularly dense cytoplasm, and wrinkled pyknotic nuclei. Progression to dysplasia is accompanied by cytological changes: an increased nuclear to cytoplasmic ratio and nuclei that are pleomorphic with nuclear chromatin hyperchromasia and clumping. Because of the prevalence of this infection and the relatively rapid progression to dysplasia, routine PAP smears are extremely important in sexually active adolescents (Emans and Goldstein, 1982; Holmes et al., 1984; Jones et al., 1984; Russo and Jones, 1984; Mitchell et al., 1986; Moscicki, 1989).

Molluscum contagiosum is caused by a DNA virus and are firm flesh-colored papules that progress to soft pearl-grey lesions with central umbilication. They can be spread by direct contact and autoinoculation and may be found in the genital areas in sexually active individuals. The diagnosis can usually be made by visual inspection, but biopsy reveals certain diagnostic histological changes (Hurwitz, 1981).

Pediculosis pubis is a louse, *Phthirus pubis*, which infects the pubic hair and causes itching. The louse lays eggs (nits) that can be seen as white material attached to the hair shaft. The excrement may leave a rust colored stain on the underlying skin. Both nits and the louse may be seen under microscopic examination (Hurwitz, 1981).

References

Braverman PK, Strasburger VC: Why adolescent gynecology?—Pediatricians and pelvic exams. *Pediatr Clin North Am* 36(3):471–478, 1989.

Comerci G, Witzke DB, Scire AJ: Adolescent medicine education in pediatric residency programs following the 1978 Task Force on Pediatric Education Report. *J Adolesc Health Care* 8:356–364, 1987.

Emans SJ, Goldstein DP: *Pediatric and Adolescent Gynecology*, ed 2. Little, Brown and Company, Boston, 1982.

Gilchrist MJ, Rauh JL: Office microscopic examination for sexually transmitted diseases. *J Adolesc Health Care* 6:311–320, 1985.

Hatcher RA, Guest F, Steward F, et al: *Contraceptive Technology 1988–1989*, ed 15. Irving Publishers, New York, 1988.

Holmes KK, Mardh P-A, Sparling PF, et al: *Sexually Transmitted Diseases*. McGraw-Hill, New York, 1984.

Huffman JW, Dewhurst CJ, Capraro VJ: *The Gynecology of Childhood and Adolescence*, ed 2. W.B. Saunders, Philadelphia, 1981.

Hurwitz S: *Clinical Pediatric Dermatology*. W.B. Saunders, Philadelphia, 1981.

Jones DE, Russo JF, Dombrowski RA, et al: Cervical intraepithelial neoplasia in adolescents. *J Adolesc Health Care* 5:243–247, 1984.

Mitchell H, Drake M, Medley G: Prospective evaluation of risk of cervical cancer after cytological evidence of human Papillomavirus infection. *Lancet* i:573–575, 1986.

Morbidity and Mortality Weekly Report: *Chlamydia trachomatis* infections, policy guidelines for prevention and control. *MMWR* 34(3S), August 23, 1985.

Moscicki B: HPV infections: an old STD revisited. *Contemp Pediatr* 6:12–48, 1989.

Neinstein LS, Shapiro JR: Pediatrician's self-evaluation of adolescent care training, skills and interest. *J Adolesc Health Care* 7:18–21, 1986.

Russo JF, Jones DJ: Abnormal cervical cytology in sexually active adolescents. *J Adolesc Health Care* 5:269–271, 1984.

Washington AE, Sweet RL, Shafer MB: Pelvic inflammatory disease and its sequelae in adolescents. *J Adolesc Health Care* 6:298–310, 1985.

6

Vulvovaginitis

Donald E. Greydanus, Kenneth Sladkin, and Robin Rosenstock

Vulvovaginitis

Prepubertal Vaginitis

Many causes of vulvovaginitis in the adolescent are reviewed in this chapter. Table 6–1 outlines some of these causes. Before discussing these etiologic factors, a few introductory comments are given on prepubertal vaginitis. With the increasing awareness of sexual abuse, as well as the increasing openness in discussing sexual information in some families, there are a number of prepubertal girls who present with complaints of vaginal discharge, vaginal itching, or dysuria (Adler, 1984). There are factors that distinguish prepubertal vaginitis from pubertal or postpubertal vaginitis. Vulvitis is common because the vulva is relatively exposed secondary to small labia majora, no hair, and thin vulvar skin (Emans, 1986). These same factors contribute to the development of vaginitis. In addition, the nonestrogenized vaginal epithelium (Fig. 5–12) is thin and atrophic with a neutral pH and without glycogen stored in the cells (Wald, 1984).

Other factors that can be problematic for the prepubertal girl include poor hygiene, especially fecal contamination from wiping back to front (Wald, 1984). Many girls this age are involved in dance and gymnastics and therefore spend long periods of time wearing tight fitting clothes that do not allow air to circulate well. In the younger prepubertal girl or in the mentally retarded, foreign bodies must be considered. Secondary to masturbation or exploration of the genital area can be infection with respiratory pathogens (Wald, 1984; Emans, 1986) or nonspecific vaginitis. Bubble baths and excessive rubbing with harsh soaps have long been recognized as irritants that can lead to nonspecific vaginitis.

The physical exam of the young girl, depending upon the age, the relationship between the girl and the examiner, and her prior experience can be easy or difficult. Some girls may need to be examined in the frog leg position on the mother's lap. Others may be examined on the exam table either in the frog leg position or the knee chest position. As the girl relaxes, the hymenal ring relaxes and the examiner should be able to see much of the vagina (Figs. 5–22 and 5–23), assuming there is a perforation in the hymen (Fig. 5–21). Various light sources can be used. An otoscope with a large speculum or a veterinary otoscope can be used for a close look. A colposcope, when available, can be a valuable aid, especially when evaluating the possibility of sexual abuse. In the more usual case, a lamp or flashlight may be adequate. In cases where the entire vagina must be visualized, such as suspected foreign body, the speculum most suited to the prepubertal girl is the Huffman (Fig. 5–1). In some instances the exam will

Table 6–1   Causes of Vulvovaginitis

1. Leukorrhea and/or vaginitis
   a. Physiologic leukorrhea
   b. *Trichomonas vaginalis* vaginitis
   c. *Haemophilus vaginalis* (*Gardnerella vaginalis*) vaginitis (bacterial vaginosis)
   d. *Candida albicans* vaginitis
2. Cervicitis due to
   a. *Neisseria gonorrhoeae*
   b. Herpes simplex virus
   c. *Chlamydia trachomatis*
3. Miscellaneous
   a. Foreign body vaginitis
   b. Allergic vulvovaginitis
   c. Vulvar ulcerations
      (syphilis, herpes, chancroid, granuloma inguinale, lymphogranuloma venereum, amebiasis, Behçet's syndrome, others)
   d. Vulvitis
      (psoriasis, tinea, molluscum contagiosum, condyloma accuminata, scabies, pediculosis, furunculosis, pruritus vulvae, others)

need to be done under general anesthetic, and for this also the Huffman speculum should be used (Altchek, 1984) (Fig. 5–1).

The few laboratory tests that are useful are pH, requiring only some pH paper, and a microscopic exam (Mead et al., 1987). The discharge should be mixed with some sterile saline, looking for polymorphonuclear cells, epithelial cells (Fig. 5–13), bacteria, and *Trichomonas* (Fig. 5–35). Potassium hydroxide (KOH), in a 10% solution can help identify yeast by the hyphae (Fig. 5–47) that appear when it is added (to the discharge). A gram stain may be useful when a bacterial pathogen is suspected (Fig. 5–28), although this is less common in preadolescents. It may be useful when enteric or respiratory flora are possibilities. Access to a laboratory that can incubate and evaluate cultures is important both when considering gonorrhea and when looking for respiratory bacteria such as group A streptococcus.

When considering nonspecific vaginitis, if the girl is already pubertal, physiologic leukorrhea may be the cause (McAnarney and Greydanus, 1987). The discharge is clear to white, sticky and nonirritating and comes from the vulvovaginal and cervical glands. The pH will be 3.5. Under the microscope, a saline wet mount will show some epithelial cells and few leukocytes or bacteria, in spite of the name (Fig. 5–11). Reassurance, a discussion of impending menarche, and the use of cotton underwear are all that are necessary. In nonspecific vaginitis due to poor hygiene or tight, nonporous clothing, the girl will present with a similar picture to the physiologic leukorrhea, except that the girl is prepubertal. The discharge is nonpurulent and does not have an odor. The pH is neutral. Microscopic exam will not show polymorphonuclear cells.

Masturbation is common in preadolescents but is very difficult for most parents and children to discuss. Many children will vehemently deny masturbating because they have been taught that it is wrong. Since this will probably not elicit a positive response, it can be addressed in general terms as a possible cause along with all the other possibilities.

Treatment of nonspecific vaginitis consists primarily of reassurance. An explanation of the normal exam and normal laboratory tests should be given. Then a discussion of the wide variety of causes along with a discussion of good hygiene and healthy clothing can ensue. Symptomatically, a sitz bath may make the girl more comfortable.

When looking for a foreign body, the primary distinguishing symptoms will be vaginal bleeding and an unpleasant odor (Paradise and Willis, 1985). An obvious discharge is less likely to be present if there is a foreign body and more likely to be present with more specific etiologies. Since toilet paper is the most common foreign body and is radiopaque, it is imperative that the entire vagina is visualized, using the otoscope, the Huffman speculum, or a colposcope.

After nonspecific vaginitis, the common causes of vaginitis are specific bacteria. However, it must be recognized that some organisms are found in asymptomatic girls. According to Hammerschlag, in decreasing frequency, the following organisms were found: diphtheroids, *Staphylococcus epidermidis*, α-hemolytic streptococcus, lactobacilli, nonhemolytic streptococcus, and coliforms (Hammerschlag et al., 1978). Specific respiratory pathogens, such as pneumococcus, meningococcus, group A β-hemolytic streptococcus, and *Haemophilus influenzae*, are commonly implicated and may either follow infection present in another site, such as the throat, or be found simultaneously. *Shigella* has been reported to cause a purulent, bloody vaginal discharge that may occur without concurrent diarrhea. *Yersinia* has also been identified as a pathogenic organism in vaginitis (Watkins and Guan, 1986). These may be examined in a gram stain, cultured on the appropriate media, and treated with an oral antibiotic.

Candida albicans is much less common in the preadolescent than in the pubertal and postpubertal girl. However, it does occur and can be carried by poor hygiene from the intestinal tract to the vagina. It may colonize and be asymptomatic. When symptomatic, it will cause a thick, white, irritating discharge, pruritus, and dysuria. Clinically the pH may be acidic, and a KOH mount may show hyphae and spores. A culture may be done on Sabouraud's or Biggy agar. Treatment should be with topical antifungal cream. Intravaginal application should rarely be necessary. Because candidal infection is uncommon in the unestrogenized vagina, repeat episodes should be investigated for an underlying cause, such as recent antibiotic use, diabetes mellitus, or immunodeficiency.

Vesicles seen on the labia or vulva should always be cultured. They may be the initial site of chickenpox, and further lesions may appear later in the course. Herpes simplex type I may be spread from oral lesions by fingers. However, since sexual abuse has become more widely investigated, Herpes simplex type II spread by sexual contact must be ruled out. Molluscum contagiosum may have a similar appearance and frequently is spread by sexual contact also. It can usually be recognized by the dimple in the center of the vesicle. Dermatologists have the most experience in treating this entity with removal of the central core.

There has been controversy about the prevalence of *Gardnerella vaginalis* in the prepubertal girl who has not been sexually abused. The most recent article by Hammerschlag, looking at clue cells on wet mount and the odor after addition of 10% KOH, found only 1 of 23 nonabused children (4%) had the typical odor, but none had any clue cells visible (Hammerschlag et al., 1985). While only one of the abused children who were examined within 48 hours after the incident had possible vaginitis, there were more definite signs and symptoms at the one week follow-up. At this time 4 of 31 children (13%) had developed definite bacterial vaginosis, and 4 of 31 children (13%) had either clue cells or positive Whiff tests, but not both.

Trichomonas is another organism that prefers the estrogenized vagina. Unfortunately, most of the studies of prevalence in prepubertal girls were done prior to the current awareness of sexual abuse. If these motile organisms are seen on a wet mount, a referral for investigation of sexual abuse must be made (Jones et al., 1985).

Another pathogen that causes vaginitis and must raise the suspicion of sexual abuse is *Chlamydia trachomatis*. Recent investigations have found this in 4%–6% of asymptomatic, sexually abused, prepubertal girls (Bump, 1985). As with adults, *Chlamydia* will be found concurrently in about one-third of those with gonorrhea. Because of the difference in cell types between the estrogenized and nonestrogenized vaginal epithelium, *Chlamydia* can be cultured from a swab of the vagina instead of the endocervix.

Neisseria gonorrhoeae is another organism for which an investigation of possible sexual abuse is mandatory. Children are frequently asymptomatic, with a vaginal discharge which may be present for weeks before it is cultured and identified. However, there are reports of asymptomatic carriage for as long as six months without treatment (White et al., 1983). Because of this, even though a child presents several months after an alleged incident of abuse, a culture for gonorrhea should be done.

In the prepubertal girl in whom all laboratory examinations have been negative and treatment for nonspecific vaginitis has not helped the symptoms to resolve, application of a topical estrogen cream may be given a clinical trial. First, however, careful and detailed education of both the parents and child on good hygiene, wiping technique after using the toilet, and good handwashing is important. It cannot be assumed that because the parents are older that they understand what good hygiene entails. Sitz baths may be used once or twice a day with mild, nonallergenic soap. Underwear should be white and made of cotton and may need to be changed more often than once a day. All tight fitting clothing, including leotards, tights, pantyhose, and jeans should be avoided. If there is no change with these methods, an estrogen cream, such as Premarin, may be tried. It can be used around the opening to the vagina instead of actually inserting it into the vagina. Used at bedtime for 2–3 weeks it should cause the epithelium to thicken and become more resistant to irritation. Potential problems are a candidal infection and mild gynecomastia with some breast tenderness. The yeast infection can be treated with antifungal cream, and the gynecomastia will resolve when the estrogen is stopped. Sometimes a trial with a broad spectrum antibiotic, such as amoxicillin or a cephalosporin, may help since a specific agent may be missed among the bacteria normally found in the vagina.

In summary, when a prepubertal child presents with complaints of dysuria without pyuria, vaginal discharge or itching or rash, it should be thoroughly investigated. Although nonspecific vaginitis is the most common etiology, using a few simple tests, the likelihood of a specific treatable cause can be determined. With a specific bacterial or fungal pathogen, the specific therapy should be used. When an organism that prefers the estrogenized vaginal epithelium and is known to be sexually transmitted is found, a referral for investigation of sexual abuse must be made. Reassurance and education still remain the primary treatment in nonspecific vaginitis.

Pubertal Vaginitis

Estrogen-effect on the genital tract occurs at puberty. This results in a longer, thicker vagina with a pH in the acidic range (often 5.0–5.5). This acidic pH is partially due to the action of lactobacilli on epithelial cell glycogen, causing lactic acid production. This thickened, acidic effect produces some protection against infection and also accounts for the observation that vulvovaginitis in adolescents is ''specific'' in nature—that is, due to a specific, usually identifiable agent. With puberty comes an alteration in the vaginal cell count: 60% superficial cells, 40% intermediate, and 9% parabasal (as noted in adults) (Gray and Kotcher, 1961).

The normal vaginal flora contains various microbes: Doderlein's lactobacilli, Enterobacteriaceae, *Bacteroides fragilis*, *Neisseria sicca*, various staphylococci, streptococci (including group B), various diphtheroids, *C. albicans*, other yeasts, other anaerobic bacteria, and other microbes (Hunter and Long, 1958; Banner, 1974; Corbishley, 1977). If certain potential pathogens (as *Trichomonas vaginalis*, *G. vaginalis*, *C. albicans*, or *N. gonorrhoeae*) are present, this does not always suggest that a symptomatic *infection* is occurring. A triggering mechanism, often of unclear causation, may be important to change the *presence* of an organism into an acute infection with characteristic symptomatology (Mendel and Haberman, 1965). There are many causes of vulvovaginitis in the adolescent, which can be divided into vaginitis, cervicitis, and vulvitis (Table 6–1). Many of these causes are also sexually transmitted disease (STD) agents in youth as well (Table 6–2).

Physiologic Leukorrhea

This identifies the normal or "physiologic" increase in vaginal discharge (leukorrhea) secondary to estrogen stimulation. It is often described in the first few days or weeks of newborn life and during early adolescence, particularly around menarche. There are numerous causes of this fluid increase, such as fluid transudation through the vaginal wall, stimulation of sebaceous, sweet, and Bartholin's glands, as well as mucus secretion of the cervical columnar epithelium. Classically this secretion starts several weeks or months before the onset of menses and it may cease or reduce at menarche as well as continue until regular menstruation occurs (Altchek, 1972, 1986).

Symptoms and Signs

A variable amount of leukorrhea develops that is usually clear, sticky, and nonirritating. Some individuals describe an increase during sexual excitement and/or pregnancy.

Table 6–2   STD Agents in Adolescence

N. gonorrhoeae
C. trachomatis
Herpes simplex
T. vaginalis
G. vaginalis
Treponema pallidum (syphilis)
Donovania granulomatis (granuloma inguinale)
Haemophilus ducreyi (chancroid)
Molluscum contagiosum
Condyloma acuminata
Human immunodeficiency virus (HIV) (AIDS)
Behçet's disease
Reiter's syndrome
Pediculosis pubis
Sarcoptes scabiei (scabies)
Others

Diagnostic Procedures

Microscopic study of a vaginal aspirate reveals normal vaginal cytology without leukocytes or pathogenic bacteria (Fig. 5–11). Cultures for bacteria and fungi are usually not indicated and are essentially negative.

Treatment

One should reassure the teenager that this is normal. Some youth may feel the discharge suggests a sexually transmitted disease or genital injury. Frequent changes of cotton undergarments will help absorb the discharge, and it should be noted that nylon absorbs poorly. Good perineal hygiene (as frequent baths) is important. Medication is avoided since it is not helpful and may lead to complications, such as dermatitis medicamentosa.

(Haemophilus) Vaginalis Vaginitis (Bacterial Vaginosis)

In 1954 Gardner and Dukes described this gram-negative facultative anaerobe as an important cause of vaginitis (Gardner and Dukes, 1954, 1955). It is now identified as a common cause of vaginitis in sexually active individuals (Dunkelberg et al., 1970; Dunkelberg, 1977; Amsel et al., 1983). Previously this microbe was called *Corynebacterium vaginale* or *Haemophilus vaginalis*; it is now called *Gardnerella vaginalis*. Most experts now state that it is transmitted sexually, and the male is frequently the asymptomatic carrier. The organism is a surface parasite which rarely causes gross vulvovaginal changes—but the female may develop a mild vaginitis. It is identified as a cause in 90% or more of the previously called "nonspecific" vaginitis cases (termed bacterial vaginosis) and has recently been described in prepubertal individuals as well.

Symptoms and Signs

G. vaginalis causes a vaginitis in which there is a gray-white, nonpruritic, frothy malodorous vaginal discharge (Editorial, 1978). Overt cervical or bladder infection is not noted, while the vaginal pH is usually 5.0–5.5. Transient *G. vaginalis* bacteremia has recently been reported, usually associated with delivery or abortion.

Diagnostic Procedures

A saline preparation or gram stain (Fig. 5–39) of the leukorrhea identifies "clue cells"—epithelial cells covered ("studded") with many gram-negative bacilli (Fig. 5–38) (Gilchrist and Rauh, 1986). Such clue cells should constitute at least 20% of the vaginal epithelial cells of the saline preparation. A less proven test is producing an amine-like odor when a small amount of this discharge is mixed with 10% potassium hydroxide (KOH) solution (whiff test) (Pheifer et al., 1978). Some laboratories have a specific fluorescent antibody test for *G. vaginalis* and also culture media, such as blood agar incubated in a CO_2 environment or thioglycolate broth. The vaginal flora contains a predominance of *G. vaginalis* and anaerobic bacteria (such as *Bacteroides* and *Peptococcus* species). Bacterial vaginosis is the current term used to describe this symptom complex.

Treatment

G. vaginalis is now considered to be part of the normal vaginal flora, and treatment is not recommended unless overt, symptomatic vaginitis is present. Effective treatment should reduce the high level of anaerobic bacteria which are present (Spiegel et al., 1980). Seven days of metronidazole (500 mg BID orally) is very effective, while the pregnant youth may benefit from ampicillin (500 mg QID for 7 days)—though the latter is not effective in all cases (Schneider, 1983). A single 2-g dose of metronidazole results in a 60%–70% cure rate versus 80%–90% with the seven day course. Other antibiotics include 7 days of cephradine (250 mg QID), cephalexin (500 mg QID), and tetracycline (500 mg QID). Though previously used, application of various vaginal creams (AVC, triple sulfa, sulfisoxazole) are ineffective and not recommended. Whether or not the asymptomatic male sex partner should be treated remains controversial. Treatment is often recommended for the sex partner if the female develops recurrent disease.

C. Albicans Vaginitis

C. albicans (*Monilia albicans, Endomyces albicans, Oidium albicans*) is a dimorphous fungus which can occur as a saphrophyte or pathogen in humans. *Cryptococcus* and *Saccharomyces* are the other two fungi genera in the vagina, but they usually do not cause disease. Other *Candida* species (such as *tropicalis, pseudotropicalis, guillermondii, stellatoidea, parkrusei,* and *krusei*) are also not associated with symptoms. *Torulopsis glabrata* can infrequently produce a candida-like vaginitis. *C. albicans* is ubiquitous, often noted on the foreskin, fingernails, or other skin parts. It can also be found in the vagina, rectum, mouth, semen, and prostatic secretions. Though noted in children, its incidence in the general adult population is 20% and in pregnant individuals, 50%. Some reports identify it in 50% of vaginitis series, whether alone or in combination.

Numerous factors, often with interrelated mechanisms, can precipitate monilial vaginitis. For example, there may be reduction of host defense mechanisms (as with severe iron deficiency anemia, steroids, chronic illness, aging), chronic *Candida* exposure (as with an intestinal reservoir, infected sex partner, contaminated soaps), removal of normal vaginal flora with *Candida* overgrowth due to broad spectrum antibiotic use, increase in glycogen content of vaginal epithelial cells which lowers the pH (as with pregnancy, diabetes, or oral contraceptives), increase in heat or moisture with obesity or tight nylon undergarments, and others (Drake and Maibach, 1973; Singleton, 1980) (Table 6–3).

Symptoms and Signs

Candida vaginitis frequently has pruritic vaginovulvar erythema, a whitish, cheese-like leukorrhea (Fig. 5–45), and a pH of 3.8–5.0 (Paradise et al., 1982). Less discharge and more pruritus with erythema is noted if antibiotics precipitate the infection. If pregnancy precipitates it, the leukorrhea may be more prominent. There may be improvement during menstruation and worsening before as well as after menstruation. Dysuria, urinary frequency, and dyspareunia are not uncommon. Chronic infection is suggested by the presence of labial or groin skin which is thickened, bronzed, or dull

Table 6–3   Precipitating Factors for *C. albicans* Vaginitis

Common factors	Other factors
Diabetes	Iron deficiency anemia
Pregnancy	Renal glycosuria
Broad-spectrum antibiotics	Endocrinopathies (hyperthyroidism, hypothyroidism;
Metronidazole	Addison's disease
Oral contraceptives	Immunosuppressive drugs
Obesity	Malignancy
Corticosteroids	Blood dyscrasias (including leukemia, agranulocytosis,
Age (over 50)	aplastic anemia)
	Pancreatitis
	Other host-factor deficiencies (as lack of transfer factor)
	Malabsorption and poor hygiene
	Large reservoir for *Candida* (skin, vagina, GI tract, mouth, semen)
	Allergic predisposition and hypersensitivity
	Tight nylon undergarments
	Increased sexual activity (including cunnilingus)
	Drug addiction (especially heroin)
	Trauma to skin or vagina
	Infected soaps, douche bags, or other toilet articles
	Removal of protective bacteria by antiseptic soaps
	Intravenous infusions (indwelling catheters)
	Use of broad-spectrum antibiotics by male partner (as tetracycline for acne vulgaris) resulting in an antibiotic level in the ejaculate
	? Emotional factors

red. Secondary bacterial infection, fissuring, and lichenification can also occur. The infection can include the inguinocrural, intercrural, or perineal areas. The infection can also involve the endocervical glands and Skene glands. Dermatophytids (Monilids) can develop as very pruritic but sterile lesions at the sides of the fingers and hands.

Diagnostic Procedures

A drop of the leukorrhea is added to a drop of 10%–20% potassium hydroxide solution. A microscopic evaluation notes that *Candida* is the only yeast present in the vagina in two forms; hyphae (also called filaments or pseudomycelia) and spores (also called yeast buds or conidia (Fig. 5–47). In addition, numerous lactobacilli are seen in the potassium hydroxide preparation. A culture can be obtained and may prove useful in atypical cases (Fig. 5–46).

Treatment

Numerous antifungal agents are effective (Dunlop, 1977; Sanfilippo, 1986; Med Lett, 1988a). Currently used imidazole drugs are miconazole nitrate (Monistat), clotrimazole (Gyne-Lotrimin, Mycelex-G), and butoconazole nitrate (Femstat).

A triazole agent, terconazole, marketed in the United States since 1988, has cited advantages over the imidazoles. These include faster systemic relief and a reduction in such side effects as itching and burning. Terconazole also has demonstrated a broad spectrum of activity against *Candida tropicalis* and *Tinea globrata*.

Table 6–4   Treatment for Vaginal Moniliasis

Active ingredient	Trade name	Form	Regimen
Imidazole agent			
Miconazole nitrate	Monistat	100-mg suppositories	1 h.s. for 3 days
		2% cream	1 applicator h.s. for 7 days
Clotrimazole	Gyne-Lotrimin	100-mg tabs	1 h.s. for 7 days
	Mycelex-G	500-mg tabs	1 h.s.
		1% cream	1 applicator for 7–14 days
Butoconazole	Femstat	2% cream	1 applicator for 3 days
Triazole agent			
Terconazole	Terazol	80-mg suppositories	1 h.s. for 3 days
		Cream	1 applicator h.s. for 7 days

Regimens for the imidazoles and terconazole are noted in Table 6–4. Another medication to consider is Nystatin vaginal tablets. These tablets are effective but require longer treatment—twice daily for two weeks. Severe, resistant vaginal candidiasis or disseminated candida infection has been treated with ketoconazole, though its major side effects lead some to caution against its use in youth. The use of warm sitz baths with baking soda and hydrocortisone ointment is therapeutic for acute candidal vulvitis.

The youth with recurrent vaginal moniliasis needs a thorough evaluation for underlying precipitants, including oral contraception, antibiotics, endocrinopathies (as diabetes), sexual activity with an infected partner, tight nylon undergarments, and others. Sometimes treating for an entire month is helpful. Some clinicians have recommended white vinegar douches when pruritus occurs. If the sex partner is infected, use of a condom as well as treatment of the male genital area (including the foreskin in uncircumcised males) with antifungal ointment can be helpful. Some recommend oral Nystatin (500,000 units BID-TID for 10 days) for both partners to reduce the gastrointestinal reservoir, though its efficacy is not proven.

T. Vaginalis Vaginitis

T. vaginalis is a unicellular, flagellated protozoan first identified in 1836 by Donné (Catterall, 1972). It is described in 10% of private gynecologic patients, 30% of general clinic patients, 38% of sexually transmitted disease clinic individuals, and 85% of women prisoners. Many of the estimated 3 million annual cases in the United States are in teenagers. It is often found with such disorders as gonorrhea and Condyloma accuminata (Schneider and Geary, 1971).

Three *trichomonas* species are described—*Trichomonas buccalis* in the mouth, *Trichomonas hominis* in the gastrointestinal tract, and *T. vaginalis* in the genital tract. *T. vaginalis* is spread sexually, including with close genital contact. It has been noted to survive for a few hours in wet towels. The incubation period is 4–30 days, after which genital tract infection occurs involving the vagina, cervix, bladder, urethra, Skene's (periurethral) and Bartholin's glands.

Symptoms and Signs

Usually there is a vaginitis and cervicitis with secondary vulvitis. The vagina is erythematous and contains a profuse, greenish (or gray), frothy ("bubbly") or malodorous discharge (Fig. 5–35). It is intensely pruritic with a pH of 5.0–5.5 or higher. A mucopurulent or turbid vaginal discharge may be noted, but this can also be seen with Herpes simplex infection, *Chlamydia* infection, and gonorrhea. "Strawberry marks" (vaginocervical ecchymosis) and swollen vaginal papillae are classic for trichomoniasis (Fig. 5–36). There may be vaginal bleeding, with genital trauma at coitus or even at touching the genital area with a cotton swab. Dysuria is frequent, and severe cases may present with low abdominal pain as well as excoriation of the vulva or inner thighs.

Adolescents may be more prone to severe symptomatology than adults. Postpartum trichomoniasis has been noted with fever, leukorrhea, and endometritis. A prolonged carrier state is possible and may be associated with menses-induced, acute exacerbations, as well as chronic pelvic congestion, dysmenorrhea, and menorrhagia.

Diagnostic Procedures

The saline drop, Papanicolaou smear, and/or culture can aid with the diagnosis (McLennan et al., 1972). The presence of the leukorrhea or cervical infection is not enough for a diagnosis. For example, what appears as an "inflamed" cervix may be benign cervical erosion in which the endocervical columnar epithelium spreads out of the cervical canal, forming a border around the external os.

A saline preparation reveals numerous pear-shaped, motile microbes which are unicellular flagellated organisms twice the size of a white blood cell (Fig. 5–37). These microbes may not be seen in chronic carriers if urine is the sample study or if the patient used a chemical douche prior to the exam. The lubricant used on the speculum can also hinder this test result.

These organisms can be noted in urine samples or on Papanicolaou smears. However, the Pap smear can result in false-negative as well as false-positive results. Cultures are possible in some laboratories; these are helpful in suspicious cases with multiple negative saline preparations.

Treatment

Metronidazole is the current treatment of choice and can be given as a single 2-g dose (eight 250-mg tablets) or as a 7-day course (250 mg TID) (Fleury et al., 1977; Dykers, 1978; Lefrock and Molavi, 1981; Gilly, 1986). A single 1.5-g dose has also been shown to be effective. It is not given during pregnancy (especially the first trimester due to its feared teratogenic potential). Lactating women can be given the 2-g dose, if breast feeding is stopped for 1–2 days and then resumed. Though a carcinogenic potential has been implied by some authors, recent studies do not confirm any association between metronidazole and cancer. Current recommendations are to use metronidazole for the treatment of trichomoniasis. If the patient is pregnant, clotrimazole (100-mg tablet, intravaginally for 7 nights) can be used to reduce symptoms, but cure is unlikely. The patient's sex partner should be evaluated and treated with the 2-g, single-dose metronidazole plan. Rare cases of resistance have been described to the single dose regimen; the full 7-day course is then recommended.

Metronidazole does have numerous side effects, including monilial vaginitis, lethargy, minor gastrointestinal disturbances, headache, dizziness, transient neutropenia, bitter aftertaste, dermatitis, dry mucosal surfaces, and possible depression. Nausea with emesis occurs when metronidazole is combined with alcohol due to a disulfiram effect. The single 2-g dose may reduce many of the side effects for the disulfiram effect.

Other antitrichomonal treatments which have been used include flunidazole tablets (200 mg TID for 5 days), povidone-iodine (solution, vaginal gel, or douche), diiodohydroxyquinoline-hydrocortisone topical preparation, and others.

N. Gonorrhoeae Cervicitis

There is currently an epidemic of disease due to *N. gonorrhoeae*, a gram-negative diplococcus (Hansfield, 1982). The current prevalence rate in the United States is 465.9 per 100,00 population, with one-fourth of the cases occurring in the 10–19 year age group. In 1980 male youth (ages 15–19) had a rate of 930 gonorrheal cases per 100,000 population. It is disturbing to note that the overall rise in gonorrhea is greatest in adolescents aged 15–19. Gonorrhea, known to Huang Ti in 2167 B.C., to Hippocrates in 400 B.C., and named by Galen in 180 A.D. is still a major sexually transmitted disease in the 1980s. It is transmitted sexually, and the female has virtually a 100% chance of acquiring it from an infected male, while the male has a one in four chance of acquiring it from an infected female.

Symptoms and Signs

Classically this organism produces a vaginitis in prepubertal girls and a cervicitis (with or without salpingitis) in pubescent girls and adult women (Hook and Holmes, 1985; Med Lett, 1988b). The majority of women (80% or more) are asymptomatic, after acquiring it via sexual activity. It has a tendency to infect the columnar epithelium of the cervical canal and the urethra, where a carrier state can last for months to years. The symptomatology is protean but usually there is a yellowish-green, mucopurulent endocervical discharge (Fig. 5–27) associated with minimal pruritus and with possible tenderness noted on cervical motion (Asgeirsson and Wientzen, 1986). Purulent endocervical discharge is a hallmark of gonorrhea, but this can be noted with trichomoniasis (Fig. 5–35), chlamydial infection (Fig. 5–31), and herpes simplex infection. Abnormal uterine bleeding and urinary tract infection symptoms are also typical of gonorrhea.

Gonorrhea can also cause the following:

1. Inflammation of Skene's glands (skenitis): a pea-sized, tender nodule is noted at the base of the urethral meatus; dysuria may occur.
2. Inflammation of a Bartholin's gland duct: a unilateral, 2.0–7.0 cm tender mass which is located in the labia majora (Fig. 5–29).
3. Urethritis: red urethral meatus with a mucopurulent discharge (often seen with milking the urethra). Subacute or chronic disease can occur without early treatment.
4. Proctitis: usually not a major infection, since it is due to the close anatomical relationship between the vulva and rectum. Direct introduction of the gonococcus into the rectum through rectal sex can result in a more serious "primary" proctitis.

5. Pelvic inflammatory disease.
6. 1%–2.5% of patients with gonorrhea may develop septicemia, with evidence of dermatitis, arthritis (or tenosynovitis), perihepatitis, meningitis, endocarditis, and others. This is called the disseminated gonococcal infection or gonococcal arthritis dermatitis syndrome.

The presence of various host factors, such as serum complement levels, serum IgG, or secretory IgA, are important factors determining which infections remain asymptomatic, which cause local infection, and which cause disseminated disease. Also important are the virulence of the strain and whether recent coitus has occurred: organisms with pili can adhere to tissues, including sperm, and thus be carried up into the genital tract.

Diagnostic Procedures

Gram stain of cervical secretions may reveal many pairs of gram-negative kidney bean-shaped diplococci in the polyps (Fig. 5–28). Since normal vaginal flora include other *Neisseria* (such as *meningitidis, sicca, subflava, flavescens*, and *mucosa*) a cervical culture using Thayer-Martin medium (Fig. 5–4) in a 10% carbon dioxide environment is mandatory to correctly identify the *N. gonorrhoeae* infection. A rectal culture will add 5% to the positive cultures, when the cervical culture is negative. If oral sex occurs, the throat culture should also be done. When gonorrhea is present, other sexually transmitted diseases should be considered, as mixed venereal diseases are often seen (including syphilis) (Table 6–1).

Treatment

Standard therapy for uncomplicated gonorrhea include (Table 6–5):

a. Ceftriaxone, 250 mg IM (Centers for Disease Control (C.D.C.), 1988—Drug of Choice).
b. Aqueous procaine penicillin G, 4.8 million units intramuscularly with 1 g of probenecid by mouth).
c. Ampicillin, 3.5 g, or Amoxicillin, 3.0 g by mouth and 1 g probenecid by mouth.
d. Tetracycline hydrochloride, 500 mg QID for five days.

If penicillinase-producing *N. gonorrhoeae* causes such symptoms, treatment is best with ceftriaxone (Table 6–6) (MMWR, 1987).

Recent studies note that this new extended-spectrum cephalosporin, ceftriaxone, is the recommended drug for uncomplicated gonorrhea, for gonorrhea of the pharynx as well as rectum, and for penicillinase-producing gonorrhea. It is given as a single 250-mg intramuscular dose. Other regimens which can be used in this situation include cefoxitin (2 g IM with 1 g p.o. of probenecid) or cefotaxime (1 g IM). In an attempt to prevent postcervicitis salpingitis, these regimens for simple or uncomplicated gonorrhea should be followed with a 7-day course of tetracycline (500 mg QID p.o.) or doxycycline (100 mg BID). This is also important in view of the frequent association of gonorrhea and chlamydia. Pregnant patients can be given erythromycin (500 mg QID) instead of tetracycline or doxycycline. Follow-up cervical and rectal cultures are important regardless of the specific treatment plan used.

Table 6–5   Treatment of Gonococcal Urethritis

1. 250 mg ceftriaxone IM (C.D.C. 1988 schedule: Drug of Choice)
2. 4.8 million units aqueous penicillin G, IM, with 1 g of oral probenecid
3. 3.5 g ampicillin or 3.0 g amoxicillin by mouth with 1 g probenecid by mouth
4. If allergic to penicillin, tetracycline hydrochloride 500 mg QID for 5 days
5. 2 g of cefoxitin IM with 1 g probenecid or 1 g cefotaxime IM without probenecid

All regimens should be followed with 7 days of tetracycline (500 mg QID), doxycycline (100 mg BID), or erythromycin (500 mg QID) to cover for the possibility of coexisting chlamydial infection.

Table 6–6   Treatment of Penicillinase-producing Gonorrhea

1. First choice: ceftriaxone, 250 mg IM
2. Cefoxitin, 2.0 g IM with probenecid, 1.0 g p.o.
3. Cefotaxime, 1.0 g IM
4. Treatment of pharyngeal gonorrheal infection: trimethoprim (80 mg) and sulfamethoxazole (400 mg), nine tablets in one dose for 5 days

Additional treatment for chlamydia is necessary—see Table 6–5.

Other Gonococcal Disorders

Additional disorders caused by gonorrhea include perihepatitis, proctitis, disseminated gonococcal infections, gonococcal arthritis, dermatitis, endocarditis, and meningitis. These are now discussed.

Perihepatitis

The *Fitz-Hugh-Curtis* syndrome (perihepatitis) is due to inflammation of the liver capsule after genital infection with *N. gonorrhoeae* or *C. trachomatis*. There may or may not be symptomatic genital infection at the time the perihepatitis presents. Acute, severe, and knife-like right upper quadrant pain develops with or without right shoulder pain, right costal margin friction rub, and abdominal rebound or rigidity. Fever, nausea, emesis, hiccups, pleurisy, and pleuritic chest pain may also occur. The erythrocyte sedimentation rate (ESR) is elevated, while there is often a brief elevation of the liver enzymes and amylase. A laparoscopy will usually demonstrate the perihepatic inflammation and/or presence of the adhesions between the anterior abdominal wall and the liver. Many acute cases will have a positive cervical culture for gonorrhea or chlamydia.

The differential diagnosis includes other sources of right upper quadrant pathology, including cholecystitis, pancreatitis, peptic ulcer disease, hepatitis, pyelonephritis, pleurisy (with or without pneumonia), pulmonary embolism, pleurodynia, herpes zoster, and others. A rapid response to antibiotics is usually noted. Some individuals develop chronic pain due to the adhesions, requiring lysing of them for pain relief via laparoscopy. Correct diagnosis is based on a high index of suspicion in a sexually active female with right upper quadrant and gonococcal or chlamydial infection which improves with antibiotics or which is confirmed via laparoscopy.

Proctitis

Inflammation of the rectum (proctitis) may be due to *N. gonorrhoeae* or *C. trachomatis* infections as well as inflammatory bowel disease (Owen, 1985). Occasionally *Entamoeba histolytica, Shigella,* herpes simplex (herpes progenitalis), *Treponema pallidum,* lymphogranuloma venereum, and β-hemolytic streptococcus may cause proctitis. Diagnosis of gonococcal proctitis is with clinical suspicion, with a positive gram stain and a positive culture for *N. gonorrhoeae*. Currently proctitis is significantly involved in a wide variety of sexually transmitted diseases, especially among homosexual adolescent males. Complications to gonococcal proctitis include anal fistulas, fissures, abscesses, rectovaginal fistulas, and disseminated gonococcal infections. Treatment of proctitis in general is dependent on the underlying cause. If a sexually transmitted disease is diagnosed and treated, follow-up culture post therapy is important.

There is not universal agreement on treatment regimens, and it is important, as with other forms of gonorrhea, to demonstrate a cure with a follow-up culture 5–7 days after therapy is completed. Failure rates up to 35% are reported and may be due to reinfection, low tissue, or intracellular concentration of antibiotics, luminal location of antibiotics, large numbers of gastrointestinal microbes which can inactivate penicillin, and other factors.

Disseminated Gonococcal Infections (DGI)

DGI occurs in 2%–3% of women with gonorrhea and 0.5%–1.0% of men with gonorrhea. The presence of DGI may be related to host factors (as reduced serum complement, presence of secretory IgA or serum IgA) or the virulence of the gonococcal strain (as those which produce a protease or contain pili). The majority of the strains which cause DGI are classified as an AHU-auxotype, requiring arginine, hypoxanthine, and uracil for growth. They seem resistant to complement-mediated bacteriolysis of normal human serum. Septicemia eventually results, with various types of DGI occurring. DGI can result from gonorrhea in the urethra, cervix, rectum, pharynx, or conjunctiva.

Gonococcal Arthritis

A polyarthritis or monoarthritis has been described, but the pattern is variable. Many joints may be involved, including the knee, ankle, wrist, small joints of the hands or feet, sternoclavicular joints, and others. The monoarticular type often affects the knee. The joint fluid is often opaque or slightly cloudy, has a poor mucin clot, increased protein, and variable leukocytosis ($10,000–100,000/mm^3$). Gonococcal dermatitis (next section) and elevated erythrocyte sedimentation rate (ESR) often occur. Tenosynovitis (dorsa of hands or feet, wrists, Achilles tendon, and others) also occurs. The ESR falls with effective therapy. Joint destruction occurs without treatment. The urethral discharge may be minimal or absent when DGI symptoms appear. This gonococcal arthritis dermatitis syndrome is the main type of DGI and the main cause of bacterial arthritis in youth is infection acquired by coitus. Gonococcal osteomyelitis is a rare complication of gonococcal arthritis. Rapid response to penicillin therapy is usually noted but is slow if purulent synovial effusions are noted. Osteomyelitis requires a much longer treatment regimen. If penicillinase-producing *N. gonorrhoeae* (PPNG) are noted, the arthritis responds to ceftriaxone, 1 g IV, once a day for 7 days.

(1988 C.D.C. Treatment recommendations. Note: ceftriaxone is the drug of choice for arthritis due to nonpenicillinase strains also.)

Gonococcal Dermatitis

The most common form of dermatitis is the vesicular pustule (4 mm—2.5 cm) which is noted within 2–4 weeks of the urethral gonorrhea and is found as 2–9 lesions on the extensor surface of the hands, dorsal surface of the ankles and toes, and other areas (Fig. 5–30). They appear in crops or at different times and probably represent gonococcal embolization or an immunologically mediated vasculitis. A positive gram stain and/or culture may be noted. The pustules develop into pigmented lesions and clear without scarring in 1–2 months. Sometimes purpuric macules on the palms or soles appear, as well as hemorrhagic bullae in various areas, or a petechial rash over the hands, feet, and ankles. The oral mucosa and scalp are usually spared. Secondary lymphadenopathy does occur. Attention is directed at the associated disorder (i.e., arthritis, perihepatitis, osteomyelitis, and others).

Endocarditis

Prior to antibiotic use this was a common cause of endocarditis. Fortunately it now is a rare but still observed complication that should be considered in an individual with a pathological heart murmur and/or evidence of progressive heart disease. Normal valves are often affected, and the aortic valve is the one most commonly involved. Congestive heart failure or arterial emboli (CNS, kidney, others) can occur. Polyarthritis and/or dermatitis may also be present. Therapy consists of 20–24 million units of aqueous crystalline penicillin G IV (per day) for at least four weeks. Chloramphenicol (4–6 g/day) has also been used by some. If PPNG is present, use a high-dose third generation cephalosporin, after consulting with an expert.

Meningitis

Gonococcal meningitis may occur in rare instances as a type of DGI, usually mimicking meningococcal meningitis. Arthritis can occur and occasionally gonococcal dermatitis as well. A 10- to 14-day course of IV aqueous crystalline penicillin is used, with a dose of 20–24 million units a day. If PPNG is present, use a high-dose intravenous third generation cephalosporin.

Herpes Simplex Virus Cervicitis (Type II)

Infection with herpes simplex virus (type I) can result in herpes labialis, keratitis, eczema herpeticum, gingivostomatitis, and 10% of herpes genitalis (Corey and Holmes, 1983). Herpes simplex virus type II classically is responsible for 90% or more of herpes genital infections. A primary infection causes a disease worse than the recurrent type infection, which can occur intermittently despite serum antibodies. The incubation period is days to weeks for primary infection, and the probable reservoir is the cervix. Herpes genital infection has its highest incidence in the 15- to 19-year-old age group, with as many as 3%–12% of sexually active adolescent females having positive cultures for the herpes simplex virus type II (Rauh et al., 1977). The active lesions are very infectious, with 30%–60% of those exposed via sexual activity acquiring the infection. Two major health concerns associated with herpes genital infection are its possible link to cervical cancer and the harmful effect on the fetus.

Symptoms and Signs

This usually is seen as a cervicitis with vulvar ulcerations (Buntin, 1985) (Fig. 5–48). An area of pruritus or hyperesthesia is noted, which then develops into small-group vesicles on erythematous bases which break down within 24 hours into small shallow tender ulcers; these can last 3–14 days and then clear without scarring. The ulcers can be located on the vulva, cervix, or periurethra, but they may spread to the vagina, urethra, thighs, or buttocks. An associated cervicitis with mucopurulent discharge is also classic. Primary herpes infection produces one to several deeper ulcers with other associated symptoms (fever, headache, anorexia, general malaise), with cervicitis and enlarged, tender inguinal lymph nodes. Reported complications to herpes genital infection include meningitis, radiculomyelitis (with acute urinary retention), ascending myelitis, erythema multiforme, and even hepatic failure.

Diagnostic Procedures

A Giemsa stain or Wright stain (Tzank test) of material collected from a vesicle or ulcer will reveal "balloon cells with intranuclear bodies or multinuclear giant cells" (Fig. 5–49). The Pap smear may also show the multinuclear giant cells, which can also be seen in varicella and herpes zoster. Electron microscopy reveals viral herpetic particles, while viral serology, immunofluorescent techniques, and culture with typing are all possible (Corey, 1985) (Figs. 5–5 and 5–50).

Treatment

In general, treatment for recurrent herpes genital infection has been preventive and symptomatic. There are measures to relieve the pain which include viscous Zylocaine jelly or ointment, warm water sitz baths, petroleum jelly, or providone-iodine (Betadine) solution. The latter should be avoided in pregnancy due to the possibility of iodine absorption through the vaginal wall with potential effects on the fetus. Many treatment modalities have been tried in the past, without success; these include iododeoxyuridine, topical ether, photodynamic inactivation (using neutral red or proflavine with fluorescent light exposure), and others.

Recently 5% acyclovir ointment has been reported to be beneficial during primary herpes genital infection (Johnson, 1987; Martien and Emans, 1987). It is applied over the genital lesions every 3–4 hours (six times daily for 7 days), and it should be started within 6 days of symptom onset. It seems to reduce virus shedding and reduce symptom duration. Unfortunately, it does not prevent or help with recurrent herpes infection. Oral and intravenous forms of acyclovir are currently being used to treat both primary and recurrent episodes. It is not recommended for pregnant or lactating women, at this time. Oral acyclovir (200 mg, five times daily for 7–10 days) may shorten the duration of primary infection and has been tried in cases of severe, recurrent disease.

Prevention or treatment of secondary bacterial infection with broad-spectrum antibiotics may be helpful. A cesarean section is recommended to reduce the risk of infection for the fetus, if the female presents with active genital lesions during delivery.

Hospitalizations may be necessary for patients with very painful lesions and/or acute urinary retention. Youth with a history of herpes genital infection should have an annual Pap smear. Sexual activity is not recommended during active lesions, and condoms are useful when coitus occurs during asymptomatic periods. Herpes is one of the STDs linked to recent increases in adolescent/adult cervical intraepithelial neoplasia (CIN) and overt genital cancer.

Recent studies note that young teenagers who are sexually active and acquire certain STDs (such as herpes simplex, human *Papillomavirus* types #16 and #18) are at carcinogenic risk in adolescent and young adult years. An increased incidence for cervical intraepithelial neoplasia (CIN) and overt genital cancer is currently being reported in these age groups. Part of this increased risk is due to the adolescent cervical changes associated with puberty. At puberty the junction of the squamous and columnar epithelial cells is on the exocervix and exposed to the vagina. The columnar cells are transformed to squamous epithelial cells in the squamocolumnar epithelial zone or "T-zone." The cells in this "T-zone" are immature and probably more susceptible to carcinogens than other cells. Changes in this zone are more dramatic in utero, at menarche, and during the first pregnancy. This T-zone moves into the endocervix as the individual gets older, and it becomes less exposed to the vagina and thus to agents introduced into the vagina. Teenagers who start their sexual (coital) experience early and who have multiple partners and develop STDs seem to be at increased risk for genital cancer in the adolescent, young adult, and probably later adult years. Herpes seems to be one of the STDs worsening this risk.

C. Trachomatis Cervicitis

C. trachomatis is an obligate intracellular parasitic microbe which requires tissue culture techniques (as with McCoy cells) for culture. Two species of *Chlamydia* are recognized: *Chlamydia psittaci* (causing psittacosis) and *C. trachomatis*). The latter consists of different subspecies which can cause cervicitis, urethritis, trachoma, and/or lymphogranuloma venereum. *C. trachomatis* is now noted to be a major cause of sexually transmitted diseases (Chacko and Louchick, 1984; Wilfert and Gutman, 1986; Fusger and Neinstein, 1987; Johnson, 1987). As many as 40%–50% of women in STD clinics have a positive culture, and as many as 60% of women with gonorrhea also have *C. trachomatis*.

Symptoms and Signs

C. trachomatis cervicitis can present in various ways, but often there is vaginal mucosal erythema, hypertrophic cervical erosion, and purulent (or mucopurulent) cervical leukorrhea (Fig. 5–31) (MMWR, 1982; Faro, 1985). Mixed infections (with other STDs) are common, as are asymptomatic cases in coitally active females. This organism can cause a wide variety of infections, as outlined in Table 6–7. Dysuria associated with pyuria can be due to *C. trachomatis* (urethral syndrome). The list of infections caused by this organism continues to expand (Table 6–7).

Diagnosis

Chlamydial culture is possible, but unfortunately not available at all laboratories. Immunofluorescent monoclonal antibody tests (MicroTrak) (Fig. 5–33) and enzyme

Table 6–7   *C. trachomatis* Infections

1.	Cervicitis
2.	Urethritis
3.	Salpingitis
4.	Peritonitis
5.	Perihepatitis (Fitz-Hugh-Curtis syndrome)
6.	Urethral syndrome
7.	Epididymitis
8.	Conjunctivitis
9.	Pharyngitis
10.	Otitis media
11.	Pneumonia
12.	Endocarditis
13.	Prostatitis
14.	Proctitis (LGV stain)
15.	? Arthritis
16.	? Reiter's syndrome
17.	Others

immunoassay are also available (Figs. 5–6 and 5–7). Clinical suspicion is necessary, and it must be considered as part of the differential diagnosis in the disorders listed in Table 6–1. It is especially considered in patients who have symptoms suggestive of gonorrhea with or without negative gram stain and culture for gonorrhea.

Treatment

Recommended treatment schedules for chlamydial cervicitis include tetracycline (500 mg QID for 7 days) or doxycycline (100 mg BID p.o. for 7 days) (Lynch, 1982; Gibbs, 1983; Faro, 1985; Macgregor, 1985). This treatment is effective for both gonor-rhea and chlamydial infections. Pregnant youth can be given erythromycin (500 mg QID p.o. for 7 days). Follow-up evaluation is necessary, as is treatment of sexual contacts.

Pelvic Inflammatory Disease

Pelvic inflammatory disease (PID) defines an infection of the uterus and fallopian tubes in menstruating females (St John and Brown, 1980). It can be associated with various factors, such as instrumentation, surgery, malignancy, pregnancy, and sexually trans-mitted diseases (STD). This discussion concentrates on PID as a STD. There are over 1 million estimated PID cases, with 25%–50% being hospitalized. Many of these episodes occur in youth. The incidence of PID has been estimated at 10–13/1,000 women aged 15–39, and 20/1,000 for women aged 20–24. Most PID patients are nulliparous and are under age 25; one-third are under age 19. Risk factors for the development of PID include many sex partners, history of previous PID, presence of an intrauterine device, and/or young age. The infection is less common in pregnant women and in some women on birth control pills (Washington et al., 1985a).

There are many microbial causes (Table 6–8). Primary causes of PID seem to be *N. gonorrhoeae*, *C. trachomatis*, and *Mycoplasma hominis* (King, 1987). Con-tinued infection, often with fallopian tube injury, leads to infection with multiple bac-teria, including gram-negative and anaerobic microbes. It is this polymicrobial

Table 6–8   Bacterial Agents of Pelvic Inflammatory Disease

C. trachomatis
N. gonorrhoeae
Mycoplasma hominis
Group A β-hemolytic streptococcus
Neisseria meningitidis
Coliform bacteria: *Enterobacteriaceae*
B. fragilis
Streptococcus faecalis
Other anaerobic microbes
Other aerobic microbes

infection which causes some major PID complications. Gonorrhea often starts the infection and is cultured in 30%–80% of PID case studies. Classic studies note that 10%–17% of cases of untreated cervical gonorrhea eventually develop into PID, and approximately two-thirds of gonococcal PID result within 7 days of the menstrual period. Chlamydia is the other major precipitant to PID.

Clinical Aspects

PID should be considered in the sexually active youth who has low abdominal (''pelvic'') pain (Eschenbach, 1980). Most will have cervicoadnexal tenderness, but only one-half present with obvious leukorrhea. There is variable symptomatology, depending on which organism(s) is involved and how long the infection has lasted. ''Classic'' aspects of gonococcal-induced PID include vaginal discharge, adnexal tenderness, fever, and elevated white blood count, as well as elevated erythrocyte sedimentation rate; however, this combination will be noted in only one in five of gonococcal-induced PID cases. Overt adnexal swelling is found in only 25% and a tuboovarian abscess in 10% of these cases. PID caused by *C. trachomatis* will have much fewer classic features and may even be silent.

Diagnosis

Thus, clinicians must observe that low abdominal pain (particularly with adnexal tenderness) strongly indicates PID in a sexually active female patient. The differential diagnosis of PID is listed in Table 6–9. This diagnosis is difficult even for the most

Table 6–9   Differential Diagnosis of Pelvic Inflammatory Disease

Appendicitis
Endometriosis
Ectopic pregnancy
Ovarian cyst (with or without torsion or rupture (Fig. 5–62)
Pyelonephritis
Mesenteric lymphadenitis
Inflammatory bowel disease
Henoch-Schönlein syndrome
Hemolytic-uremic syndrome
Gastroenteritis (as due to *Yersinia enterocolitica* or *Campylobacter fetus*)
Acute intermittent porphyria
Other

experienced clinician. A misdiagnosis is not unusual if the diagnosis is made solely on the basis of history, abdominal examination, and pelvic evaluation. This should always be remembered when evaluating a patient suspected of having PID.

There are many procedures which can be used in this regard (Shafer et al., 1982; Swinker, 1985). Leukocytosis is variable, while a high erythrocyte sedimentation rate frequently is noted. Specific culture results depend on the site which is used (as rectum, fallopian tube, cervix, or peritoneum) and the symptom duration. *N. gonorrhoeae* may not be cultured from the cervix many days after the symptoms develop, but the toxin-induced fallopian tube injury may have occurred already (causing the polymicrobial infection). Culdocentesis and ultrasound may be needed in some PID cases. A negative serum pregnancy test essentially eliminates the possibility of an ectopic pregnancy. Most clinicians now note that laparoscopy is an excellent procedure in these cases (Fig. 5–34), particularly if it is an atypical or silent PID case.

Early diagnosis and therapy is important to lessen the many complications of PID (Washington et al., 1985b). Many teenagers develop tubal occlusion because of PID, with resultant infertility. Classic papers describe a 13% infertility rate after one severe episode of gonococcal-induced PID; this becomes 35% with the second infection, and then the rate is over 70% with three or more episodes. An estimated 20% develop recurrent PID, and unfortunately a large number of teenagers are sterilized each year because of this major STD. The recently observed tripling of ectopic pregnancy is mostly due to PID. Other sequelae of PID include dysmenorrhea, dysfunctional uterine bleeding, chronic abdominal pain, Fitz-Hugh-Curtis syndrome, and others.

Treatment

Numerous therapy plans have been offered for the treatment of PID (Swinker, 1985; King, 1987). Complicating the decision of what therapy plan to use is the fact that the exact microbiologic etiology is often unclear. Also complicating this problem is the possibility that PID may be in part an autoimmune phenomenon. However, all agree that early diagnosis and treatment is vital to lower the PID-associated morbidity.

Outpatient plans can be used for mild cases and are designed for treatment of gonorrhea and/or chlamydial infections (Tables 6–5 and 6–6). Further treatments for PID involve the combination of metronidazole (500–750 mg TID) with tetracycline (500 mg QID) or doxycycline (100 mg BID) for 7–14 days. Failure to improve with such oral plans and suspicion of severe PID are good reasons to hospitalize young women with this disorder. Other reasons for hospitalization include patients who have an adnexal mass, pregnancy, peritoneal signs, inability to take pills, and those with an uncertain diagnosis. Hospitalized teenagers can be offered one of the plans outlined in Table 6–10. Adequate coverage for the numerous microbial causes of PID must be provided—with particular attention to the anerobic bacteria, as *B. fragilis*. Metronidazole has become advocated for its superior antiaerobic coverage.

These medications are continued for at least 2–4 days after improvement. An oral outpatient antibiotic regimen can then be prescribed (as doxycycline or tetracycline) to finish a 10- to 14-day course of therapy. Careful follow-up is recommended.

Vulvitis

Inflammation and or infection of the vulva may cause many diverse disorders in the adolescent, especially if she is sexually active (Ridley, 1972). According to Young,

Table 6–10   Intravenous Anti-PID Antibiotic Therapy Plans

1. Doxycycline (100 mg BID) with cefoxitin (2 g QID) for at least 4 days; this is followed by doxycycline (100 mg BID, orally) to complete a 10- to 14-day course.
2. Doxycycline (100 mg BID) with metronidazole (1 g BID) for at least 4 days; this is followed by the same oral doses of both to complete a 10- to 14-day course.
3. Clindamycin (600 mg QID) with gentamicin (2 mg/kg once, followed by a dose of 1.5 mg/kg TID) until improvement; this is followed by clindamycin (450 mg QID) orally to complete a 10- to 14-day course.
5. Aqueous crystalline penicillin G (20 million units/day) with gentamicin or tobramycin (2 mg/kg initially, followed by 1.5 mg/kg TID). Clindamycin can be added in 1–2 days if clinical improvement does not occur.
6. Others

161 of 375 patients (43%) at a vulvitis clinic (primarily for adult women) had a sexually transmitted disease (Young et al., 1977). General treatment includes adequate perineal hygiene (including the use of Tuck's pads), plain warm sitz baths, frequent changes of white cotton undergarments (if vaginal discharge is present), and use of hydrocortisone ointment or cream for severe inflammation (Olansky et al., 1976). Cooling compresses with Burrow's solution or colloidal bath compresses may be very helpful. Treatment of secondary bacterial infection is important. Also, overtreatment resulting in sensitization, dermatitis medicamentosa, secondary eczema, or *Monilia vaginitis* should be avoided.

Table 6–11 lists some causes of vulvar erosions or ulcerations which may be observed in teenage or adult women. Some of these disorders are briefly described in this chapter. It should also be remembered that more than one sexually transmitted disease (STD) can occur at the same time; thus, if one is found, always look for others.

Syphilis

Evaluation of a vulvar (or vaginal) ulcer (Fig. 5–40) must always include the possibility of primary syphilis if it is a single, punched-out, nontender sore with a serous discharge in association with inguinal lymphadenopathy (Fiumara and Calhour, 1982). A darkfield examination for *T. pallidum* (Fig. 5–44) on three successive days is recommended, as well as serological testing for syphilis at the time the ulcer is noted, 6 weeks later, and at a 3-month follow-up evaluation (Lugar et al., 1980). Secondary

Table 6–11   Vulvitis: Miscellaneous

1. Molluscum contagiosum
2. Condyloma acuminata
3. Scabies
4. Pediculosis (Fig. 5–58)
5. Tinea
6. Psoriasis
7. Furunculosis
8. Hidradenitis (Fig. 5–16)
9. Intertrigo
10. Hemangiomas
11. Herpes zoster
12. Erythema multiforme
13. Pruritis vulvae
14. Others

syphilis should be considered if influenza-like symptoms are associated with generalized lymphadenopathy and a generalized skin and mucous membrane rash (Figs. 5–41 and 5–42). The manifestations of secondary syphilis are very diverse, including vulvar swelling as the present symptom.

Treatment

Standard treatment of primary or secondary syphilis is with 2.4 million units of penicillin G benzathine intramuscularly (Siegel and Washington, 1987). The Jarisch-Herxheimer reaction is quite common after the penicillin treatment of secondary syphilis and less common with primary syphilis. Alternate treatment plans include 30 days of tetracycline or erythromycin at a dose of 500 mg QID.

Chancroid

This venereal disease is due to *Haemophilus ducreyi*, a gram-negative coccobacillus with an incubation period of 3–5 days (Gaisin and Heaton, 1975). Though usually dismissed as a tropical infection, recent studies note that it may occur in temperate climates also. Our current computerized jet age with so many individuals traveling about the world is certainly one reason for its widespread occurrence.

Symptoms and Signs

Tender, shallow, purulent, sharply circumcised ulcer(s) of the vulva or cervix with inflamed inguinal lymph nodes (buboes) develop. Secondary bacterial infection and autoinoculation producing multiple lesions may be observed. The differential diagnosis includes syphilis, herpes, lymphogranuloma venereum, granuloma inguinale, traumatic ulcers, and others (see Table 6–11).

Diagnostic Procedures

A gram stain or Giemsa stain of ulcer or lymph node material reveals gram-negative, pleomorphic organisms in clusters (Hammond et al., 1978). Biopsy of the ulcer, skin testing, complement fixation titers, and culture may be helpful. Culture techniques have recently improved so that this is considered by many to be the diagnostic procedure of choice for chancroid.

Treatment

Sulfisoxazole (4 g/day), tetracycline (2 g/day), or erythromycin (2 g/day) is prescribed for several weeks or until the lesions clear (Lynch, 1982; Fast et al., 1983). Combinations of antibiotics have been used in some cases, as sulfisoxazole and tetracycline, sulfisoxazole and streptomycin, or trimethoprim with sulfamethoxazole.

Lymphogranuloma Venereum (LGV)

This tropic venereal disease is due to *C. trachomatis* (different serotypes than those implicated in nongonococcal urethritis) and has an incubation period of 7–85 days

(Felman and Nikitas, 1980; Kampmeier, 1982). Approximately 25,000 cases are reported annually in the United States.

Symptoms and Signs

A painful ulcer of the vulva, vagina, or cervix results which disappears in a few days and is followed in 2–6 weeks by suppurative inguinal buboes. Inguinal or femoral lymphadenopathy may be the only presenting sign. If both these lymph node areas are noted together, separated by inguinal ligament, this is called the ''groove sign'' and is characteristic of LGV. Other conditions that may be noted include fever, arthralgias, erythema nodosum, headache, conjunctivitis, and proctitis. Healing may be delayed with resultant scarring and stricture of the urethra and/or rectum. In addition, an increased incidence of carcinoma in these patients has been suggested by some authors.

Diagnostic Procedures

Though the Frei test was previously used, it is not currently available, and serial LGV complement fixation testing is currently the diagnostic procedure of choice. A 1:64 titer is considered diagnostic. Other procedures are possible, including immunofluorescence, counterimmunoelectrophoresis, and culture (though difficult). Lymphography may be useful to monitor some of the sequelae.

Treatment

Various antibiotics have been used, which are given for a 2- to 4-week period. These include sulfisoxazole, erythromycin, tetracycline, minocycline, and doxycycline.

Granuloma Inguinale

This is due to *Calymmatobacterium* (Donovania) *granulomatosis*, a gram-negative coccobacillus which has an incubation period of approximately 8–12 weeks (Kuberski, 1980; Felman and Nikitas, 1981). Though it should be considered in the differential diagnosis of genital ulcers, it is a relatively rare STD in most parts of the United States.

Symptoms and Signs

Painful ulcers of the vulva, vagina, or cervix develop, which appear as classic red granulation tissue. Inguinal lymph nodes enlarge when there is secondary bacterial infection. Sclerosing types are described, and vaginal lesions may cause vaginal bleeding as a presenting sign.

Diagnostic Procedures

A Wright or Giemsa stain reveals Donovan bodies, while a biopsy shows granulation tissue. Culture of the organism is difficult.

Treatment

The usual treatment includes oral tetracycline, oral erythromycin, or parenteral gentamicin (40 mg BID for 14 days). Chloramphenicol, streptomycin, and trimethoprim-sulfamethoxazole have also been used.

Amebiasis

Vulvar ulcerations can be due to *E. histolytica* infection in rare situations.

Symptoms and Signs

This starts as an ulcer with a raised thickened edge and white membranous flora. It slowly develops into a very painful, foul-smelling eschar, associated with a blood-stained, malodorous leukorrhea and amebic enteritis (Heiniz, 1973; Tranowitz, 1974). Oral-ano-genital sex can be an important precipitating factor in amebiasis, as well as giardiasis and shigellosis, especially among homosexual individuals. Other *parasitic* gynecologic diseases include schistosomiasis, trichomoniasis, and even pinworm infection (*Enterobius vermicularis*).

Diagnostic Procedures

This organism may be identified by wet (saline) preparation from the ulcer or vaginal secretion, from a Pap smear, or from a biopsy of the eschar or cervix.

Treatment

Therapy with metronidazole (750 mg TID p.o. for 7–10 days) has been suggested.

Behçet's Disease

This disorder (mostly found in Eastern Mediterranean countries and Japan) refers to a classic triad of symptoms (recurrent genital ulcers, iritis or uveitis, and recurrent aphthous stomatitis) often in association with a variety of other conditions such as: thrombophlebitis, vasculitis, ulcerative colitis, epididymitis, arthritis (arthralgias), pyodermas, erythema multiforme, and meningoencephalitis (Ammann et al., 1985; Silber, 1986). Psychiatric manifestations have also been described. Theories regarding the etiology of Behçet's disease (as environmental pollutants or viruses) are unproven.

Symptoms and Signs

The hallmark of Behçet's disease is the oral aphthous ulcer that is painful, single or multiple, and has the appearance of a canker sore. Genital lesions are of a protean nature: red macules, papules, follicles, pustules, or 1- to 2-cm aphthous-like ulcers which generally heal within 1–2 weeks. Blister formation or an inflammatory reaction may occur at the site of a venipuncture or scratch in some of these individuals. A poor prognosis may occur with chronic eye disease or central nervous system manifestations.

Diagnosis

Some disagree regarding the exact definition of Behçet's disease, but the combination of recurrent oral ulcers with two or more of the above mentioned signs, is consistent with this diagnosis. An increase in HLA-B5 antigen has been noted in many patients. Behcet's disease has also been classified in a group of arthritis disorders which are sero-negative for rheumatoid factor; this includes ulcerative colitis, Crohn's disease, ankylosing spondylitis, psoriatic arthritis, and Reiter's disease. Differentiation from recurrent herpes simplex infection may require careful evaluation.

Treatment

There is currently no proven therapy. Oral prednisone or oral contraceptives have been tried, as well as a wide variety of other drugs: chlorambucil, cyclophosphamide, levamisol, tetracycline, azathioprine, 6-mercaptopurine, colchicine, and others.

Miscellaneous Disorders Affecting the Vulva

Table 6–11 lists various disorders which can affect the vulva in the course of their disease processes. A few of these are now described.

Molluscum Contagiosum

This is due to a large pox virus with an incubation period of 3–6 weeks (Brown et al., 1981; Smith and Rainer, 1982). It is spread by close contact and tends to affect the skin and/or mucous membrane of the trunk, abdomen, and genitals. Chronic molluscum contagiosum infection may be noted in some patients with impaired cellular immunity.

Symptoms and Signs   Discrete, flesh-colored or pearly gray papules, 1–6 mm in diameter, with central umbilication are classic (Fig. 5–57). Plaques can develop due to several papules coalescing. These lesions commonly last 4–6 months, but occasionally may be present for years.

Diagnostic Procedures   Potassium hydroxide preparations of curetted specimens pressed between a slide and coverslip demonstrate diagnostic intracytoplasmic inclusions (Lipschutz cells). Wright, Giemsa, Gram, or Papanicolaou staining of the specimen is helpful, while biopsy is confirmatory. Differentiation must be made from epidermal cysts, eruptive xanthomas, flat warts, and others.

Treatment   Open each papule and apply phenol, trichloracetic acid, liquid nitrogen, podophyllin, carbolic acid, tretinoin, or even cantharidin. Curettage and electrodesiccation has also been used in some cases, as well as silver nitrate applications. Griseofulvin therapy has been used for extensive lesions.

Condyloma Acuminata

These wart-like lesions (Figs. 5–51 to 5–54) are due to infection with human *Papillomavirus* (HPV) which has an incubation period of a few weeks to several months (Kinghorn, 1978; Moore et al., 1978). It is sexually transmitted and is often associated with other STDs (as trichomonal vaginitis, monilial vaginitis, and gonococcal cervicitis). As many as 70% of the patient's sex partners have or have had these warts. The potential of the HPV types 16 and 18 for possible malignant changes is recently noted by many authors (Sanz and Gurdian, 1986) (Figs. 5–8 and 5–9).

Symptoms and Signs   Condyloma acuminata may involve any part of the genitals (including vagina, urethra, bladder, or anal canal) and can be very extensive. They seem to worsen in individuals with vaginal discharge, poor hygiene, heavy perspiration, and pregnancy. Lesions resistant to treatment are reported in some individuals with insulin-dependent diabetes mellitus and with immunosuppression disorders.

Diagnostic Procedures   The presence of squamous papillomas in moist mucocutaneous areas of the external genitalia and perianal regions is usually sufficient for its diagnosis (Fig. 5–51). Biopsy is confirmatory (Fig. 5–55) and mandatory if lesions are resistant to podophyllin therapy. Voiding cystourethrography will demonstrate if intraurethral spread has occurred.

Treatment   Therapy for concomitant venereal disease and using 3%–25% tincture of podophyllin (podophyllum resin in tincture of benzoin) on the lesions is often helpful, especially if the areas are less than 2 cm in diameter (Simmonds, 1981). White petrolatum jelly is then added, and this mixture of podophyllin and white petrolatum jelly is thoroughly washed off in 2–4 hours. There are other techniques for using podophyllin, but they all stress that normal tissue must be protected from the caustic podophyllin. Weekly applications may be necessary and seem to be most effective with moist, fleshy, sessile genital warts. The role of more frequent application is under study. Podophyllin is not used for cervical warts or for pregnant patients. If there is not regression after four weekly trials, other methods are used. The use of topical chemotherapeutic agents (as trichloroacetic acid or 5-fluorouracil) has been used as a supplement to topical podophyllin treatment. Methods which have been recommended as alternatives to podophyllin therapy include curettage, electrodesiccation, surgical excision, and cryotherapy (with liquid nitrogen or solid carbon dioxide). Immunotherapy with an autogenous vaccine (prepared from excised warts) has been attempted but is without proven success. Laser treatment has also been used with success.

Scabies and Pediculosis

Scabies   *Sarcoptes scabiei* var. *hominis* causes this pruritic dermatitis, which is spread by intimate contact and involves an incubation period of up to two months. It is currently occurring in epidemic proportions in this country. Atopic dermatitis, contact dermatitis, and neurodermatitis are often confused with scabies.

Symptoms and signs   When burrow lesions or nodular areas are found in the genital area, scabies should be considered. Excoriated papules may also be found in the webs of fingers, flexural surfaces of the elbows, axillary folds, and buttocks. Generalized, persistent, severe pruritus is noted. Secondary infection or secondary eczema may also be seen. Acute glomerulonephritis due to nephritogenic streptocococcal strains has been reported. Other sexually transmitted diseases, such as syphilis and gonorrhea, may be found. Steroids may lessen the symptoms and signs, making the diagnosis more difficult.

Diagnostic procedures   The scrapings from a suspected lesion are placed on a slide with mineral oil or 10% potassium hydroxide, and the observer uses a microscope to look for the mites, eggs, or fecal pellets (scybala). A biopsy may also reveal mites.

Treatment Effective medications include gamma benzene hexachloride, 1% cream or lotion; crotamiton, 10% cream or lotion; 25% benzyl benzoate emulsion; or 5%–10% precipitated sulfur in petrolatum. The entire family and sexual partners as well as fomites (underwear, pajamas, shorts, and pillowcases) should be treated or cleaned. A hypersensitivity state producing pruritus can last several days or weeks after all the mites are dead. Overuse of the medication should be avoided.

Pediculosis Pubis (Phthirus pubis) (Fig. 5–59) Pubic lice are also being seen in epidemic proportions among teenagers. It is spread by close contact and is often found with other venereal diseases.

Symptoms and signs This condition should be suspected when there is intense pruritus in hairy parts of the body, especially the genitals.

Diagnostic procedures Careful examination may reveal nits (ova) (Fig. 5–58) attached by cement-like material to hair and/or maculae ceruleae (sky-blue spots), transient blue maculae on the trunk or thighs which represent blood pigment or excretion. Severe pruritus caused by secondary allergic sensitization and excoriation with pyodermas caused by scratching may develop.

Treatment Gamma benzene hexachloride (shampoo and cream or lotion), 25% benzyl benzoate lotion, or DDT powder can be used. Family members should be treated if necessary and the clothes cleaned. The adolescent should be evaluated for other sexually transmitted diseases.

Miscellaneous

Table 6–2 lists other disorders that can affect the vulva. It should be noted that Reiter's syndrome (a sexually transmitted disorder usually diagnosed in males with arthritis, urethritis, conjunctivitis, and HLA-B27 tissue-typing antigen), infrequently is observed in females. In these cases, vaginal and cervical discharge, vulvar erosions, or erythema nodosum have been reported (McMillan, 1975; Thamber et al., 1977; Daunt et al., 1982).

When vulvar itching is a presenting symptom, the term pruritus vulvae is used, and as listed in Table 6–12, may be due to many disorders (Kaufman, 1975; Fish, 1976). A related condition is pruritus ani which may present as or cause pruritus vulvae (Smith, 1977; Turell, 1977).

Because of the current large numbers of sexually transmitted diseases and also pregnancy in teenagers, the practitioners inevitably will see both these conditions in the same teenage patient (McAnarney and Greydanus, 1981). Indeed, certain sexually transmitted diseases, such as monilial vaginitis, condyloma acuminata, and possibly gonococcal arthritis, may develop or worsen during pregnancy. Treatment must be tempered with awareness of which medications are contraindicated in pregnancy and which may be safe. Physicians must constantly review the safety of any medications given to the pregnant individual.

Finally, other lesions, including true neoplasms of the lower genital tract in adolescent girls, are rare. However, lichen sclerosis et atrophicus, leukoplakia, hidradenoma (Fig. 5–16), vulvar sarcoma or carcinomas, diethylstilbestrol (DES)-induced vaginal adenosis, or DES-induced vaginal or clear cell adenocarcinoma, sarcoma botryoid, and other lesions (Fig. 5–56) are occasionally seen in teenage girls. An excellent review is provided by Underwood and Kreutner (1978). If there is a history of DES use by the patient's mother, if atrophic changes or unusual lesions of the lower genital tract are noted, or if the more common causes of vulvovaginitis presented by this

Table 6–12   Pruritus Vulvae

A. Systemic causes
    1. Diabetes mellitus
    2. Seborrheic dermatitis
    3. Part of systemic drug reaction
    4. Lichen planus
    5. Leukemia
    6. Psoriasis
    7. Disorders with jaundice
    8. Rhus dermatitis
    9. Severe anemia
   10. Avitaminosis A
   11. Psychosomatic pruritus vulvae

B. Local causes
    1. Infections
       a. Cutaneous candidiasis (diabetic vulvitis)
       b. Pediculosis pubis (Fig. 5–58)
       c. Sarcoptes scabiei
       d. Tinea cruris (Epidermophyton floccosum; Trichophyton mentagrophytes; Trichophyton rubrum)
       e. *Enterobius vermicularis*
       f. Other: flea, tick, mosquito, bed bug, chigger
    2. Contact vulvovaginitis
    3. Dermatitis medicamentosa
    4. Neurodermatitis
    5. Pruritus ani
    6. Lichen sclerosis et atrophica
    7. Vulvar dystrophies
    8. Carcinoma in situ
    9. Fox-Fordyce disease
   10. Atrophic vulvovaginitis
   11. Others

discussion are refractory to standard treatment, referral to a gynecologist and/or dermatologist is indicated. Also, the clinician must constantly be aware of the ever-expanding range of STDs noted in sexually active individuals. Recent interest in the acquired immunodeficiency syndrome (AIDS) is a clear example of this principle.

References

Adler J: Diagnosis of dysuria in adolescent girls. *Postgrad Med* 76(8):206–209, 212–214, 1984.

Altchek A: Adolescent vulvovaginitis. *Pediatr Clin North Am* 19:735, 1972.

Altchek A: Pediatric vulvovaginitis. *J Reprod Med* 29(6):359–375, 1984.

Altchek A: Recognizing and controlling vulvovaginitis in children. *Contemp Pediatr* 3:59–70, 1986.

Ammann AJ, Johnson A, Fyfe GA, et al: Behçet syndrome. *J Pediatr* 107:41, 1985.

Amsel R, Totten PA, Spiegel CA, et al: Non-specific vaginitis. *Am J Med* 74:14–22, 1983.

Asgeirsson G, Wientzen RL: Epidemiology and pathophysiology of Neisseria gonorrhoeae infection. *Semin Adolesc Med* 2(2):99–105, 1986.

Banner EA: Vaginitis. *Med Clin North Am* 58:759, 1974.

Brown ST, Nallery JF, Kraus SJ: Molluscum contagiosum. *Sex Transm Dis* 8:227–234, 1981.

Bump RC: Chlamydia trachomatis as a cause of prepubertal vaginitis. *Obstet Gynecol* 65(3):384–388, 1985.

Buntin DM: Cutaneous features of sexually transmitted diseases. *Postgrad Med* 78(7):121–128, 1985.

Catterall RD: Trichomonal infections of the genital tract. *Med Clin North Am* 56:1203, 1972.

Chacko MR, Louchik J: Chlamydia trachomatis infection in sexually active adolescents: Prevalence and risk factors. *Pediatrics* 73:836–840, 1984.

Corbishley CM: Microbial flora of the vagina and cervix. *J Clin Pathol* 30:745, 1977.

Corey L: Diagnosis of genital Herpes simplex virus infections. *J Reprod Med* 30(3):262–268, 1985.

Corey L, Holmes KK: Genital herpes simplex virus infections. Current concepts in diagnosis, therapy and prevention. *Ann Intern Med* 98:973–983, 1983.

Daunt S, Kotowski KE, O'Reilley AP, et al: Ulcerative vulvitis in Reiter's syndrome. A case report. *Br J Vener Dis* 58:405–407, 1982.

Drake TE, Maibach HI: Candida and candidiasis. I. Cultural conditions, epidemiology and pathogenesis. *Postgrad Med* 58:83, 1973.

Dunkelberg WE: Corynebacterium vaginale. *Sex Transm Dis* 4:69, 1977.

Dunkelberg WE, Skaggs R, Kellog DS, Domescik GK: Relative incidence of Corynebacterium vaginale (Haemophilus vaginalis), Neisseria gonorrhoeae and Trichomonas spp among women attending a venereal disease clinic. *Br J Vener Dis* 46:187, 1970.

Dunlop EMC: Sexually transmitted diseases. *Clin Obstet Gynecol* 4:451, 1977.

Dykers JR: Single-dose metronidazole for trichomonal vaginitis: patient and consort. *Am J Obstet Gynecol* 132:579, 1978.

Editorial: Haemophilus vaginalis in non-specific vaginitis. *Lancet* 2:459, 1978.

Emans SJ: Vulvovaginitis in the child and adolescent. *Pediatr Rev* 8(1):12–19, 1986.

Eschenbach DA: Epidemiology and diagnosis of acute pelvic inflammatory disease. *Obstet Gynecol* 55(5):142(S), 1980 (Suppl).

Faro S: Chlamydia trachomatis infection in women. *J Reprod Med* 30:273–278, 1985.

Fast MV, NSanze H, D'Costa LJ, et al: Antimicrobial therapy of chancroid: An evaluation of five treatment regimens correlated with *in vitro* sensitivity. *Sex Transm Dis* 10(1):1–6, 1983.

Felman YM, Nikitas JA: Lymphogranuloma venereum. *Cutis* 26:464–477, 1980.

Felman YM, Nikitas JA: Granuloma inguinale. *Cutis* 27:364–377, 1981.

Fish SA: Special problems in managing vulvar disease. *Consultant (Phila)* 16(7):155–160, 1976.

Fiumara NJ, Calhour J: Multiple sexually transmitted diseases. *Sex Transm Dis* 9(2):98–99, 1982.

Fleury FJ, Van Bergen WS, Prentice RL, et al: Single dose of two grams of metronidazole for Trichomonas vaginalis infection. *Am J Obstet Gynecol* 128:320, 1977.

Fusger CD, Neinstein LS: Vaginal chlamydia trachomatis prevalence in sexually abused prepubertal girls. *Pediatrics* 79(2):235–238, 1987.

Gaisin A, Heaton CL: Chancroid: Alias the soft chancre. *Int J Dermatol* 14:188–196, 1975.

Gardner HS, Dukes CD: New etiologic agent in non-specific bacterial vaginitis. *Science* 120:853, 1954.

Gardner HS, Dukes CD: Haemophilus vaginilis. A newly defined specific infection previously classified "nonspecific" vaginitis. *Am J Obstet Gynecol* 69:962, 1955.

Gibbs RS: Sexually transmitted diseases in the female. *Med Clin North Am* 67(1):221–234, 1983.

Gilchrist MJR, Rauh JL: Office microscopic evaluation for sexually transmitted diseases: A tool to lower costs. *J Adolesc Health Care* 6(4):311–320, 1986.

Gilly PA: Vaginal discharge: Its cause and cures. *Postgrad Med* 80(8):231–237, 1986.

Gray LA, Kotcher E: Vaginitis in childhood. *Am J Obstet Gynecol* 82:530, 1961.

Hammerschalg MR, Alpert S, Rosner I, et al: Microbiology of the vagina in children: Normal and potentially pathogenic organisms. *Pediatrics* 62:57–62, 1978.

Hammerschlag MR, Cummings M, Doraiswamy B, Cox P, McComack WM: Nonspecific vaginitis following sexual abuse in children. *Pediatrics* 75(6):1028–1031, 1985.

Hammond GW, Lian CJ, Wilt JC, Ronald AR: Comparison of specimen collection and laboratory techniques for isolation of Haemophilus ducreyi. *J Clin Microbiol* 7(1):39–43, 1978.

Hansfield HH:Sexually transmitted diseases. *Hosp Pract* 17(1):99–116, 1982.

Heiniz KPW: Amoebic infection of the female genital tract. *S Afr Med J* 43:1795–1798, 1973.

Hook EW III, Holmes KK: Gonococcal infections. *Ann Intern Med* 102:229–243, 1985.

Hunter CA, Long KR: A study of the microbiological flora of the vagina. *Am J Obstet Gynecol* 75:865, 1958.

Johnson J: Sexually transmitted diseases in adolescents. *Primary Care* 14(1):101–120, 1987.

Jones JG, Yamauchi T, Lambert B: Trichomonas vaginalis infestation in sexually abused girls. *Am J Dis Child* 139(8):846–847, 1985.

Kampmeier RH: The establishment of lymphogranuloma inguinale (lymphopathia venereum) as a sexually transmitted disease. *Sex Transm Dis* 9:146–148, 1982.

Kaufman RH: The many causes of pruritis vulvae. *Consultant (Phila)* 15(11):182–196, 1975.

King LA: Pelvic inflammatory disease: Its pathogenesis, diagnosis and treatment. *Postgrad Med* 81(4):105–112, 1987.

Kinghorn GR: Genital warts: Incidence of associated genital infections. *Br J Dermatol* 99:405–409, 1978.

Kuberski T: Granuloma inguinale (Donovanosis). *Sex Transm Dis* 7:29–36, 1980.

Lefrock JL, Molavi A: Metronidazole. *Am Fam Phys* 24(1):185, 1981.

Lugar A, Schmidt B, Spendlingwimmer I, et al: Recent observations on the serology of syphilis. *Br J Vener Dis* 56:12, 1980.

Lynch PJ: Therapy of sexually transmitted diseases. *Med Clin North Am* 66(4):915–926, 1982.

Macgregor JA: Adolescent misadventures with urethritis and cervicitis. *J Adolesc Health Care* 6:286–297, 1985.

Martien KM, Emans SJ: Treatment of common genital infections in adolescents. *J Adolesc Health Care* 8:129–136, 1987.

McAnarney ER, Greydanus DE (eds): Adolescent pregnancy: A high risk condition? *Semin Perinatol* 5(1):1–101, 1981.

McAnarney ER, Greydanus DE: Adolescence, in Kempe CH, Silver HA, O'Brien D (eds): *Current Pediatric Diagnosis & Treatment*, 9th ed. (pp. 246–248). Appleton and Lange Publications, Los Altos, CA, 1987.

McLennan MT, Smith JM, McLennan CE: Diagnosis of vaginal mycosis and trichomoniasis. Reliability of cytologic smear, wet smear, and culture. *Obstet Gynecol* 40:231, 1972.

McMillan A: Reiter's disease in a female presenting as erythema nodosum. *Br J Vener Dis* 51: 345–347, 1975.

Mead PB, Miller D, Tomason J: A thorough workup for vaginitis. *Patient Care* 21:178–191, 1987.

Med Lett: Terconazole for Candida vaginitis. *Med Lett Drugs Ther* 30:118–119, 1988a.

Med Lett: Treatment of sexually transmitted diseases. *Med Lett Drugs Ther* 30:5, 1988b.

Mendel EB, Haberman S: The vaginal ecology and its relationship to symptoms in vaginitis. *South Med J* 58:734, 1965.

MMWR: Sexually transmitted diseases treatment guidelines, 1982. *MMWR Week Rep* 31:33S–60S, 1982.

MMWR: Antibiotic-resistant strains of Neisseria gonorrhoeae. *MMWR* 36(SS):1–18, 1987.

Moore GE, North LW, Meiselbaught DM: Condyloma. A new epidemic. *Arch Surg* 113 (5): 630–631, 1978.

Olansky S, Rogers WG, Anthony WC: Diagnosis of anogenital ulcers. *Cutis* 17:705–708, 1976.

Owen WF: Medical problems of the homosexual adolescent. *J Adolesc Health Care* 6:278–285, 1985.

Paradise JE, Campos JM, Friedman HM, et al: Vulvovaginitis in premenarcheal girls: Clinical features and diagnostic evaluation. *Pediatrics* 70(2):193–198, 1982.

Paradise JE, Willis ED: Probability of vaginal foreign body in girls with genital complaints. *Am J Dis Child* 139(5):472–476, 1985.

Pheifer TA, Forsyth PS, Durfee MA, et al: Non-specific vaginitis. Role of Haemophilus vaginalis and treatment with metronidazole. *N Engl J Med* 298:1429, 1978.

Rauh JL, Brookman RR, Schiff GM: Genital viral surveillance among sexually active adolescent girls. *J Pediatr* 90:844, 1977.

Ridley CM: A review of the recent literature on diseases of the vulva-Part II. Vulvitis: Infections. *Br J Dermatol* 87:58–69, 1972.

Sanfilippo JS: Adolescent girls with vaginal discharge. *Pediatr Ann* 15(7):509–519, 1986.

Sanz LE, Gurdian J: Human papillomavirus and cervical intraepithelial neoplasia as sexually transmitted diseases. *Semin Adolesc Med* 2(2):121–124, 1986.

Schneider GT: Vaginal infections. *Postgrad Med* 73(2):255–262, 1983.

Schneider GT, Geary WL: Vaginitis in adolescent girls. *Clin Obstet Gynecol* 14:1507, 1971.

Shafer MB, Irwin CE, Sweet RL: Acute salpingitis in the adolescent. *J Pediatr* 100(3): 339–350, 1982.

Siegel D, Washington AE: Syphilis: Updated approach to an old disease. *Postgrad Med* 81:83–90, 1987.

Silber TJ: Genital ulcer syndrome. *Semin Adolesc Med* 2(2):155–1622, 1986.

Simmonds PD: Podophyllin 10% and 25% in the treatment of ano-genital warts. *Br J Vener Dis* 57:209–219, 1981.

Singleton AF: Vaginal discharge in children and adolescents. *Clin Pediatr* 19(12): 799–804, 1980.

Smith EB, Rainer SS: Common viral infections of the skin and their treatment. *Med Clin North Am* 66(4):807–818, 1982.

Smith L: The long-standing problem of anal itching. *Consultant (Phila)* 17(11):115–118, 1977.

Spiegel CA, Amstel R, Eschenbach, et al: Anaerobic bacteria in non-specific vaginitis. *N Engl J Med* 303(11):601–606, 1980.

St. John RK, Brown ST (eds): International symposium on pelvic inflammatory disease. *Am J Obstet Gynecol* 138(7):845–1112, 1980 (Part 2, Dec. 1).

Swinker ML: Salpingitis and pelvic inflammatory disease. *Am Fam Phys* 31(1):143–149, 1985.

Thamber IV, Dunlop R, Thin RN, Huskisson EC: Circinate vulvitis in Reiter's syndrome. *Br J Vener Dis* 53:260–262, 1977.

Tranowitz HB: Parasitic gynecologic diseases. *Med Aspects Human Sex* 8:45–63, 1974.

Turell R: Intolerable pruritis ani. *Consultant (Phila)* 17(5):61–64, 1977.

Underwood PB, Kreutner A: Neoplasms and tumorous conditions of the lower genital tract and uterus, in Kreutner AK, Hollingworth DR (eds): *Adolescent Obstetrics and Gynecology* (pp. 479–502). Year Book, Chicago, 1978.

Vaginal candidosis, editorial. *Br Med J* 1:357, 1978.

Wald ER: Gynecologic infections in the pediatric age group. *Pediatric Infect Dis* 3(3 Suppl): S10–13, 1984.

Washington AE, Gove S, Schachter J, et al: Oral contraceptives, Chlamydia trachomatis infection, and pelvic inflammatory disease. A word of caution about protection. *JAMA* 253(15): 2246–2250, 1985a.

Washington AE, Sweet RL, Shafer MB: Pelvic inflammatory disease and its sequelae in adolescents. *J Adolesc Health Care* 6:293–310, 1985b.

Watkins S, Guan L: Vulvovaginitis caused by Yersinia enterocolitica. *Pediatr Infect Dis* 3(5): 444–445, 1986.

White ST, Loda FA, Ingram DL, Pearson A: Sexually transmitted diseases in sexually abused children. *Pediatrics* 72(1):16–21, 1983.

Wilfert CM, Gutman LT: Chlamydia trachomatis infection of infants and children. *Adv Pediatr* 33:49–70, 1986.

Young AW, Tovell HMM, Sadri K: Erosions and ulcers of the vulva. Diagnosis, incidence, and management. *Obstet Gynecol* 50(1):35–39, 1977.

7

Breast Disorders

Col. Manuel Schydlower, Lt. Col. Walter K. Imai, Maj. Elisabeth M. Stafford, and Maj. Alan G. Getts

This chapter provides the physician caring for adolescent females with an overview of breast conditions presenting in this patient population. A basic understanding of normal breast development and its variations is essential to sound management. Sensitivity to the potential impact of a breast disorder on an individual's emerging psychosexual identity during adolescence is critical to provision of total patient care.

Development

The mammary gland or breast is derived primarily from the epidermis with some contribution from the mesoderm. As early as the 5th fetal week, the milk line develops, extending from the axilla to the anterior aspect of the groin (Drukker and Pfeffer, 1984; Rehman, 1978). Rarely, the milk line may extend cephalad to the axilla and caudally to the labia or the buttocks (Osborne, 1987). Multiple papillae evolve along the milk line and then normally regress by the 9th fetal week. One papilla is left on each side at the level of the 5th intercostal space in the midclavicular line, which ultimately progresses to full breast development during puberty (Drukker and Pfeffer, 1984; Rehman, 1978).

At birth, transient mammary gland hyperplasia and colostrum production occur in response to the transplacental transfer of maternal hormones. This process subsides over a 3- to 4-week period.

Breast tissue, for the most part, remains fairly quiescent until the onset of puberty. Thelarche, or breast budding, is usually the first sign to herald the onset of pubertal maturation (Rehman, 1978). This occurs between the ages of 8 and 14 years. Both precocious onset of development prior to 8 years, or failure to initiate development by 14 years, are distinctly abnormal and warrant further investigation.

Weight, percentage of body fat, nutrition, and genetic predisposition all appear to impact on the initiation of hormonal changes that trigger the onset of puberty (Drukker and Pfeffer, 1984). Under the influence of gonadotropin-releasing hormone, the pituitary gland secretes increasing levels of FSH and LH. These hormones, in turn, affect changes in the ovary which lead to increased production of estrogen and eventually progesterone. Early puberty is characterized by anovulatory cycles in the ovary, and at this time the breast is mainly affected by estrogen. This leads to elongation and branching of the ductal system. Once ovulation is established, progesterone, secreted by the corpus luteum, promotes development of the breast's

---

The opinions or assertions contained herein are the private views of the authors and are not to be construed as official or as reflecting the views of the Department of the Army or Department of Defense.

lobuloalveolar structure (Rehman, 1978). Prolactin, glucocorticoids, and growth hormone play a role in ductal growth. Insulin and thyroid hormone appear to exhibit permissive effects leading to full breast development (Jacobs and Horton, 1982; Shingleton and McCarty, 1987). Exposure to adult male physiologic levels of testosterone will inhibit ductal growth. Further ductal-lobular-alveolar development continues in response to cyclic hormonal fluxes until approximately 30 years of age (Georgiade and Lanier, 1984).

Breast development from childhood through pubertal maturation has been divided into five stages as described by Marshall and Tanner (1969) (Fig. 7–1).

It is of note that in longitudinal studies, some females bypass stage IV. Tanner has reported stage IV breast development to be present in 50%, slight in 25%, and absent in 25% of individuals (Tanner, 1962). The rate of breast development in adolescence varies as well. Some may pass from stage II through V in 2–3 years, while others may not complete development until their early 20s (Pietsch, 1985).

Recently, nipple/areolar changes have been described in relation to sexual maturity rating based on breast development and pubic hair distribution and in relation to menarche. The greatest increase in areolar diameter occurs between breast stages III–V and pubic hair stages IV–V, and from 2 years prior to and 1 year after menarche (Rohn, 1987).

Premature thelarche is defined as onset of breast development before the age of 8 in the absence of other signs of sexual development. Such patients should be monitored closely. In most cases, breast development reaches a plateau and remains stationary or regresses slightly until onset of puberty. Occasionally, growth of the breast continues throughout childhood until completion at puberty. Extensive workup generally is not warranted for these patients, unless there are signs and symptoms suggestive of a source accounting for the secretion of excess estrogen.

Premature thelarche, however, may be the first sign of precocious puberty, referring to generalized sexual development prior to the age of 8. The idiopathic form is most commonly encountered, but it can be associated with Albright's syndrome and certain intracranial lesions. Such patients have the typical progression of hormonal changes seen over the course of puberty.

In pseudoprecocious puberty, the gonads remain immature or undergo only partial development. Ovulation does not occur. Most common etiologies for this are ovarian and adrenal tumors and long-term exposure to exogenous estrogens (Dewhurst, 1981; Huffman et al., 1981; Seashore, 1975).

Anomalies of Development

Polythelia, an accessory nipple, is the most frequently encountered breast anomaly (Fig. 7–2) (Osborne, 1987). This is found in approximately 2% of the population. An accessory nipple may be found anywhere along the milk line, but occurs most commonly just proximal to or inferior and medial to the normal nipple position. It may be mistaken for a pigmented nevus. No intervention is needed unless the patient finds the lesion to be cosmetically problematic. In this case, the lesion can be surgically removed, leaving little scar. Renal anomalies have been previously reported in association with polythelia, and screening renal ultrasonography has been recommended for these patients (Meggyvessy and Mehes, 1987). More recent reports suggest that in otherwise normal appearing individuals, polythelia is not an indication for urinary tract investigation (Hersh et al., 1987; Kenney et al., 1987).

Stage	Age	Physical Changes	
Stage I:	pre-pubertal	Preadolescent elevation of the nipple with no palpable glandular tissue or areolar pigmentation.	
Stage II	11.1 + 1.1 yrs	Presence of glandular tissue in the subareolar region. The nipple and breast project as a single mound from the chest wall.	
Stage III	12.1 + 1.09 yrs	Increase in the amount of readily palpable glandular tissue with enlargement of the breast and increased diameter and pigmentation of the areola. The contour of the breast and nipple remain in a single plane.	
Stage IV	13.1 + 1.15 yrs	Enlargement of the areola and increased areolar pigmentation. The nipple and areola form a secondary mound above the level of the breast.	
Stage V	15.3 + 1.7 yrs	Final adolescent development of a smooth contour with no projection of the areola and nipple.	

7–1 Tanner stages of breast development.

Polymastia, an accessory true mammary gland, is a rare anomaly, most commonly found in the axilla (Fig. 7–3). During pregnancy and lactation, as well as premenstrually, the patient may experience swelling and discomfort. The accessory breast may occasionally be functional if it has an associated nipple, and should be subject to routine screening breast examination (Osborne, 1987).

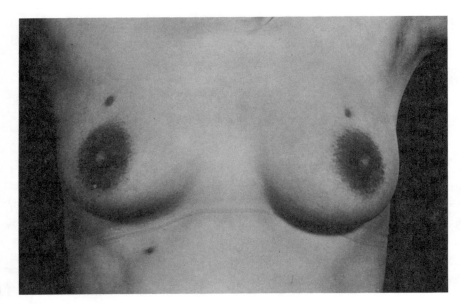

7–2 Patient with polythelia.

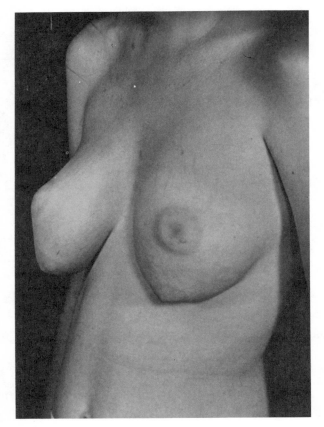

7–3 Patient with polymastia.

Amastia, congenital absence of the breast, is quite rare and occurs unilaterally most often. It has been associated with the inhibited growth of other reproductive organs and with Poland's syndrome (Fig. 7–4). *Athelia,* absence of a nipple, is also rare and may or may not be associated with absent breast tissue. When breast tissue is absent, but the nipple is present, the condition is termed *amazia.* Amazia is most often of iatrogenic cause, resulting most frequently from the injudicious biopsy of a breast bud (Georgiade and Lanier, 1984; Osborne, 1987).

Hypomastia, absent or poor breast growth, is divided into three categories. Most patients fall into a category of delayed and slow growth of a normal breast (Fig. 7–5). Positive family history is helpful in establishing this diagnosis. In such cases, support and reassurance can be given. A second group includes disorders causing ovarian failure or suppression inhibiting normal breast development. These disorders include chromosomal abnormalities, androgen-producing tumors, adrenal hyperplasia, and gonadal dysgenesis. Treatment of the underlying disorder often promotes normal breast development. Finally, individuals with partial end organ responsiveness fall into a third group. Breasts are small but function normally. One must carefully assess the emotional impact of hypomastia on the adolescent female. If psychic distress is such that augmentation is recommended, it should be delayed if possible until breast development is complete. Growth is assumed to be complete when breast measurements remain unchanged for a period of 6 months and the patient is beyond the age of 17 years (Huffman et al., 1981; Pietsch, 1985). Hypomastia has been found in association with mitral valve prolapse (Rosenberg et al., 1983).

Tuberous breasts are characterized by an excessive dumbbell-shaped growth involving the nipple areolar area and underlying breast tissue (Fig. 7–6). It is often associated with hypomastia. Surgical intervention aims to modify the areolar contour and augment breast tissue as needed (Georgiade and Lanier, 1984).

Macromastia, or massive breast enlargement, is referred to as virginal hypertrophy when it occurs during puberty, provided that the patient is not pregnant

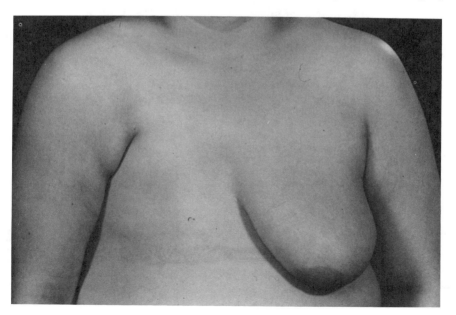

7–4 Patient with amastia associated with Poland syndrome.

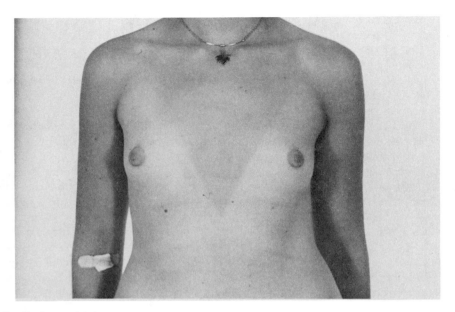

7–5   Patient with hypomastia.

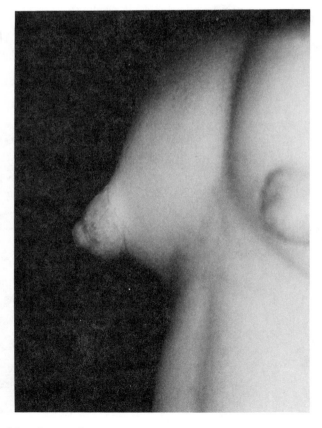

7–6   Patient with tuberous breast.

(Fig. 7–7). The underlying etiology is at this time undetermined; however, a 66% familial incidence has been reported. It is usually bilateral and causes not only physical discomfort, but significant emotional distress for many patients. Increased size and weight may lead to postural problems, backache, severe premenstrual mastalgia, and thoracic outlet syndrome. Of equal, if not greater import, is the associated psychologic morbidity leading to negative self-image and interfering with development of healthy peer relationships. Treatment of choice is reduction mammoplasty, delayed until late adolescence to allow completion of breast development. Delay may be difficult, with persistent pressure for surgical intervention from the patient and parents. Emotional support must be provided during this period. The patient must be counseled that although satisfactory cosmetic results can be achieved, the procedure may lead to decreased sensation and altered lactation. Breast-feeding is not recommended for such patients. An alternative to surgical intervention is medical management with danazol. This modality is currently under investigation (Huffman et al., 1981; Jacobs and Horton, 1982; Pietsch, 1985).

Inverted nipples are occasionally seen with the completion of breast development. Surgical intervention may be undertaken. However, this will greatly decrease the probability of successful breast-feeding (Pietsch, 1985).

Atrophy of the breast is almost uniformly secondary to nutritional deprivation as seen with crash dieting, anorexia nervosa, and chronic organic illness (Fig. 7–8). In such cases, adequate nutritional support leads to reversal of atrophy. Scleroderma involving the breast may lead to atrophy and most often requires surgical intervention for correction (Pietsch, 1985).

Breast development may be unequal early in the phase of rapid growth (Tanner stages II–IV). This asymmetry generally becomes much less apparent as development progresses further. Occasionally, asymmetry is so marked that the adolescent suffers significant emotional distress (Fig. 7–9). The patient can be counseled for future breast augmentation or reduction with the completion of breast development. In the interven-

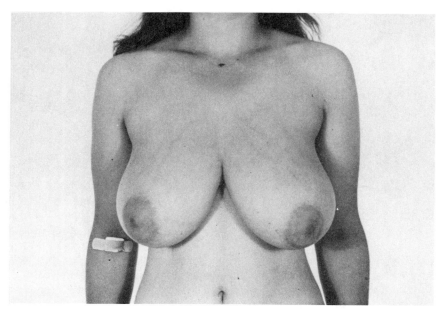

7–7   Patient with virginal hypertrophy.

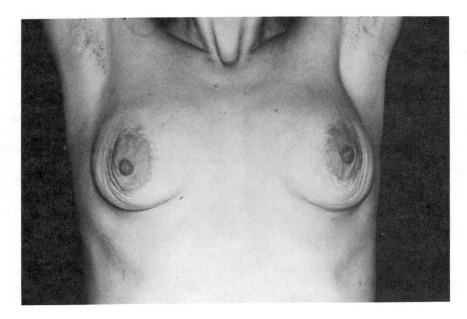

7–8   Patient with atrophied breasts.

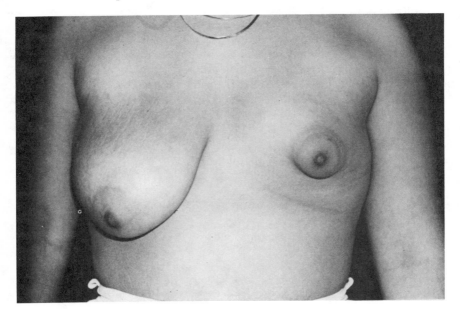

7–9   Patient with breast asymmetry.

ing period, ongoing emotional support is imperative. The patient may elect to wear a cosmetic prosthesis on the affected side. Inequality of breast size that persists for 2 or more years in the adolescent who has reached Tanner stage V breast development is unlikely to resolve (Hoffman, 1983).

Breast Masses

The abnormalities most frequently found during breast examinations of adolescents are breast masses. The discovery of such a mass creates much anxiety for the adolescent and her family due to the publicity and emotions surrounding the topic of breast cancer. It is, therefore, important to place the finding of a breast mass in perspective for the adolescent. Rarely are adolescent breast masses malignant. However, many types of these breast masses may require aspiration, biopsy, or excision. Physicians must keep in mind that adolescents can be very proficient in finding breast masses themselves, even without prior breast self-examination (BSE) training (Daniel and Mathews, 1968; Hein et al., 1982; Ligon et al., 1980). Thus, when an adolescent patient presents with the complaint of a breast lump, a thorough breast examination is needed to verify her findings and to reassure her, if appropriate, of the lesion's benign nature.

This section discusses the etiology and management of adolescent breast masses. The different types of lesions are classified as benign, neoplastic, and inflammatory masses. Unique management aspects of each type of mass are discussed after the description of the lesion. General comments regarding the management of adolescent breast masses are presented at the end of the section.

Benign Masses

Breast buds, marking the female's onset of puberty, are the most common "breast masses" in children. Virtually all females will develop breast buds (thelarche), as part of their pubertal development. The average age of thelarche in the United States is 11.2 years (Schydlower, 1982). It may normally occur, however, as early as age 8 or as late as age 14 years. Conditions such as precocious puberty and premature thelarche may cause significant breast growth at even earlier ages. Often one breast will develop before the other, and the tissue growth may be painful. It is potentially tragic to mistake a normal breast bud for a pathologic lesion. Misguided concern can cause undue patient anxiety and mistakenly lead to unnecessary surgery or biopsy. The result could be permanent disfigurement or absence of further growth in the affected breast. Vigilance against such clinical errors must be maintained when any pre- or early pubertal female complains of a breast lump or pain.

Fibroadenomas are the most frequently biopsied breast mass among adolescents (Daniel and Mathews, 1968; Diehl and Kaplan, 1985; Goldstein and Miller, 1982; Hein et al., 1982; Ligon et al., 1980; Rosenberg et al., 1983; Stone et al., 1977). Typically fibroadenomas are smooth, well-demarcated, rubbery, and highly mobile masses that occur most commonly in black females and in the upper-outer quadrant of the breast. A fibroadenomatous mass usually presents in the late teen years as a solitary, slow-growing lump. They can, however, appear at any age after the onset of puberty. Uncommonly, multiple fibroadenomas occur simultaneously in the same patient. Fibroadenomas generally do not vary in size during the menstrual cycle and most do not grow beyond 4 cm in diameter; however, lesions up to 15 cm are possible. If physically comparable to an already biopsied primary lesion, very small fibroadenomas that do not change in size may not need excision (Dudgeon, 1985; Harris et al., 1987). To avoid unnecessary procedures, it is prudent to observe a mass that is clinically consistent with a fibroadenoma for 2–3 months before a biopsy is performed. During that time some masses will regress or disappear, obviating the need for surgery (Beach, 1987).

In the past it has been advocated that all fibroadenomas be excised due to their potential for malignant degeneration in adult women (Seashore, 1975). However, reviews on this subject have found an occurrence of carcinoma in less than 0.5% of fibroadenomas (Harris et al., 1987).

New fibroadenomas may occur at any time during puberty, but they are most common in the mid- to late teen years. Therefore, to prevent disfigurement, it is recommended that multiple fibroadenomas be excised only after full breast development has occurred. This will decrease the number of repeated operative procedures when subsequent lesions appear during late pubertal growth (Schydlower, 1982; Seashore, 1975).

When excised, fibroadenomas appear as well demarcated, round or oval, grey-white masses. Microscopically they consist of mixed epithelial and stromal (connective tissue) elements. The epithelial components are well-defined, gland-like, and duct-like spaces with cuboidal or columnar cell linings (Harris et al., 1987).

Fibrocystic changes of the breast are another common finding in adolescent breast examinations. Reports on the relative frequency of fibrocystic changes versus fibroadenomas are conflicting. Those studies that report only biopsied breast masses note fibroadenomas to be the most common breast lesion (Daniel and Mathews, 1968; Stone et al., 1977; Ligon et al., 1980; Goldstein and Miller, 1982; Hein et al., 1982). Very few studies have evaluated adolescent breast lesions without selecting biopsied versus nonbiopsied lesions. Diehl and Kaplan (1985) has reported that in one outpatient clinic (patient ages 13–21 years), 51% of the breast lesions evaluated were clinically diagnosed as fibrocystic in nature, while only 15% were clinically diagnosed as fibroadenomas. All other breast lesions were less common. Therefore, although data are scant, it seems probable that fibrocystic disorders are more common, yet due to their cyclical symptomatology, they are more clinically apparent and are biopsied less often.

The spectrum of fibrocystic breast changes, also called fibrocystic mastopathies or fibrocystic breast disease, is broad and includes many different types of breast changes. It is likely that many adolescent females have symptoms of cyclic mastodynia due to nonpathologic amounts of fibrous and/or microcystic areas of the breast. In this regard some authors have considered fibrocystic "disease" as a difference in quantity of otherwise normal cyclical breast changes, not a difference of quality (Love et al., 1982). Other entities frequently included in this group are: large solitary breast cysts (also known as "blue-domed" cysts), single simple cysts, and galactoceles (Rosenberg et al., 1983). Clinical distinction of these lesions is often not possible and will probably not be necessary as long as one has a logical approach to the patient with a breast mass.

Several theories have been proposed to explain the pathophysiology of fibrocystic mastopathies. The common theme of these theories is that there seems to be a neuroendocrine disorder that causes a low progestin to estrogen ratio during the luteal phase of the menstrual cycle. This hormonal imbalance has been associated with cystic breast changes in humans and other animals (Harris et al., 1987).

The typical clinical scenario is that of a menstruating, pubertally mature female with breast pain, with or without noticeable breast lumps, whose symptoms worsen during the few days before each menses and relent during or towards the end of the menstrual flow. On examination the breasts will vary in texture, depending on the phase of the menstrual cycle. During the time of symptoms the breasts may be fuller and with more dense fibrous or cystic areas. The lesions are more common on the right and in the upper and outer quadrants (Daniel and Mathews, 1968; Hein et al., 1982), and are reported more frequently in white than in nonwhite females (Diehl and Kaplan, 1985; Harris et al., 1987). During asymptomatic periods, the breast examination may be entirely normal or reveal only a painless, increased fibrous nature of the breast. With this in mind it is necessary to caution against overdiagnosing fibrocystic mastopathies in many adolescents who have an increased proportion of fibrous breast tissue yet remain asymptomatic and should be considered normal. Many cystic breast lesions will resolve after 1–3 months (Dudgeon, 1985; Beach, 1987). This clinical marker plays a significant role in determining the actions taken when managing an adolescent with a breast mass. (See "Management of Breast Masses" below).

As one might expect, the common nature of this disorder and the lack of thorough understanding of its pathophysiology have caused a multitude of recommendations for treatment. Most of these recommendations are derived from research in adult women. Their usefulness in adolescents has not been determined.

The most benign recommendations for treating fibrocystic mastopathies or cyclic mastodynia include the use of heat, firm support bras, and mild analgesics, and are worth a trial in adolescents with symptoms. The most commonly used pharmacologic therapy in young adult women has been supplemental progestins, often in the form of oral contraceptives, to suppress ovarian function and restore a normal progestin to estrogen balance. Results of this treatment in adults have been favorable, and this may be a reasonable choice for adolescents (Humphrey, 1983; Harris et al., 1987). The relative risks of using oral contraceptives must be weighed against the potential gain *and* the patient's need for effective contraception. It must be remembered that while supplemental hormones treat and prevent some forms of fibrocystic mastopathies, only the nonpremalignant forms of fibrocystic disorders have been shown to be responsive. Oral contraceptives have not been shown to protect women from premalignant fibrocystic disorders (LiVolsi et al., 1978).

Dietary manipulations have received much lay attention for relieving symptoms of fibrocystic breast symptoms. The most popularly mentioned are methylxanthine restriction and the use of vitamins E, A, B1, C, and oil of evening primrose. In reviews of these methods none have been found more effective than placebos, when careful clinical studies were performed (Humphrey, 1983; Harris et al., 1987). Hence, they do not seem justified as recommendations for adolescents.

Recently, danazol has been advocated as specific treatment for fibrocystic breast disease in adult women. Danazol acts by interrupting the hypothalamic-pituitary axis for gonadotropin release. Danazol has other endocrine effects, the most significant of which is a direct, mild androgen-like activity on end organs. Studies have shown danazol to be effective in reducing breast pain and nodularity of fibrocystic mastopathy in 70%–80% of treated patients (Humphrey, 1983; Harris et al., 1987; Huff, 1987). However, experience with danazol in adolescents is very limited, and some of the virilizing effects can be irreversible. Therefore, danazol may be a useful therapy when an adolescent with significant breast discomfort or nodularity has already tried other reasonable treatment alternatives and symptoms persist. It is advisable that the patients be forewarned of the possible side effects and the lack of experience of this medication in adolescents before danazol therapy is begun. Also, since danazol does not thoroughly suppress ovarian function, other contraceptive measures must be used if contraception is needed.

Other modes of therapy for fibrocystic mastopathy which are not recommended in adolescents include diuretics, bromocriptine, thyroxine, and tamoxifen treatment (Humphrey, 1983; Harris et al., 1987). Surgical therapy for fibrocystic mastopathy is generally not plausible due to the diffuse nature of the breast changes.

Many misconceptions exist regarding the relationship of fibrocystic mastopathies and breast cancer. It has been reported that females with fibrocystic breast disorders have a 2- to 6-fold increase in the risk of subsequent breast carcinoma. However, only the duct epithelial hyperplasia with atypia and the apocrine metaplasia with atypia forms of fibrocystic disorders appear to be precancerous. Other histologic forms of fibrocystic disorders, which are more common, appear to have no bearing on an individual's risk for breast cancer (Brooks, 1982).

When a breast mass consistent with fibrocystic mastopathy either persists, grows rapidly, or demonstrates other changes suspicious for neoplasia, a surgical approach is indicated. (See "Management of Breast Masses" below).

Juvenile giant fibroadenomas are a rapidly growing variant of fibroadenomas that occur primarily in black adolescent females. These lesions are somewhat softer and less well defined than normal fibroadenomas. Occasionally they are accompanied by overlying venous distention of the superficial vessels. These lesions are always benign. Surgical excision is curative and often necessary to prevent significant disfigurement. Occasionally the juvenile giant fibroadenoma will, by virtue of its size, compress and cause atrophy of the involved breast tissue. In such cases, early excision may prevent disfigurement and the later need for a breast prosthesis (Dudgeon, 1985).

Intraductal papillomas are uncommon in adolescents, representing only 2.8% of biopsied breast masses in one study (Stone et al., 1977). The intraductal papilloma lesion is generally small, subareolar, and painless (Seashore, 1975). A bloody nipple discharge is a common clinical finding. When an intraductal papilloma is suspected, localization of the mass can be done by palpating around the areola and observing which ductal area produces the nipple discharge upon compression (Diehl and Kaplan, 1985). Surgical excision of the mass and the involved ductal segment is curative. Malignant degeneration is rare (Harris et al., 1987).

Cystosarcoma phyllodes is another uncommon cause of adolescent breast masses, accounting for 1%–2% of biopsied masses (Stone et al., 1977; Hein et al., 1982). This lesion occurs more often in black adolescent females and commonly exhibits nipple discharges or overlying skin changes. Axillary lymph node involvement is rare. In adolescents, cystosarcoma phyllodes tumors tend to grow rapidly and may be clinically indistinguishable from juvenile giant fibroadenomas. Sizes of up to 40 cm have been reported (Amerson, 1970). At excision a 2-cm margin is recommended to prevent otherwise frequent local recurrence (Harris et al., 1987). On histologic examination cystosarcoma phyllodes is very similar to fibroadenomas, and some controversy exists as to whether cystosarcoma phyllodes arises from preexisting fibroadenomas. Malignant disease arising from cystosarcoma phyllodes is rare but possible in adolescents and adults (Dudgeon, 1985; Harris et al., 1987). Total excision of this lesion is the treatment of choice, while total mastectomy is not usually required (Dudgeon, 1985).

Trauma-induced breast masses are uncommon and always benign. As discussed in the "Trauma and Sports" section below, trauma to the breast during sports is infrequent. Occasionally, hematomas of the breast skin or mammary tissue or fat necrosis of the superficial mammary structures does occur; however, usually the adolescent will not recall the occurrence of any breast trauma. While these lesions are harmless they often cause concern because of their clinical characteristics. The masses are often ill-defined without clear borders, and the healing processes can cause fixation to other breast structures and/or skin dimpling and retraction (Seashore, 1975). The management of these lesions and the indications for their biopsy are the same as for other persistent lesions. Diagnosis is often made only after biopsy.

Granular cell myoblastomas are rare (<1% of breast masses in adolescents) breast lesions that are derived from neural crest tissue (Stone et al., 1977). These lesions are characteristic for their rock hard consistency. Their location is usually in the superficial soft tissue over the breast. Diagnosis is made at biopsy, and caution must be exercised not to let the hardness nor the unusual histologic nature of the lesion lead to erroneous mastectomy based upon inaccurate suspicions of malignancy (Seashore, 1975).

Multiple other types of breast lesions have been reported in adolescents. All are less common than the lesions listed above (Table 7–1).

Neoplastic Masses

Malignant breast diseases are among the most rare causes of breast masses in adolescent females. In reviews of biopsied specimens from adolescents, malignant disease has been found in far less than 1% of all masses (Stone et al., 1977; Gallager et al., 1978). An estimated 150 cases of breast cancer occur annually in patients less than 25 years of age (McSweeney and Egan, 1984). Only a small percent of these occur in adolescents.

The largest review of pediatric breast cancers included 74 cases in patients ranging from 3 to 20 years of age (Ashikari et al., 1977). Ninety percent of these lesions presented as breast masses. Other presenting symptoms included arm swelling, leg swelling, pleural effusion, hepatomegaly, dyspnea, and back pain. Of 44 lesions with known histologic type, 18 (40.9%) were adenocarcinomas and 10 (22.7%) were secretory carcinomas. Other forms were less common. The prognosis was excellent for those adolescents with secretory carcinoma, which presents relatively more often in adolescents than in adults. Other histologic types had a poorer prognosis, especially if axillary lymph node spread had occurred by the time of diagnosis. Simple mastectomy or wide excision was the treatment of choice, with radical mastectomy rarely needed. In this study, no predisposing factors could be identified that indicated high risk for breast cancer in adolescence (Ashikari et al., 1977). Well known risk factors for breast cancer in adults, such as family history of breast cancer, did not seem to play a role in the rare occurrence of adolescent breast cancer (Sattin et al., 1985; Shingleton and McCarty,

Table 7–1   Breast Masses in Female Adolescents

Masses associated with puberty
  Breast buds

Benign tumors
  Fibradenomas
  Fibrocystic disease
  Cystosarcoma phyllodes
  Intraductal papilloma
  Lipoma
  Fibroma
  Keratoma
  Papilloma
  Myoblastoma
  Hemangioma
  Lymphangioma
  Galactocele

Inflammatory masses
  Abscess and cellulitis

Breast cancer
  Adenocarcinoma
  Secretory carcinoma

1987). No doubt more information is needed regarding adolescent breast cancer, and further reporting of cases is encouraged.

Older adolescent patients will often inquire about the risk of malignant breast disease in their adult life. Therefore, the physician caring for adolescents must have an understanding of breast cancer statistics in adults. The incidence of breast cancer is rising in the United States and in Western Europe. For unknown reasons it is more common in white than in black females (Shingleton and McCarty, 1987). Known risk factors for adult breast cancer are shown in Table 7–2. It is prudent to address the increased risk for future breast cancer with those adolescents who are at high risk. These patients should be encouraged to perform monthly breast self-examination and obtain yearly routine physician exams, aiming at early detection of breast cancer.

Inflammatory Masses

Inflammatory breast masses in adolescents may take the form of either breast cellulitis or abscesses. Breast infections are more common during times of hormonal stimulation of the breast, especially during the neonatal period and during lactation. The next most common period for infections is adolescence. In surveys of biopsied breast masses, abscesses and mastitis make up 2%–12% of the lesions (Sandison and Walker, 1968; Stone et al., 1977; Hein et al., 1982). The frequency of breast infection in any survey will be dependent upon the age of the study subjects due to the age dependency of this type of lesion.

It has been hypothesized that duct obstruction is the primary problem leading to mastitis; however, this is controversial (Ekland and Zeigler, 1973). Some lesions may be initiated by shaving or plucking periareolar hair (Emans and Goldstein, 1982). There is no evidence indicating that female athletes are at increased risk for breast infections due to breast trauma (Rosenberg et al., 1983).

In developed breasts most abscesses are found in the subareolar area (Ekland and Zeigler, 1973). The lesions are most often caused by staphylococcal infections, and they respond well to heat and systemic penicillinase-resistant antibiotics. While sub-areolar abscesses, in adolescent and adult breasts, have an incidence of recurrence as high as 39%, peripheral breast abscesses are less common and recur infrequently (Ekland and Zeigler, 1973).

The typical clinical scenario of a breast infection in adolescence is that of a rapidly growing, warm, tender breast lump, usually in the subareolar area. Fever and other systemic symptoms occasionally occur. The mass may become fluctuant within 2–3 days, requiring incision and drainage. Systemic antibiotics are indicated in all cases. If the lesion is a subareolar abscess, treatment for 3–4 weeks is recommended due to the high recurrence rate. In recurrent difficult lesions it may become necessary to surgically excise the involved ductal system (Seashore, 1975), always with attention to preventing significant disfigurement or scarring.

After any breast infection, abscess incision, or ductal excision, some sub-cutaneous scarring may occur which results in a palpable lump. When such lumps occur

Table 7–2   Risk Factors for Breast Cancer in Adult Women

First degree relative with breast cancer
First child after age 35 or nulliparous
Anovulatory menstrual cycles
Obesity
Diabetes mellitus
High fat diet

From Sattin et al., 1985.

at the same site as a previous infection they do not need to be biopsied, unless they appear suspicious of another process.

Management of Breast Masses

When managing the care of an adolescent with a breast mass it is important to have a well thought out plan for diagnosis and treatment. Most adolescents in this situation will be very anxious. The physician who is hesitant or indecisive will augment this anxiety and, worse, may lead himself and the patient toward an inappropriate choice. Physicians caring for both adult and adolescent females will have the additional burden of separating their approach to adult breast masses from their approach to the same problem in adolescents. The adolescent breast mass has a much lower chance of representing malignant disease and, therefore, deserves a more conservative approach. The goals of management will be first to make an accurate diagnosis without causing unnecessary surgery and second, to do so without missing serious pathology.

The very best diagnostic tools for assessing adolescent breast masses are an accurate history and a careful physical examination. Once a breast mass is found, any history of inciting agents (e.g., medications, marijuana, opiates) (Dudgeon, 1985) should be sought and their use terminated if possible. The nature of the breast symptoms and their timing with relation to the menstrual cycle are crucial to the evaluation. During the examination the mass should be carefully measured and a diagram of its location in the breast drawn in the chart. Occasionally, photographs of the lesion are more helpful. Other features to be noted are the site of the lesion, demarcation of borders, cystic or solid nature, tenderness, mobility, distortion of overlying tissue, associated breast discharge or lymph nodes, and rate of growth. The latter feature may need to be tracked over one to several months to be gauged accurately. In general, the available technology rests in the examiner's fingers, followed by occasional breast aspiration, ultrasound, and/or local excision or biopsy (Emans and Goldstein, 1982; Dudgeon, 1985; Beach, 1987).

Based upon clinical features the physician can categorize adolescent breast lesions as either cystic, solid benign-appearing, or suspicious for malignancy. Cystic lesions most often represent fibrocystic mastopathies. Benign solid lesions will usually turn out to be fibroadenomas, infectious lesions, traumatic lesions, or intraductal papillomas. The third category includes rapidly growing or distorting lesions and those lesions with associated lymphadenopathy. Many benign entities will fall into this third category; however, their clinical distinction from malignancy is difficult and hence their management is initially the same.

Cystic breast lesions should all be reexamined following the patient's next menses. Many cysts will resolve at this time or change enough in nature to assure their diagnosis as fibrocystic mastopathy. Cysts that advance in size and symptoms or that do not resolve after a menstrual period should be further examined by ultrasound or aspiration (Dudgeon, 1985; Beach, 1987). Ultrasonography can be useful if the radiologist can clearly determine the cystic or solid nature of a persistent lump. Cystic lesions can then be considered benign, and no further therapy is necessary unless they persist longer than three months or enlarge (Dudgeon, 1985; Beach, 1987). In the event that breast ultrasonography is not available or that the sonogram reveals a solid or undetermined nature of the lesion, aspiration is indicated. An excellent review of the technique for cyst aspiration is described by Vorherr (1984). All fluid and tissue aspirated is histologically examined. Lesions suspicious for malignancy histologically are then referred for excisional biopsy. Breast aspiration cannot, however, totally rule out the possibility of a breast malignancy. A benign aspirate histology coupled with a lesion that collapses after aspiration virtually assures a cystic disorder (Emans and Goldstein, 1982). The breast mass that does not collapse after aspiration must be referred for excisional biopsy to rule out malignancy.

If a benign cystic disorder is diagnosed, no further intervention is necessary. The patient should be reexamined in approximately 10 weeks and periodically thereafter based upon further findings. Treatment is based upon symptoms as discussed above.

Solid benign-appearing lesions should also be reexamined in 1 month, preferably after menstruation, to note hormonally induced change. Provided the lesion improves or does not change, follow-up is then indicated after 2–3 more months. At that time persistent lesions should be biopsied for diagnosis (Dudgeon, 1985; Beach, 1987; Marks and Fisher, 1987). Many of these lesions, especially fibroadenomas, may occur in clusters or may recur after excision. After the diagnosis is assured in the first lesion, subsequent similar lesions may be observed over time, provided they have no additional features suspicious for malignancy and are small enough not to be disfiguring. Observing such lesions until the end of breast maturation will prevent repeated surgical excisions. After breast maturity is reached, fibroadenomas, single or multiple, should be excised to prevent later cosmetic problems (Seashore, 1975).

Lesions suspicious for malignancy or that at discovery are of sufficient size to cause disfigurement should be promptly referred for local excision. In nearly all cases a local excisional biopsy can be performed on an outpatient basis, utilizing local anesthesia. In no instance should the diagnosis of breast malignancy be made based upon rapid frozen sections. Occasionally the unusual histology of adolescent breast lesions will be misread due to inexperienced pathologists or confusing histologic appearances (Ligon et al., 1980; Drukker and Pfeffer, 1984). The rarity of adolescent breast carcinomas must make one cautious in their diagnosis. Any surgical approach should always attend to the need for good cosmetic results, because of crucial concerns experienced by the adolescent regarding her self-image and peer acceptance.

After biopsy, benign disorders are followed up at periodic intervals appropriate to the underlying disorder. When malignancy is diagnosed referral for oncologic care is needed. Many malignant conditions in adolescents will be treated the same as in adults. However, adolescents' prognosis after simple mastectomy or local excision is excellent for some types of lesions (Ashikari et al., 1977). For that reason surgical and medical treatment should be performed only by physicians familiar with breast cancer in adolescents.

In summary, managing adolescent breast masses requires an assuring personality and awareness of the differences between adolescent and adult breast diseases. Conservative management is the rule; however, vigilance must be carried out in observance for the occasional malignant or disfiguring benign lesion. Generally, the indications for local excisional biopsy in adolescents are: 1) to establish the diagnosis in persistent or suspicious lesions, 2) to allay excessive patient or family fears about malignancy, and 3) to correct an obvious or highly likely cosmetic deformity (Table 7–3) (Turbey et al., 1975; Dudgeon, 1985).

Table 7–3   Indications for Breast Biopsy in Adolescents

1. To establish diagnosis.
2. To correct cosmetic deformity.
3. To allay excessive patient anxiety.

From Turbey et al., 1975.

Breast Examination

Due to the mystique and eroticism often ascribed to the breast, adolescents, and frequently their health care providers, experience embarrassment and anxiety during the breast examination. It is therefore crucial that the breast examination be approached with sensitivity and tact. As always, the adolescent's modesty should be protected to the greatest extent possible without compromising the evaluation. Disrobing should be done in private and as much partial cover as possible maintained with sheets, gowns, etc. Hospital-type gowns, which open to expose the chest, work well for the breast examination; however, a separate sheet or towel should be draped across the lap to cover the genital area.

Self-examination, breast disease publicity, and the underlying mystique associated with the breast make many adolescent females anxious about the potential for breast disease and disfigurement. Medically insignificant anomalies of the breasts may have been noted by the patient before coming to the physicians's office; however, anxiety frequently prevents the adolescent from mentioning such findings as a concern. For this reason, any minor anamolies noted during the breast examination (e.g., breast asymmetry, hyper- or hypomastia, areolar anomalies) should be discussed, and, if appropriate, the patient should be reassured.

Yearly check-ups during adolescence are the optimal schedule of health maintenance (Marks and Fisher, 1987). These health evaluations should include a breast examination. While some have argued that breast examinations at early pubertal ages are not cost efficient and may cause unnecessary anxiety (Frank and Mai, 1985; Goldbloom, 1985), others feel that discussing and examining the breast in these patients reassures the patient of her normalcy and provides an excellent way for the patient to begin a healthy self-exploration of her body and her sexuality (Beach, 1987). Other indications for breast examinations include the initial and annual gynecologic examinations of adolescents using oral contraceptives and at any time that the patient presents with breast-related complaints (e.g., breast discharge, pain, or lumps).

An excellent description of the adolescent breast examination is outlined in a text by Emans and Goldstein (1982). The examination starts with the patient sitting. Inspection is performed looking for breast dimpling, nipple retraction, and breast asymmetry. If there is a question of breast dimpling the contour of the breast can be augmented by having the patient contract her pectoralis muscles with her hands pressing against her hips. This maneuver will cause any dimpling to be more prominent and more easily detected. Finally, with the patient's arm lifted overhead, the undersides of the breasts are visualized and inspected for dimpling or other lesions.

After inspection the patient is next examined supine. At this time the Tanner stage of the breasts are determined and measurements are made, if needed. A convention for recording breast dimensions has been suggested by Emans and Goldstein (1982). It calls for horizontal diameters to be written first followed by vertical diameters. An example of such a record would be:

	Right	Left
Areola	2.5 × 2.5 cm	3 × 2.5 cm
Breast mound	9.0 × 8.0 cm	10 × 9.0 cm

Palpation of the breasts is also performed with the patient supine. During the examination of each breast the patient should raise the ipsilateral arm and rest it with the hand behind her head. Palpation starts at the 12 o'clock position at the perimeter of the breast mound. Light pressure is applied with the flat portion of the fingers and small circular motions are made. The examiner then proceeds radially toward the nipple moving in increments small enough to allow palpation of all breast tissue en route. Then, proceeding clockwise, similar radial examinations are made around the entire circumference of the breast. Usually six to eight radial examinations are needed, depending upon the amount of breast tissue present.

During palpation the consistency of the breast is noted and distinct masses are sought. The normal consistency for an adolescent's breast tissue has been described as like that of tapioca pudding (Emans and Goldstein, 1982). If palpation is difficult or suspicious areas of breast tissue are found, the sensitivity of the palpation can be increased by raising the ipsilateral shoulder onto a rolled towel or pillow or by placing talc powder on the surfaces of the examining fingers (Harris et al., 1987). Indications of possible breast pathology include: dense, fibrous breast tissue with or without discrete lumps; smooth, mobile nodules that tend to indicate benign breast disease; or firm, matted, and fixed masses which may indicate malignant breast disease.

The areola should also be compressed looking for subareolar masses and breast discharge.

The axillary tail of the breast is palpated in a fashion similar to that used for the other parts of the breast, remembering that this tissue may extend out to the midaxillary line and is also prone to mass formation. After locating and palpating the full extent of the breast tail, the deep axilla is palpated, looking for enlarged axillary lymph nodes which may signal other breast pathology.

At this point the ipsilateral breast examination is complete. If not done previously, the patient now raises her opposite hand behind her head and the other breast is examined in like fashion.

Breast Self-Examination

In recent years breast self-examination (BSE) has become common primarily due to physicians' advocacy of BSE and publicity from the American Cancer Society. Recent controversy has caused some authorities to no longer recommend BSE in adults (US Preventive Services Task Force, 1987). Regardless, some mention of its use in adolescents is warranted.

The primary reasons for abandoning BSE in adults is the advent of newer, more accurate diagnostic methods that are available for mass screening (e.g., mammography, thermography) and the lack of scientifically proven efficacy of BSE (Harris et al., 1987; O'Malley and Fletcher, 1987; Shingleton and McCarty, 1987; US Preventive Services Task Force, 1987). Also, it is suspected that BSE may cause unnecessary patient anxiety and eventually lead to unnecessary surgical procedures on benign lesions (Turbey et al., 1975). In adolescents, however, the newer methods of breast screening and diagnosis are not useful. The greater fibrous content of the adolescent breast makes imaging difficult to interpret (Ligon et al., 1980; Hein et al., 1982; Cohen et al., 1985; Williams et al., 1986). Also, concern exists about the safety of radiation to breasts before the age of lactation. Hence, BSE and physician exams remain the only mass screening tools available for adolescents.

Due to the relative rarity of malignant breast masses in adolescents some may wonder why have any adolescent breast screening at all? In response to this one must remember that, although uncommon, such malignancies do occur, and their treatment is most successful when begun early. In one study before the advocacy of BSE, less than 25% of surgically excised breast masses were self-discovered (Daniel and Mathews, 1968). In studies performed since BSE became common, 81% and 88% of surgically excised masses were self-detected. Up to 2% of these masses were malignant, and some malignancies occurred in adolescents (Ligon el al., 1980; Hein et al., 1982; Diehl and Kaplan, 1985).

There are other benefits derived from adolescent BSE. First, the process of BSE familiarizes the adolescent with normal breast consistency, which she may use as reference later in life when breast malignancies are a greater hazard. It is informative to have an adolescent begin BSE after a physician's examination to reassure her that her breasts are normal at that time. Also, BSE gives the adolescent an opportunity to participate in preventive medicine and self-care. These concepts will be new to most adolescents, yet they are necessary for a life-style of future health. Finally, teaching BSE offers the physician an opportunity to begin the discussion of some aspects of sexuality with the adolescent.

The recommendation remains to continue teaching BSE to adolescents and to advise that BSE be performed at monthly intervals. Practically, it is reasonable to teach and recommend monthly BSE to patients during their mid- to late adolescent years. At that stage of cognitive development, the adolescent will have developed the abstract skills required to appreciate the long-term gain of preventive health measures. Compliance with BSE, however, will vary from adolescent to adolescent. Compliance may be improved through thoughtful, sensitive teaching and by providing handout instructions that the adolescent can take home for further reference. Such handouts are available through the American Cancer Society and the National Cancer Institute.

Galactorrhea

Background

The breast is a secretory organ, and in the presence of certain hormones will produce secretions. Nipple secretion of various colors and clarity has been shown in 83% of nonpregnant women using heat and suction (Love et al., 1987). In addition, visible secretions of fluid by glands on the periphery of the areola (Montgomery's glands) have been described (Heyman and Rauh, 1983). Most of these secretions are felt to be benign, and in fact may be quite common but of insufficient quantity to be noticed more often. The presence of milky fluid, however, prompts more concern, as it may be associated with other abnormalities.

Galactorrhea, from the Greek terms meaning "milk" and "flow," is the secretion of milk-like fluid from one or both breasts not associated with pregnancy, the postpartum period, or nursing. It implies the production of fat-containing fluid by the mammary tissue. The prevalence of galactorrhea is reported at anywhere between 0.1% and 50%, reflecting the wide variation in definition and study design (Sakiyama and Quan, 1983; Rohn, 1984). It may be noted spontaneously by the patient or produced most effectively by compression of the breast from the base up towards the nipple in a "milking" fashion by the examiner. Galactorrhea appears to be more common in older women and previously parous women and less common in adolescents and nulligravid women (Sakiyama and Quan, 1983; Rohn, 1984). Within the adolescent age range, it is more common in girls and during the latter part of the teen years.

Mammogenesis in the developing female proceeds under the influence of estrogen, progesterone, insulin, thyroid hormone, adrenal steroids, and growth hormone. In the pregnant female, estrogen, progesterone, prolactin, and human placental lactogen stimulate further breast development. Estrogen also inhibits prolactin receptors on breast tissue. With the sudden decrease in estrogen and progesterone postpartum, prolactin acts unopposed, and lactation ensues (Emans and Goldstein, 1982; Sakiyama and Quan, 1983).

Prolactin, a peptide hormone produced by the anterior pituitary gland, acts on breast tissue receptors to stimulate milk protein production. Prolactin production is stimulated by thyrotropin-releasing hormone (TRH), serotonin, and other stimuli. Prolactin production is under tonic inhibitory control by prolactin inhibitory factor (PIF) in an apparent dopaminergic mechanism (Emans and Goldstein, 1982; Sakiyama and Quan, 1983; Rohn, 1984). Prolactin levels remain low in children and males. Increased levels are normally seen in women during pregnancy, the puerperium, and with lactation. However, prolactin levels normally decrease postpartum to the normal range within a few months even with continued breast-feeding. Galactorrhea, or inappropriate milk production, is associated with hyperprolactinemia in 49%–77% of cases. In contrast, only 15%–68% of patients with hyperprolactinemia develop galactorrhea (Sakiyama and Quan, 1983). Other factors, such as end organ sensitivity, cofactors, inhibiting factors, episodic variation, or biologic activity may play a role in the relationship between hyperprolactinemia and galactorrhea.

Etiology

Galactorrhea, with or without increased prolactin levels, has been associated with a myriad of conditions. Several factors may interact to produce the sign that brings the patient to medical attention. Major causative categories include pituitary tumors, drug or hormone-induced, idiopathic, and neurogenic (Table 7–4). A more extensive tabulation of the many causes of galactorrhea may be found in the review by Rohn (1984).

The most common and most important detectable cause of galactorrhea is a pituitary tumor. These tumors have been reported in 20%–85% of cases of galactorrhea. The most common of these is the prolactin-secreting pituitary adenoma, or prolactinoma, comprising about a third of pituitary tumors (Kleinberg et al., 1977; Sakiyama and Quan, 1983; Rohn, 1984). A prolactin-secreting adenoma is often associated with galactorrhea and amenorrhea. This has been termed the amenorrhea-galactorrhea syndrome, or the Forbes-Albright syndrome in the past. Even non-prolactin-secreting pituitary tumors may be associated with hyperprolactinemia by impinging on the hypothalamic stalk and impeding the flow of prolactin-inhibiting factor. Recent studies using newer techniques have revealed more information about pituitary tumors. Prolactin secretion by pituitary tumors may be more common than previously thought and difficult to detect microadenomas may be involved. Microadenomas have been reported in 2%–27% of autopsies (Zervas and Martin, 1980; Emans and Goldstein, 1982).

Hypothalamic or parapituitary lesions causing galactorrhea are rare but include craniopharyngioma, empty sella syndrome, other tumors, tuberculosis, granulomatosis, phakomatoses, trauma, and vascular lesions.

Oral contraceptive use is a relatively frequent association, occurring in 10%–14% of cases of galactorrhea. Both estrogen and progesterone may increase prolactin secretion. About 30% of birth control pill users may have elevated prolactin levels (Sakiyama and Quan, 1983). Estrogen and progesterone withdrawal in the face of elevated prolactin may make galactorrhea even more common after discontinuation of birth control pills (March et al., 1979; Taler et al., 1985). An association between birth control pill use and prolactinomas has been a topic of controversy but remains

Table 7–4   Causes of Galactorrhea

Pituitary
 Prolactinoma
 Pituitary stalk disruption
 Empty sella syndrome

Hypothalamic
 Craniopharyngioma and other tumors
 Granulomatosis
 Phakomatoses
 Trauma
 Vascular lesions
 CNS infection

Drugs
 Birth control pills
 Phenothiazines
 Butyrophenones
 Metoclopramide
 Methyldopa
 Opiates
 Cimetidine
 Isoniazid
 Amphetamines
 Verapamil
 Benzodiazepines

Endocrine
 Hypothyroidism
 Graves' disease
 Adrenal/renal tumors
 Pulmonary tumors
 Reproductive cell tumors
 Polycystic ovary syndrome

Neurogenic
 Nipple stimulation
 Chest wall surgery or trauma
 Chest wall burns
 Herpes zoster
 Psychological stress

Idiopathic

unproven. However, a history of birth control pill use in an adolescent with galactorrhea certainly does not obviate the need for further evaluation.

A large number of drugs have been associated with galactorrhea. These include phenothiazines, butyrophenones, metoclopramide, methyldopa, opiates, cimetidine, tricyclic antidepressants, insoniazid, amphetamines, verapamil, and benzodiazepines.

Hypothyroidism may be associated with 2%–6% of cases of galactorrhea. Thyrotropin-releasing hormone (TRH) is known to stimulate prolactin release, and hyperprolactinemia is found in 39% of patients with untreated primary hypothyroidism (Sakiyama and Quan, 1983). Other conditions of hormone activity, including adrenal, renal, pulmonary, or reproductive cell tumors, polycystic ovary syndrome, and Graves' disease may also cause galactorrhea (Emans and Goldstein, 1982; Sakiyama and Quan, 1983; Rohn, 1984).

Neurogenic causes of galactorrhea include nipple stimulation, chest wall surgery, burns, trauma, and herpes zoster. All of these probably have in common intercostal nerve stimulation affecting secretion of prolactin inhibitory factor in the hypothalamus (Letson and Moore, 1984). Psychologic stress has also been implicated (Greydanus, 1983; Rohn, 1984).

A large group of women have no cause of galactorrhea established after evaluation. This idiopathic group comprises 40%–50% of patients. Most of these have normal prolactin levels, and in previously parous women galactorrhea may reflect increased end organ sensitivity. Twenty to 37% of the idiopathic group may have elevated prolactin and are likely to also be amenorrheic. An unknown number of these cases may represent undetectable microadenomas (Kleinberg et al., 1977; Wiebe, 1980; Sakiyama and Quan, 1983).

Evaluation

As with any medical evaluation, a careful history is required, especially with the wide range of causes and associations described with galactorrhea. Other symptoms of a central nervous system tumor should be sought for, including polydipsia, polyuria, visual disturbance, and headache. Symptoms of hypothyroidism, such as temperature intolerance, fatigue, and weight change should be noted. A careful drug history should be obtained, going beyond the obvious birth control pills. The adolescent without amenorrhea will most likely fall into the drug-induced or idiopathic categories of galactorrhea (Emans and Goldstein, 1982). Chest wall trauma, surgery, skin conditions, or unusual stress should be kept in mind. The adolescent should also be questioned about nipple stimulation by clothing, self-manipulation, or sexual activity.

The physical examination should include visual field and fundoscopic examination, careful neurological evaluation, thyroid palpation, skin survey for hirsutism or pigmentation change, sexual maturation assessment, and pelvic examination for ovarian mass and estrogenization. Careful examination of the breasts is required to confirm and characterize the galactorrhea and to collect a specimen for laboratory analysis. Testing for fat, blood, and cytology may be helpful when the nature of the secretion is uncertain. All sections of the breasts should be stripped with bimanual pressure from the base to the nipple (Rohn, 1984; Beach, 1987).

Initial laboratory evaluation should include thyroid function tests, including thyroid-stimulating hormone (TSH) and serum prolactin level. If increased prolactin levels are found, a prolactinoma is vigorously searched for. The chances of finding a tumor increase with increasing prolactin level. A level >200 ng/ml virtually assures the presence of a tumor, while a level >100 ng/ml suggests a greater than 50% chance (Kleinberg et al., 1977; Turksoy et al., 1980; Wiebe, 1980; Zervas and Martin, 1980; Dewhurst, 1981; Sakiyama and Quan, 1983). There is reported episodic secretion of prolactin and a night-time peak associated with sleep (Boyar et al., 1976). Some investigators recommend three samples taken over an hour to avoid spurious results (Wiebe, 1980; Rohn, 1984). Others recommend a single morning sample, noting loss of the nocturnal peak and basal levels consistently above normal in patients with hyperprolactinemia (Boyar et al., 1976; Zervas and Martin, 1980; Sakiyama and Quan, 1983). Normal prolactin level is usually regarded as less than 20–25 ng/ml. Borderline levels in this range should prompt repetition, with three separate samples taken within an hour (Molitch and Reichlin, 1980).

Anteroposterior and lateral cone-down x-ray views of the sella turcica are frequently obtained as part of the initial workup. However, a more than 50% false-negative rate for tumor detection has been reported, except in patients with normal prolactin levels. Sella polytomography increases the diagnostic yield for smaller adenomas, but high resolution CT scan is supplanting the previous x-ray studies as the radiological procedure of choice (Emans and Goldstein, 1982; Sakiyama and Quan, 1983; Rohn, 1984).

Management

If the history suggests a drug-associated etiology, the medication should be discontinued if possible, with the expectation of resolution of the galactorrhea and normalization of prolactin, if elevated, within 6 months.

If hypothyroidism is diagnosed, thyroxine replacement should be instituted with the expectation of resolution within 6 months.

If prolactin and menses are normal, cone-down sella x-rays may be obtained. If these are normal, the patient should then be followed with prolactin levels measured every 6 months while symptoms persist. Any treatable associated condition should be addressed.

If prolactin is normal and menses are diminished or absent, or if prolactin is elevated, CT scan should be done. If the radiological study is normal, the patient should be followed and prolactin levels repeated every 6 months. If the radiologic study is abnormal, endocrinologic and neurosurgical consultation is suggested. Various prolactin suppression and stimulation tests have been studied to identify organic pathology. Tumors requiring surgery are more likely to be approached with newer transphenoidal microsurgical techniques when appropriate. If persistent galactorrhea is a problem, bromocriptine, a dopamine receptor agonist, may be used. Bromocriptine increases PIF secretion, thereby lowering serum prolactin and suppressing galactorrhea. It may also reinstitute normal ovulatory menstrual cycles in patients with amenorrhea and has been reported to shrink prolactinomas.

Because of the complex nature of the natural history and evaluation of prolactin-secreting tumors, patients should have continued follow-up as long as abnormalities persist or treatment continues.

Trauma and Sports

Breast conditions attributed to trauma include contusions, hematoma, fat necrosis, and abscess.

Breast abscesses are more common in the newborn and in lactating women and uncommon in adolescent females (Turbey et al., 1975; Emans and Goldstein, 1982). They accounted for between 0% and 3.9% of lesions in five multiyear reviews of adolescent breast masses (Farrow and Ashikari, 1969; Turbey et al., 1975; Stone et al., 1977; Goldstein and Miller, 1982; Diehl and Kaplan, 1985). Trauma may predispose to abrasion and skin infection or duct obstruction but is not a common antecedent to breast abscess (Turbey et al., 1975).

Trauma to the breast may cause superficial ecchymosis or deeper hematomas. Contusion from a significant force results in an indistinct, tender mass. The suspensory ligaments of the breast permit considerable mobility, and injury probably results from sufficient force to compress the breast tissue against the bony thorax. A shearing force causing movement of the breast over the pectoral fascia with resulting ecchymosis and hematoma appears to be an increasingly common mechanism with the high forces transmitted in an automobile accident with an across the breast shoulder seat belt in place (Murday, 1982; Dawes et al., 1986). Overly aggressive sexual activity might also result in sufficient compressive force to result in injury (Drukker and Pfeffer, 1984).

Fat necrosis results in a firm mass that may be tender. It is usually superficial and may be fixed to the skin. Its physical characteristics and radiologic appearance may be indistinguishable from carcinoma. It is most common in obese, pendulous breasts and may be related to continual local pressure (Wilson, 1986). In most cases, no history of trauma is given, but it certainly may result from severe trauma (Farrow and Ashikari, 1969; Gallager et al., 1978; Dudgeon, 1985). Fat necrosis may also be seen after surgery, radiation, and in conjunction with carcinoma. Excisional biopsy is usually required for accurate diagnosis. Fat necrosis is rare in adolescents, comprising from 0% to 1.7% of breast masses in five multiyear reviews (Farrow and Ashikari, 1969; Turbey et al., 1975; Stone et al., 1977; Goldstein and Miller, 1982; Diehl and Kaplan, 1985).

The breast of the adolescent female is a focus and symbol of emerging sexuality for both the adolescent and adult alike. This heightened sensitivity may have played a role in previous thinking that the breast of the adolescent was particularly susceptible to injury (Turbey et al., 1975). Perhaps undue caution in this respect played a role in restricting sports participation for females, as breast trauma might result from even "bumping the breast in normal daily activities" (Drukker and Pfeffer, 1984). However, the literature does not bear out a pattern of significant traumatic injury to the breast in normal activity or sports participation for the adolescent female. Over the past 15 years since Title IX legislation was passed, female participation in recreational and competitive sports has greatly expanded. Only recently are data addressing incidence of injury emerging. No significant injuries were reported in a 6-year review of women's sports at the college level or in marathon runners (Hale, 1984). In a study of adult women, 15% reported sports-related injuries, but these were confined to minor contusions and abrasions (Lorentzen and Lawson, 1987).

Athletes of both sexes do encounter minor injuries to the nipples. Friction from clothing results in irritation and abrasion, commonly known as "runner's" or "jogger's nipples." This is more likely to happen in the female who runs without a brassiere and can be prevented by using tape over the nipples or a protective coating of petrolatum (Levit, 1977). A similar problem results from cold injury to the nipples due to evaporation and wind chill in bicycle riders. "Bicyclist's nipples" may be prevented by using wind-resistant material over the breasts (Powell, 1983).

Excessive breast motion and resulting soreness during strenuous activity such as running can adversely affect participation and performance. This is a greater problem for the woman with larger breasts. More rigidly constructed brassieres that hold the breasts in a rounded shape close to the body are most effective in preventing excessive motion. Sports-specific design in strap construction and protective padding for contact sports are desirable (Kulund, 1982; Nirschl, 1982; Beach, 1987; Lorentzen and Lawson, 1987).

Psychosocial Aspects

When evaluating the adolescent female with breast abnormalities, it is important to address the potential impact of the condition on the psychosocial development of the patient. There are a number of milestones that an adolescent must negotiate, and a breast abnormality can prove to be a potential obstacle in achieving the following psychosocial tasks of adolescence: development of a sexual identity, development of healthy peer relationships, and acceptance of body changes during puberty (Hoffman, 1983; Neinstein, 1984).

Onset of breast development is most often the first event to herald the onset of pubertal maturation. As the breast has become a major symbol of femininity and sexual desirability in our culture, it is understandable how breast abnormalities might lead to significant emotional morbidity. There is a strong need in adolescence to be liked by peers. Any perception of being different or disliked by peers may lead to social isolation and depression. Consider the patient with failure of breast development. The psychosocial impact of this is readily apparent. The impact of minor abnormalities such as a supernumerary nipple or "slow" breast development may not be as obvious to the physician. The physician should address even minor abnormalities with the patient and assess the impact of a breast condition on the ongoing process of psychosocial maturation. Patients' concerns about minor variations of normal should not be trivialized or simply dismissed but dealt with in a sensitive and gentle manner.

Another factor that exaggerates breast concerns is the publicity that has been given to the fact that breast cancer is the most common malignancy of adult women. Although breast cancer is rare in the adolescent population, the patient who finds a mass may be reluctant to discuss this with the physician, fearing the worst. Anticipatory guidance may do much to allay fears that may arise in the future with regard to discovery of a mass.

Finally, the breast can be a highly emotionally charged area of the physical examination, both for the patient and the physician alike. The physician, caring for female patients during earlier childhood years, should make examination of the breast a practice during routine care. This practice may serve to lessen the potential embarrassment of breast examination during early adolescence and facilitate communication regarding breast development.

References

Amerson JR: Cystosarcoma phyllodes in adolescent females, a report of seven patients. *Ann Surg* 107:849–856, 1970.

Ashikari H, Jun MY, Farrow JH, et al: Breast carcinoma in children and adolescents. *Clin Bull* 7:55–62, 1977.

Beach RK: Routine breast exams: a chance to reassure, guide and protect. *Contemp Pediatr* 4:70–100, 1987.

Boyar RM, Kapen S, Weitzman ED, Hellman L: Pituitary microadenoma and hyperprolactinemia, a cause of unexplained secondary amenorrhea. *N Engl J Med* 294:263–265, 1976.

Brooks PG: Epidemiology and risk factors in breast cancer: can we change the odds? *J Reprod Med* 27:670–674, 1982.

Cohen MI, Mintzer RA, Matthies HJ, et al: Mammography in women less than 40 years of age. *Surg Gynecol Obstet* 160:220–222, 1985.

Daniel WA, Mathews MD: Tumors of the breast in adolescent females. *Pediatrics* 41:743–749, 1968.

Dawes RFH, Smallwood JA, Taylor I: Seat belt injury to the female breast. *Br J Surg* 73:106–107, 1986.

Dewhurst J: Breast disorders in children and adolescents. *Pediatr Clin North Am* 28:287–308, 1981.

Diehl T, Kaplan DW: Breast masses in adolescent females. *J Adolesc Health Care* 6:353–357, 1985.

Drukker BH, Pfeffer WH: Breast problems of teenagers. *Contemp Ob/Gyn* 11:45–56, 1984.

Dudgeon DL: Pediatric breast lesions: take the conservative approach. *Contemp Pediatr* 2:61–73, 1985.

Ekland DA, Zeigler MG: Abscess in the nonlactating breast. *Arch Surg* 107:398–401, 1973.

Emans SJH, Goldstein DP: The breast: examination and lesions, and the assessment of galactor-rhea. In *Pediatric and Adolescent Gynecology*, ed 2. Little, Brown, Boston, 1982.

Farrow JH, Ashikari H: Breast lesions in young girls. *Surg Clin North Am* 49:261–269, 1969.

Frank JW, Mai V: Breast self-examination in young women: more harm than good? *Lancet* 10:654–657, 1985.

Gallager HS, Leis HP, Snyderman RK (eds): *The Breast*. CV Mosby, St. Louis, 1978.

Georgiade GS, Lanier VC: Developmental breast abnormalities in children. In Seraphin, D, and Georgiade, NG (eds).: *Pediatric Plastic Surgery*. CV Mosby, Saint Louis, 1984.

Goldbloom RB: Self examination by adolescents. *Pediatrics* 76:126–128, 1985.

Goldstein DP, Miller V: Breast masses in adolescent females. *Clin Pediatr* 21:17–19, 1982.

Greydanus DE: The thorax: disorders of the breast. In Hoffmann, AD (ed): *Adolescent Medicine*. Addison-Wesley, Menlo Park, NJ, 1983.

Hale RW: Factors important to women engaged in vigorous physical activity. In Strauss, RH (ed): *Sports Medicine*. WB Saunders Co, Philadelphia, 1984.

Harris JR, Hellman S, Henderson IC, et al. (eds): *Breast Diseases*. JB Lippincott, Philadelphia, 1987.

Hein K, et al: Self-detection of a breast mass in adolescent females. *J Adolesc Health Care* 3:15–17, 1982.

Hersh JH, Bloom AS, Cromer AO, et al: Does a supernumerary nipple/renal field defect exist? *Am J Dis Child* 141:989–991, 1987.

Heyman RB, Rauh JL: Areolar gland discharge in adolescent females. *J Adolesc Health Care* 4:285–286, 1983.

Hoffman AD: *Adolescent Medicine*. Addison-Wesley, Reading MA, 1983.

Huff BA (ed): *Physicians' Desk Reference*. Medical Economics Co, Oradell, NJ, 1987.

Huffman JW, Dewhurst CJ, Capraro, VJ: *The Gynecology of Childhood and Adolescence*. WB Saunders, Philadelphia, 1981.

Humphrey LJ: Medical management of the fibrocystic breast. In *Proceedings of the Fibrocystic Breast, A Multidisciplinary Approach*, a symposium cosponsored by The Society for the Study of Breast Disease and Tufts University School of Medicine, May 21, 1983, Boston.

Jacobs JS, Horton CE: Macromastia in adolescence. In Hernahan, DA, et al. (eds.): *Symposium on Pediatric Plastic Surgery*. CV Mosby, Saint Louis, 1982.

Kenney RD, Flippo JL, Black EB: Supernumerary nipples and renal anomalies in neonates. *Am J Dis Child* 141:987–988. 1987.

Kleinberg DL, Noel GL, Frantz AG: Galactorrhea: a study of 235 cases, including 48 with pituitary tumors. *N Engl J Med* 296:589–600, 1977.

Kulund DN: The torso, hip, and thigh. In *The Injured Athlete*. JB Lippincott, Philadelphia, 1982.

Letson GW, Moore DC: Galactorrhea secondary to chest wall surgery in an adolescent. *J Adolesc Health Care* 4:277–278, 1984.

Levit F: Jogger's nipples. *N Engl J Med* 297:1127, 1977.

Ligon RE, Stevenson, DR, Diner W, et al: Breast masses in young women. *Am J Surg* 140:779–782, 1980.

LiVolsi VA, Stadel BV, Kelsey JL, et al: Fibrocystic breast disease in oral-contraceptive users: a histopathological evaluation of epithelial atypia. *N Engl J Med* 299:381–385, 1978.

Lorentzen D, Lawson L: Selected sports bras: a biomechanical analysis of breast motion while jogging. *Phys Sports Med* 5:128–139, 1987.

Love SM, Gelman RS, Silen W: Fibrocystic 'disease' of the breast—a nondisease? *N Engl J Med* 307:1010–1014, 1982.

Love SM, Schnitt SJ, Conolly JL, et al: Benign breast disorders. In Harris JR, Hellman S, Henderson IC, et al. (eds): *Breast Diseases*. JB Lippincott, Philadelphia, 1987.

March CM, Mishell DR, Kletzky OA, et al: Galactorrhea and pituitary tumors in postpill and non-postpill secondary amenorrhea. *Am J Obstet Gynecol* 134:45–48, 1979.

Marks A, Fisher M: Health assessment and screening during adolescence. *Pediatrics* 80:135–158, 1987.

Marshall WA, Tanner JM: Variations in pattern of pubertal changes in girls. *Arch Dis Child* 44:291, 1969.

McSweeney MB, Egan RL: Breast cancer in the younger patient. *Recent Results Cancer Res* 90:36–40, 1984.

Meggyvessy V, Mehes K: Association of supernumerary nipples with renal anomalies. *J Pediatr* 111:412–413, 1987.

Molitch ME, Reichlin S: The amenorrhea, galactorrhea and hyperprolactinemia syndromes. *Adv Intern Med* 26:37–65, 1980.

Murday AJ: Seat belt injury of the breast—a case report. *Injury* 14:276–277, 1982.

Neinstein LS: *Adolescent Health Care: A Practical Guide*, ed 2. Urban & Schwarzenberg, Baltimore, 1990.

Nirschl RP: Sports injuries. *The Female Patient* 7:43–56, 1982.

O'Malley MS, Fletcher SW: Screening for breast cancer with breast self-examination: a critical review. *JAMA* 257:2197–2203, 1987.

Osborne, MP: Breast development and anatomy. In Harris JR, Hellman S, Henderson IC, et al. (eds): *Breast Diseases*. JB Lippincott, Philadelphia, 1987.

Pietsch J: Breast disorders. In Lavery JP, Sanfilippo JS (eds): *Pediatric and Adolescent Obstetrics and Gynecology*. Springer-Verlag, New York, 1985.

Powell B: Bicyclist's nipples. *N Engl J Med* 249:2457, 1983.

Rehman I: Embryology and anatomy of the breast. In Gallager SH, Leis HP, Snyderman RK, et al. (eds): *The Breast*. CV Mosby, Saint Louis, 1978.

Rohn RD: Galactorrhea in the adolescent. *J Adolesc Health Care* 5:37–49, 1984.

Rohn RD: Nipple (papilla) development in puberty: Longitudinal observations in girls. *Pediatrics* 79:745–747, 1987.

Rosenberg CA, Gordon HD, Grabb WC, et al: Hypomastia and mitral valve prolapse. *N Engl J Med* 309:1230–1234, 1983.

Sakiyama R, Quan M: Galactorrhea and hyperprolactinemia. *Obstet Gynecol Surv* 38:689–700, 1983.

Sandison AT, Walker JC: Diseases of the adolescent female breast: A clinicopathological study. *Br J Surg* 55:443–448, 1968.

Sattin RW, Rubin GL, Webster LA, et al: Family history and the risk of breast cancer. *JAMA* 253:1908–1913, 1985.

Schydlower M: Breast masses in adolescence. *Am Fam Physician* 25:141–145, 1982.

Seashore JH: Breast enlargements in infants and children. *Pediatr Ann* 10:7–47, 1975.

Shingleton WW, McCarty KS: What you should know about breast pathology. *Contemp Ob/Gyn* 2:90–106, 1987.

Stone AM, Shenker IR, McCarthy K: Adolescent breast masses. *Am J Surg* 134:275–277, 1977.

Taler SJ, Coulam CB, Annegers JF, et al: Case-control study of galactorrhea and its relationship to the use of oral contraceptives. *Obstet Gynecol* 65:665–668, 1985.

Tanner J: *Growth at Adolescence*. Blackwell Scientific Publications, Ltd, Oxford, 1962.

Turbey WJ, Buntain WL, Dudgeon DL: The surgical management of pediatric breast masses. *Pediatrics* 56:736–739, 1975.

Turksoy RN, Farber M, Mitchell GW: Diagnostic and therapeutic modalities in women with galactorrhea. *Obstet Gynecol* 56:323–329, 1980.

US Preventive Services Task Force: Recommendations for breast cancer screening. *JAMA* 257:2196, 1987.

Vorherr H: Breast aspiration biopsy. *Am J Obstet Gynecol* 148:127–133, 1984.

Wiebe RH: Endocrine evaluation of hyperprolactinemia. *Clin Obstet Gynecol* 23:349–365, 1980.

Williams SM, Kaplan PA, Peterson JC, et al: Mammography in women under age 30. *Radiology* 161:49–51, 1986.

Wilson RE: The breast. In Sabiston DC Jr (ed): *Textbook of Surgery,* ed 13. WB Saunders, Philadelphia, 1986.

Zervas NT, Martin JB: Management of hormone-secreting pituitary adenomas. *N Engl J Med* 302:210–214, 1980.

8

Menstrual Disorders

I can state with certainty that menstruation can be, and therefore should be, free from
suffering of any kind. (Clow AES: The prevention of menstrual troubles. _Br Med J_
2:447, 1927)

Six decades later, Alice Clow's statement is close to final affirmation. This chapter is
intended to summarize current knowledge and survey recent studies that contribute to
our understanding of the process of menstruation and its disorders in adolescents and
young adults. Practical guidelines are included for the evaluation and management of
menstrual disorders in an outpatient setting.

Mean age of menarche has remained at 12.8 years with 1 standard deviation
(SD) of 1.2 years for the past four decades. Wyshak and Frisch (1982a) reviewed
218 reports on the age of menarche in Europe from 1795 to 1981 and noted that the
long-term decline in age of menarche correlated with a well-documented growth
acceleration during the past century. With an optimal growth rate, age of menarche
levels off. United States data indicate that menarche occurred at an average age of
14.75 years in 1870, 13.0 years in 1930, and 12.8 years in 1947, for a decline of
2.3 months per decade (Wyshak and Frisch, 1982b). In Europe a decline of approximately 3 years was noted from 1840 to 1940, attributed to improved nutrition with
early accumulation of body fat and control of infectious diseases (Baker, 1985).
Menarche in the United States occurs at a mean weight of 47.8 kg $\pm$ 0.5 kg, and a
mean height of 158.5 cm $\pm$ 0.5 cm (Frisch, 1984). Peak height velocity usually occurs
1 year after onset of breast budding and 1½ years before menarche. Linear growth after
menarche is limited to approximately 2–5 cm (Reindollar and McDonough, 1983;
Soules, 1987). Menarche predictably occurs within 30 months of onset of breast
budding. Occurrence of menarche by Tanner stage is listed in Table 8–1.

In the first year after menarche, 56% of cycles are anovulatory, and cycle length
averages 29.5 days, with a range of 21–40 days, a flow of 3–8 days, and estimated
blood loss of 40–100 ml. The first 10 menstrual cycles occur during the first 15 months
after menarche, and an average of 20 cycles are required before regular ovulation is
established (Altchek, 1977). The incidence of ovulatory cycles increases with both
gynecologic age and bone age. The early years postmenarche are characterized by a
high incidence of anovulatory cycles and cycles with a short luteal phase. In a study of
99 adolescents ranging in age from 13 to 16 years, Talbert et al. (1985) correlated self-
evaluation of a pubertal development index with the likelihood of ovulatory cycles
defined by a progesterone value of at least 3 ng/ml. At a gynecologic age of 18 months
(18 months postmenarche), 32% of subjects had ovulated. This increased to 61% at a
gynecologic age of at least 31 months. Breast development and pubic hair, but not
axillary hair, correlated with ovulation. Ovulation had occurred in 44% by Tanner stage
IV and in 57% by Tanner stage V for breast development, and in 35% by Tanner

Table 8–1   Incidence of Menarche by Tanner Stage

Stage	Incidence (%)
I	0
II	0
III	25
IV	65
V	10

stage IV and 60% by Tanner stage V for pubic hair development. By chronologic age, ovulatory cycles were documented in 53% at age 13 years and 66% at age 15–16 years.

In a prospective study of normal menstrual patterns in healthy students at an independent high school, Wilson et al. (1984) surveyed 327 adolescent females ranging from 13 to 18 years with a mean age of 15.5 ± 1.1 years. Age at menarche ranged from 9 to 15 years with a mean of 12.6 ± 1.1 years. At the time of the initial survey, 93.6% were postmenarchal and 6.4% premenarchal. Regular cycles were reported in 72.5%, and irregular cycles were associated with stress in 13.1% and with exercise in 12.1%. Reported duration of menstrual flow was 4–7 days in 92.8%, 3 days or less in 3.8%, and 8 days or more in 3.4%. A follow-up of menstrual calendars obtained 8–15 months later in a subgroup of 25% of the original students revealed that all adolescents whose cycles changed from regular to irregular were boarding students, thus suggesting that separation from home was a significant stress.

In a study of symptoms related to menstruation in Swiss adolescents, Flug et al. (1985) reported data obtained from 1954 through 1980 in the Zurich Longitudinal Study of Growth and Development. A standardized questionnaire was administered every 6 months to 140 adolescent females followed for 6 years after menarche. The questionnaire specifically addressed the symptoms of abdominal pain, headache, and "general discomfort" associated with menses. The prevalance of dysmenorrhea peaked at 64% at 3 years postmenarche, but less than 5% of this group reported premenstrual headache or general discomfort during menstruation in any of the 6 years postmenarche. General discomfort was defined as nausea, loss of appetite, and other poorly defined symptoms.

Venturoli et al. (1987) recently studied 95 adolescents with menstrual irregularities since menarche. Within this group, 75 reported long cycles of greater than 35 days, and 20 reported short cycles of less than 26 days. Endocrinologic evaluation revealed persistent irregular anovulatory cycles associated with low estrogen levels, high LH, low FSH, high androgens, and enlarged ovaries on ultrasound evaluation. The study concluded that the appearance of enlarged multifollicular ovaries associated with increased LH and hyperandrogenism may be transitory and reversible and represent a slow maturational process in some adolescents whose menstrual pattern will normalize with maturity.

Sandler et al. (1984) analyzed longitudinal data from the Menstrual and Reproductive Health Study which correlated age at menarche with subsequent reproductive performance. Age at menarche correlated with age at first marriage and first conception, but was unrelated to total number of pregnancies, stillbirths, or induced abortions. There was an increased risk of spontaneous abortion with menarche under age 11 years and a three-fold increased risk of ectopic pregnancy with menarche before age 12 years or at age 15 years or older.

Gardner (1983), in analyzing historical data obtained in a longitudinal study initiated in the 1930s, correlated adolescent menstrual characteristics with subsequent gynecologic health and concluded that the risk of "poor gynecologic health" was greatly increased with both dysmenorrhea and irregular menses in the first 4–8 years postmenarche. The sample size was not sufficient to relate early menstrual characteristics to specific gynecologic diagnoses, such as endometriosis, but adverse outcomes appeared to be associated with early maturation.

Both health education and family attitudes toward menses are likely to significantly affect the adolescent's response both to normal menses and menstrual disorders. In evaluating data obtained in the 1960s from the National Health Examination Survey, Klein and Litt (1981) reported that 16.5% of white females with menarche at or before age 11 years and 10% of all black females were given no information about menstruation prior to menarche. In a study of menstrual folklore, Snow and Johnson (1977) questioned 40 multiethnic females ranging in age from 17 to 41 years to assess their knowledge and beliefs about menstruation. Among these women, the majority lacked accurate information concerning onset of menses, cessation of menses, and origin of menstrual flow. Most lacked basic anatomic knowledge about the location and function of the uterus, tubes, and ovaries. They believed that menstruating women should change their behavior (62.5%), avoid intercourse (62.5%), avoid water and cold air (37.5%), change their diet (22.5%), avoid climbing and exercise (17.5%), and might be attacked by reptiles due to menstrual flow (12.5%). Despite recent inroads in health education, it is apparent that many adolescents lack even a basic understanding of normal menstrual physiology, the timing of ovulation, and its relationship to fertility.

Obtaining a menstrual history is the first step in evaluating adolescent menstrual disorders. Suggested topics are included in Table 8–2. The use of a menstrual calendar (Fig. 8–1) will often help to clarify the presence of irregular menses, since a surprising number of adolescents believe that their menstrual periods begin on the same chronologic day each month. In discussing menstrual hygiene, both pads and tampons can be safely recommended for use by adolescents. Although there is an increased risk of toxic shock syndrome among adolescents using tampons, this risk can be minimized by avoidance of super absorbent tampons, frequent changing, and the use of pads overnight. Tampon use has the potential advantage of reducing the discomfort of the first pelvic examination and enhancing compliance with barrier methods of contraception, such as the diaphragm or vaginal sponge.

Amenorrhea and Oligomenorrhea

We must supply the place of the menstrual evacuations, until the system be habituated to the suppression, by local bleedings at the perinaeum, the anus, or the vulva, and we shall take care that the abstraction of blood correspond with the menstrual periods. General bleeding should likewise, in some cases, be employed. . .

The woman should in the meantime avoid all the causes of excitement, which might act upon an organ affected with inflammation, or disposed to become so; such are

Table 8–2   Menstrual History

Age of onset of menses	Use of pads or tampons
Frequency of menses	Use of contraceptives
Duration of flow	Family history of menarche
Quantity of flow	Attitude toward menses
Presence of cramps	

	1	2	3	4	5	6	7	8	9	10	11	12	13	14	15	16	17	18	19	20	21	22	23	24	25	26	27	28	29	30	31
Jan																															
Feb																															
Mar																															
Apr																															
May																															
Jun																															
Jul																															
Aug																															
Sep																															
Oct																															
Nov																															
Dec																															

8–1   Sample menstrual calendar. Record days of bleeding with ● and days of spotting with X.

> frequent venereal indulgence, violent passions, and every thing that can prevent the movement of the blood towards the periphery of the body, crowd it upon the viscera, and create congestion in them, such as cold, corsets, belts, or other parts of dress worn too tight. (Coster J: *The Practice of Medicine*. Carey & Lea, Philadelphia, 1831, p. 217)

In a study to determine the prevalence of menstrual disorders in a college population, Bachmann and Kemmann (1982) conducted a questionnaire survey of 991 students, age 17–23 years, with a mean age of 19.2 years. Oligomenorrhea, defined as menstrual cycles with intervals of 35–90 days, was reported by 11.3%, and amenorrhea, defined as menses less than every 3 months, was reported by 2.6%. Amenorrhea was especially common in students with weight loss of greater than 20 pounds or participation in jogging. Students with oligomenorrhea and amenorrhea had significantly later menarche than students with regular cycles, and the menstrual irregularity usually developed immediately after menarche rather than during the college years. Menstrual disorders were not significantly correlated with measures of psychologic stress, perception of an excessive academic load, or the usage of medications or illicit drugs.

Normal pubertal progression in the female has been attributed to increased gonadotropin release as the hypothalamus becomes less sensitive to the negative feedback of adrenal and ovarian hormones (Soules, 1987). An initial rise in follicle-stimulating hormone (FSH) is followed by nightly episodic elevations of luteinizing hormone (LH), resulting in rising estrogen levels (Reindollar and McDonough, 1981). Recent evidence suggests that the primary control mechanisms for the initiation of puberty are related to neurotransmitters in the central nervous system that signal secretion of gonadotropin-releasing hormone (GnRH) independent of gonadal steroid secretion (Soules, 1987). Dopamine is known to inhibit GnRH and result in decreased FSH and LH release while norepinephrine stimulates GnRH. Excess secretion of β-endorphin, as seen in stress, affects gonadotropin release by decreasing the pulse generation, amplitude, or availability of GnRH. Gonadotropin-releasing hormone must be released in a pulsatile fashion for menstruation, ovulation, and ovarian steroid synthesis to occur (Kase, 1983). Maturation is complete when the hypothalamic pituitary axis is capable of a positive feedback response to estrogen, resulting in an ovulation-inducing LH surge. In luteal phase deficiency, progesterone production after ovulation is inadequate, and cycles tend to occur at regular intervals of less than 25 days. Estradiol (E_2) from the ovary is needed for complete breast development. Estrone (E_1) from the adrenals can lead to the onset of puberty and result in Tanner stage II–III early breast development and mature pubic hair development (Soules, 1987).

Primary amenorrhea, secondary amenorrhea, and oligomenorrhea will be addressed as they most commonly present during adolescence; however, considerable overlap may occur, depending upon the timing, manifestations, and severity of the disorder that is influencing the menstrual cycle. For example, vigorous athletic activity may result in primary amenorrhea if training begins prior to menarche, secondary amenorrhea if training begins after menarche, and oligomenorrhea or luteal phase deficiency as an intermediate stage.

Primary Amenorrhea

Delayed menarche is defined as the absence of uterine withdrawal bleeding by age 16 years, approximately 2 SDs beyond the mean age of menarche. Indications for evaluation of primary amenorrhea are included in Table 8–3.

Reindollar and McDonough (1981, 1983) reported on the etiology of delayed sexual development in 252 patients studied at the Medical College of Georgia. Hypergonadotropic hypogonadism associated with primary ovarian failure was noted in 43%. A chromosomal abnormality was present in 63% of this subgroup. Hypogonadotropic hypogonadism was found in 31%, including physiologic delay in 14% and congenital deficiency syndromes in 8%. The remaining 26% of patients with eugonadism included 18% with anatomic malformations and 7% with probable polycystic ovary syndrome. In a summary of common causes of primary amenorrhea, Soules (1987) noted gonadal dysgenesis in 33%, Mullerian anomalies in 20%, hypothalamic-pituitary causes in 15%, constitutional delay in 10%, and other causes in the remaining 22%.

Primary amenorrhea associated with elevated gonadotropin levels is most commonly associated with gonadal dysgenesis and its variants. Mosaicism is more common than classic Turner syndrome, and marked variation is noted in the presence of physical anomalies. Deficiency in the X chromosome often results in short stature and a phenotypic appearance characterized by high arched palate, webbing of the neck, shield chest, cubitus valgus, shortened fourth metacarpals, and hypoplastic nails. Gonadal dysgenesis is also associated with coarctation of the aorta and horseshoe kidneys; thus, cardiovascular and renal evaluations are indicated. Gonadotropin levels may be normal prior to puberty in this disorder, and adolescents with mosaicism may actually experience brief menstrual cycles prior to the onset of prolonged amenorrhea

Table 8–3   Indications for Evaluation of Primary Amenorrhea

Absence of menses at age 16 years

Absence of breast development at age 14 years

Absence of pubic hair at age 14 years

Absence of menses more than 3 years after onset of breast development

Height below the third percentile for age in adolescence

Weight below the third percentile for age in adolescence

Cyclic lower abdominal pain or midline suprapubic mass in the absence of menses

(Reindollar and McDonough, 1981). In contrast, patients wth ovarian failure and normal chromosomes may present as taller than average, since their epiphyses remain open due to the lack of sex steroids. Etiologies include radiation or chemotherapy, viral or infiltrative disease, or an autoimmune endocrine disorder which may be associated with myasthenia gravis, Addison's disease, or Hashimoto's thyroiditis (Mansfield and Emans, 1984).

In the Georgia series, physiologic delay was noted in 46% of patients with hypogonadotropic hypogonadism and was often associated with a family history of pubertal delay. Gonadotropin levels were found to be low or normal, and bone age was delayed. Hypogonadism with delayed menarche may also be seen with prepubertal onset of systemic diseases, such as hypothyroidism, congenital adrenal hyperplasia, Cushing's syndrome, regional enteritis, ulcerative colitis, anorexia nervosa, and other causes of weight loss (Reindollar and McDonough, 1981, 1983). Sadeghi-Nejad et al. (1981) reported three patients with primary amenorrhea associated with hyperprolactinemia. All had normal onset and progression of puberty, and none had a history of galactorrhea, but galactorrhea was elicited on physical examination in each case. Hughes and Garner (1987) also reported four patients presenting with primary amenorrhea at ages 17–22 years associated with hyperprolactinemia in the absence of galactorrhea, each with normal architecture of the sella. Most cases of hyperprolactinemia are associated with secondary rather than primary amenorrhea, and primary cases likely account for only 3% of the total incidence of this disorder.

Frisch et al. (1981) reported delayed menarche in college athletes related to age at onset of training. Runners and swimmers who began intense physical training before menarche attained menarche more than 2 years later than teammates who began training after menarche. Menarche occurred in an average of 15.1 years ± 0.5 years as a result of inadequate adiposity in relation to lean body mass and the effect of the stress of training on adrenal catecholamines that influence hypothalamic control of gonadotropin release. Hypogonadotropic hypogonadism is also associated with congenital deficiencies, the most common of which is Kallmann syndrome, the congenital absence of endogenous hypothalamic GnRH, often associated with anosmia (Reindollar and McDonough, 1981; Soules, 1987).

Eugonadism with normal phenotypic appearance of breast development with or without pubic hair is most commonly associated with anatomic anomalies (Reindollar and McDonough, 1981). Rokitansky-Kuster-Hauser syndrome consists of complete absence of the vagina, a rudimentary duplex uterus, shortened fallopian tubes, and normally functioning ovaries (Harkins et al., 1981). Renal evaluation is indicated since there is a 30% incidence of associated urinary tract anomalies. A karyotype should be done to rule out the presence of a Y chromosome. Ultrasonography and/or laparoscopy may be needed to confirm the diagnosis. Management includes creation of a neovagina via mechanical dilatation or surgery. Causes of genital tract obstruction include transverse vaginal septum and less commonly, imperforate hymen (Reindollar and McDonough, 1981; Mansfield and Emans, 1984; Soules, 1987). Patients present with normal breasts and pubic hair, cyclic abdominal pain, and a midline mass. Hematocolpos is defined as accumulation of menstrual blood in the vagina, hematometra is accumulation of menstrual blood in the uterus, and hematocolpometra is accumulation of menstrual blood in the vagina and uterus. Associated malformations are less common, but management is relatively urgent since outflow obstruction leads to retrograde flow and an increased likelihood of endometriosis and adhesions with potential impairment of fertility (Soules, 1987). Asherman syndrome consists of uterine synechiae following trauma or postabortal infection (Mansfield and Emans, 1984).

Testicular feminization syndrome due to androgen insensitivity presents with a normal external female phenotype, mature breast development, absent pubic hair, and no uterus, tubes, or upper vagina (Mansfield and Emans, 1984; Soules, 1987). Endocrine evaluation reveals normal male levels of testosterone, and inguinal or abdominal testes are present. Surgical removal of the gonads is indicated after breast development is complete, followed by replacement therapy (Harkins et al., 1981).

Reproductive prognosis in primary amenorrhea is related to etiology. In the Georgia study, 59% of the patients had absolute barriers to fertility, 16% required induction of ovulation, 11% had remediable medical or surgical disorders, and 14% experienced physiologic delay with a normal reproductive prognosis (Reindollar and McDonough, 1981).

A summary of common etiologies for primary amenorrhea is presented in Table 8–4 followed by a suggested approach to diagnostic evaluation in Table 8–5.

Table 8–4   Causes of Primary Amenorrhea

Hypothalamic
    Physiologic delay, often familial
    Prepubertal onset of rigorous athletic exercise
    Prepubertal onset of systemic disease
    Kallmann syndrome
    Laurence-Moon-Bardet-Biedl syndrome
    Prader-Labhart-Willi syndrome
    Drugs
Gonadal
    Turner syndrome and mosaicism
    Pure gonadal dysgenesis
    Testicular feminization syndrome
    Hermaphroditism
    Ovarian failure
Anatomic
    Rokitansky-Kuster-Hauser syndrome
    Transverse vaginal septum
    Imperforate hymen
    Asherman syndrome

Table 8–5   Sequential Evaluation of Primary Amenorrhea

1. Complete history, including family, chronic illness, stress, diet, exercise, drug, sexual, and contraceptive
2. Complete physical examination, including Tanner staging of secondary sexual development
3. Pelvic examination
4. Ultrasound examination, if necessary to define pelvic anatomy
5. FSH, LH, prolactin, testosterone
6. Bone age films
7. Karyotype

Secondary Amenorrhea

Secondary amenorrhea is defined as the prolonged absence of menstrual bleeding at any time after menarche. Proposed criteria for the duration of amenorrhea range from as few as 3 months to as many as 12 months (Soules, 1987). Common etiologies are summarized in Table 8–6. In practice, once pregnancy has been ruled out, a detailed diagnostic evaluation might be deferred until the amenorrhea has persisted for 4–6 months. This is particularly true of a young postmenarchal adolescent in whom menstrual periods are frequently irregular. Pregnancy should always be the first consideration in the differential diagnosis of secondary amenorrhea. Urine or serum assay for the beta subunit of human chorionic gonadotropin (HCG) should be obtained, even given a negative history of sexual activity. In the absence of pregnancy, an induction trial with Provera may be attempted prior to proceeding with the sequential evaluation suggested in Table 8–7.

Adolescents may report amenorrhea or menstrual irregularity in association with times of situational stress, such as family conflict, academic examinations, and fear of pregnancy due to unprotected sexual activity. This effect is attributed to the influence of adrenal catecholamines on central neurotransmitters and the hypothalamic control of gonadotropin release (Kase, 1983). Simple weight loss and eating disorders are also commonly associated with secondary amenorrhea. Cessation of menses is expected with a 15% weight loss (Frisch et al., 1981). In anorexia nervosa, secondary amenorrhea occurs in 71% of patients either before or coinciding with onset of weight loss (Fears et al., 1983). Many patients fail to resume menstruation after regaining sufficient weight, and persistence of a prepubertal or pubertal pattern of LH secretion has been noted in patients who have maintained their abnormal eating behavior. Frisch concludes that fatness is necessary but may not be sufficient for menses to resume and that the effects of both exercise and stress must be involved. Amenorrhea has also been associated with carotenemia, seen both in anorexia nervosa due to impaired metabolism of carotenes and vegetarian diets in which there may be excessive ingestion of carotene-rich vegetables unassociated with weight loss. Kemmann et al. (1983) demonstrated that modification of diet and reduction of serum carotenes resulted in improved menstrual function. Supportive evidence for this association includes menstrual disorders associated with excessive use of carotene pills as tanning agents. Mechanism of action is unknown but thought to be either a peripheral antiestrogenic effect or central hypothalamic effect of carotenes.

Amenorrhea associated with athletic participation has been extensively studied during the past decade. The prevalence of amenorrhea or oligomenorrhea in the general population is estimated at 5%, in exercising women at 20%, and in competitive athletes at 50%. The spectrum of menstrual disorders in female athletes includes luteal phase deficiency, anovulatory cycles, and hypoestrogenic amenorrhea. Even in female athletes with apparently normal regular menses, it is estimated that one-third are anovulatory, one-third have luteal deficiencies, and one-third have normal luteal function (Shangold, 1985a,b). Sanborn et al. (1982) found a higher prevalence of amenorrhea among runners (25.7%) than among swimmers (12.3%) and cyclists (12.1%). In runners, amenorrhea correlated with the number of miles of training per week, but there was no correlation with training among swimmers or cyclists. The prevalence of amenorrhea increased as the percentage of body fat of all athletes decreased. In a comparison study of amenorrheic runners, regular menstruating runners and nonrunning controls, Schwartz et al. (1981) found that the runners with amenorrhea had a higher incidence of prior menstrual irregularity, weighed less, had a lower

Table 8–6   Causes of Secondary Amenorrhea

Pregnancy

Stress

Exercise

Weight loss/eating disorders

Systemic disease

Regional enteritis	Cushing syndrome
Ulcerative colitis	Diabetes mellitus
Hyperthyroidism	Renal failure
Congenital adrenal hyperplasia	Cystic fibrosis

Drugs

Cytotoxins	Sex steroids
Phenothiazines	Isotretinoin
Opiates	Amphetamines

Polycystic ovary syndrome

Hyperprolactinemia/pituitary adenoma

Partial gonadal dysgenesis

Ovarian failure

Adrenal/ovarian tumor

Asherman syndrome

Carotenemia

Lactation

Post-oral contraceptive pill

Table 8–7   Sequential Evaluation of Secondary Amenorrhea

1. Complete history, including family, chronic illness, stress, diet, exercise, drug, sexual, and contraceptive

2. Complete physical examination, including Tanner staging of secondary sexual development

3. Pelvic examination

4. Pregnancy test—urine or serum HCG

5. Induction trial with Provera, 10 mg BID $\times$ 5 days

6. Complete blood count, sedimentation rate, urinalysis, serum carotenes

7. FSH, LH, prolactin

8. Thyroid function—thyroxine (T4), T3 uptake, thyroid-stimulating hormone (TSH)

9. Androgens—free testosterone, androstenedione, DHEA, DHEA-S, 17-OH-progesterone

10. Pelvic ultrasound examination

percentage of body fat, were faster runners, reported greater weight loss, and associated more stress with running than reported by the normally menstruating runners. In a study of young ballet dancers, Frisch et al. (1980) found primary amenorrhea in 22%, secondary amenorrhea in 15%, irregular cycles in 30%, and regular cycles in 33%. Dancers with amenorrhea and irregular cycles were significantly leaner than dancers with regular cycles. Bullen et al. (1985) demonstrated induction of menstrual disorders by strenuous exercise in untrained young women. They prospectively studied subjects with a mean age of 22 years and an initial body fat of 26% and followed them through a 2-month cycle of exercise training associated with either weight maintenance or weight loss. All had prior normal menstrual cycles. Only 4 of 28 subjects had a normal cycle during exercise training, and only 5 of 53 cycles were normal. Amenorrhea and loss of the LH surge was significantly more likely in the weight loss group, and a high incidence of anovulation and luteal disorders was noted. In contrast, Russell et al. (1984) studied adolescent swimmers, adult runners, and young adult controls and concluded that the amount of exercise and training appeared to be the critical factor in cessation of menstrual cycles, not the percentage of body fat or the amount of weight loss. In all three groups, the initial percentage of body fat was less than the 22% hypothesized by Frisch to be necessary for maintenance of ovulatory cycles. They hypothesized that with exercise, catecholamines and β-endorphin interact to suppress norepinephrine stimulation of GnRH in the hypothalamus and thus suppress LH release.

Gadpaille et al. (1987) recently studied young adult runners and found a clustering of eating and affective disorders in runners with amenorrhea. Among 19 runners with regular menses, no eating or major affective disorders were noted, but one runner had first-degree relatives with major affective disorders. In contrast, among 13 amenorrheic runners, 11 (85%) reported major affective disorders in themselves or first- and second-degree relatives, and 8 (62%) reported eating disorders in themselves. Twelve of the 13 amenorrheic runners were vegetarians compared with 3 of the 19 with regular menses. There was no significant difference in percentage body fat between the regularly menstruating and amenorrheic runners; however, those with amenorrhea were more likely to report low food intake, ritualized dietary habits, heightened energy and activity, and compulsive behavior associated with anorexia nervosa. Athletic amenorrhea may therefore represent a variant of anorexia nervosa or a major affective disorder, perhaps due to a neurotransmitter disorder of the central nervous system.

At present, the menstrual disorders associated with athletic training appear readily reversible by decreasing training or increasing dietary intake and body weight; however, concern has been expressed that the prolonged estrogen deficiency associated with amenorrhea may result in osteoporosis and atrophic vaginitis. Estrogen acts to decrease bone resorption of calcium, increase intestinal absorption of calcium, and increase renal tubular reabsorption of calcium (Shangold, 1985a). Exercise enhances bone density but is not sufficient to overcome the effects of estrogen deficit (Shangold, 1985b). Drinkwater et al. (1984) studied the bone mineral content of amenorrheic and normally menstruating athletes and documented a decrease in mineral density of the lumbar vertebrae in those with amenorrhea. Mean percentage body fat did not differ significantly, but the amenorrheic athletes ran nearly twice as many miles per week as those with normal menses. In a survey of ballet dancers, Warren et al. (1986) found delayed menarche and prolonged intervals of amenorrhea associated with a 24% incidence of scoliosis and 61% incidence of stress fractures reflecting prolonged hypoestrogenism. The incidence of both scoliosis and stress fractures rose with increasing age at menarche and with increasing prevalence of secondary amenorrhea. Finally, it should be emphasized that athletic amenorrhea is most commonly associated with strenuous athletic training in competitive runners, dancers, and gymnasts. Wilson et al. (1984) surveyed female high school students participating in a normal athletic program. Mean age was 15 years, and the students reported exercising a mean of 1.5 hours ± 0.8 hours per day. Only dancing, among 12 sports studied, was more likely to be associated with irregular menses.

Hyperprolactinemia due to pituitary microadenoma should be considered in the evaluation of secondary amenorrhea even in the absence of a history or physical evidence of galactorrhea. Koppelman et al. (1984) reported on the natural history of hyperprolactinemia in untreated patients followed for a mean of 11.3 years. At presentation 16 of 25 had both galactorrhea and a menstrual disorder, six had amenorrhea alone, and three had galactorrhea alone. In seven patients menses resumed spontaneously, and galactorrhea resolved completely in 6 of 19. Galactorrhea was spontaneous in 9 and elicited with breast massage in 10. The onset of hyperprolactinemia was spontaneous in 11, followed oral contraceptive use in 10, and followed pregnancy in 4. The clinical course was benign. No patient worsened clinically, and the mean prolactin level had actually fallen at the time of reevaluation. Conservative management is recommended with no surgical intervention unless growth of the adenoma beyond the sella is noted on serial computerized axial tomography scanning.

"Post pill" amenorrhea associated with discontinuing oral contraception is estimated to occur in 1/1,000 users. The mechanism is thought to be interference with cycle initiation, and there is no increased risk of primary ovarian failure, hyperprolactinemia, or pituitary tumor associated with oral contraceptive use (Hull et al., 1981). In a follow-up study of 96 patients with post pill amenorrhea, Soltan and Hancock (1982) reported an overall pregnancy rate of 82% of those not excluded for other reasons. One-third conceived after spontaneous ovulation and two-thirds after induced ovulation. The pregnancy rate was nearly identical in patients with previous regular or irregular cycles prior to initiation of oral contraception. Alternative causes for amenorrhea should be sought, but if the evaluation is negative, oral contraception can be safely resumed even in patients with irregular menses or amenorrhea. Post pill amenorrhea is more likely to occur in thin women below ideal body weight; thus, an attempt at weight gain might be the first step in management prior to conducting an extensive evaluation (Wentz, 1980).

Having noted initially that secondary amenorrhea is commonly associated with pregnancy, it should also be mentioned that postpartum amenorrhea persists for 1½–4 months in the absence of lactation and that unrestricted breast-feeding results in an average of 11 months of postpartum amenorrhea (Ojofeitimi, 1982). The longer the mother breast-feeds her baby, the longer menstruation is delayed, since high levels of maternal prolactin inhibit both estrogen and progesterone.

Polycystic ovary syndrome associated with obesity, virilization, and hyperandrogenism most often presents with oligomenorrhea or secondary amenorrhea followed by a pattern of dysfunctional uterine bleeding. Finally, secondary amenorrhea is associated with chronic illnesses such as inflammatory bowel disease, celiac disease, cystic fibrosis, renal failure, hyperthyroidism, and diabetes mellitus, as well as drug therapy with cytotoxic agents, phenothiazines, or opiates (Wentz, 1980). Amenorrhea has also been reported during isotretinoin therapy for nodulocystic acne (Cox, 1988).

Oligomenorrhea

Oligomenorrhea refers to markedly diminished menstrual flow, usually manifested as scanty irregular bleeding. More precise definitions include more than two cycles of greater than 37 days duration during the previous 6–12 months (Siegberg et al., 1986) and one to six cycles per year in an adolescent at least 2 years postmenarche (Emans et al., 1980).

Siegberg et al. (1986) studied 45 oligomenorrheic adolescents and found increased LH, androstenedione, dehydroepiandrosterone sulfate (DHEA-S), free testosterone, and lower sex hormone-binding globulin (SHBG) compared with 28 adolescents with regular menstrual cycles. The oligomenorrheic adolescents were not obese, had mild or absent acne or hirsutism, and most had never had regular menses, yet 66% of the oligomenorrheic cycles were ovulatory. Since ovulation occurred in the majority, oligomenorrhea was not attributed to an inadequate LH response to estrogen but rather to elevated levels of androgens and LH as seen in adult polycystic ovary disease. A comparison of LH:FSH ratios revealed a mean of 1.3 in normally menstruating females, 2.3 in adolescents with oligomenorrhea, and 3.7 in adults with polycystic ovary disease. Siegberg and colleagues theorized that in a subgroup of normal adolescents, oligomenorrhea may represent a transient condition that resolves with maturation, and in some adolescents represents an early form of polycystic ovary disease which will progress to persistent anovulation and clinical signs of hyperandrogenism. They advocate oral contraceptive use in oligomenorrhea, which accomplishes the dual purpose of lowering androgen levels and providing effective contraception since ovulation is likely.

In a study of 42 oligomenorrheic adolescents with a mean age of 17.3 years, Emans et al. (1980) found 19 with androgen excess and 23 with hypothalamic suppression and normal androgen levels. Among the 19 (45%) with androgen excess, 12 had polycystic ovary syndrome, 5 had adrenal and ovarian androgen overproduction, and 2 had an adrenal enzyme block. The differential diagnosis of hyperandrogenism includes an arrhenoblastoma, a virilizing ovarian tumor which produces very high testosterone, androstenedione, and dehydroepiandrosterone (DHEA) levels, which fail to suppress with dexamethasone. The LH to FSH ratio is usually normal in contrast to polycystic ovary syndrome (Mansfield and Emans, 1984). Other causes of hyperandrogenism include Cushing's disease and congenital adrenal hyperplasia. As many as 25% of adolescents with congenital adrenal hyperplasia have oligomenorrhea or amenorrhea. Primary objectives in treatment include achievement of normal adult height, suppression of virilization, and maintenance of normal menses and fertility (Granoff, 1981). Adolescents may require a switch from hydrocortisone to prednisone or dexamethasone, which are longer acting and provide better adrenal suppression with resultant initiation or regulation of the menstrual cycle (Granoff, 1981; Birnbaum and Rose, 1984). Diagnosis of late-onset congenital adrenal hyperplasia, usually due to 21-hydroxylase deficiency, requires an ACTH stimulation test with measurement of serum 17-hydroxyprogesterone (Birnbaum and Rose, 1984; Mansfield and Emans, 1984).

Dysfunctional Uterine Bleeding

> If the haemorrhage threatens to become abundant, and the patient is strong and plethoric, general blood-letting: if on the contrary, the woman be of a debilitated constitution, and if nevertheless there are signs of strong uterine irritation, the application of leeches to the hypogastric region. . . If the abundance of the haemorrhage is such as to require it to be arrested with great promptitude, dry cups to the abdomen, and even upon the breasts; cold and astringent injections; plugging with lint, wet with an astringent liquor, or the introduction, as far as the neck of the womb, of a lemon deprived of its rind. (Coster J: *The Practice of Medicine.* Carey & Lea, Philadelphia, 1831, pp. 202–203)

Dysfunctional uterine bleeding is defined as abnormal uterine bleeding without apparent gross local anatomic cause (Altchek, 1977; Gidwani, 1984). This condition incorporates menorrhagia or excessive uterine bleeding occurring at regular intervals, menometrorrhagia or excessive uterine bleeding occurring at irregular intervals, and metrorrhagia or uterine bleeding in normal amounts occurring at irregular intervals. Alternate definitions include uterine bleeding in cycles of less than 20 days or more than 40 days, lasting greater than 8 days, with blood loss greater than 80 ml, or associated with anemia (Anderson et al., 1986).

The diagnosis of dysfunctional bleeding is complicated by the subjective perceptions of menstrual blood loss reported by patients. Frequency of changing pads or tampons has been traditionally used as an indicator of menstrual flow; however, no significant correlation has been demonstrated between the number of pads or tampons used and actual measured blood loss (Mishell, 1984). Fraser et al. (1984) suggested that frequency of changing pads or tampons is influenced by beliefs about hygiene, age, race, education, climate, physical activity, urinary frequency or diarrhea, availability of toilet facilities, and concern about toxic shock syndrome and tampon use. In a study of therapy for menorrhagia, only 43% of patients with a convincing history of excessive flow demonstrated objective menorrhagia with measured menstrual blood loss of greater than 80 ml (Fraser et al., 1981). The mean amount of menstrual blood loss is estimated at 35 ml per cycle and 20 ml per cycle in patients on oral contraceptives. In 95% of women, monthly blood loss is less than 60 ml. Cyclic menstrual loss of greater than 80 ml is consistently associated with a high risk of anemia (Mishell, 1984). In a study comparing perceived daily blood loss with objective volume measurements, women who described blood loss as spotting averaged 2.5 ml with a range of 0.1–15.5 ml. Light flow averaged 5.7 ml with a range of 0.1–63.1 ml, moderate flow averaged 16.1 ml with a range of 0.5–108.6 ml, and very heavy flow averaged 22.0 ml with a range of 1.4–215.8 ml. Subjects 26 years of age or younger were significantly more likely than women 37 years of age or older to regard moderate loss as very heavy loss (Fraser et al., 1984).

Etiology

In contrast to older women in whom dysfunctional bleeding may be the first sign of gynecologic malignancy, approximately 95% of such bleeding in adolescents may be attributed to anovulatory cycles (Gidwani, 1984). Normal menses in ovulatory cycles occur regularly at 26- to 38-day intervals, with flow lasting 4–7 days. After ovulation, progesterone from the corpus luteum controls maturation from a proliferative to secretory endometrium. With regression of the corpus luteum late in the cycle, progesterone levels fall dramatically, and shrinkage of endometrial spiral arterioles, ischemia, necrosis, and hemorrhage ensue, resulting in uniform endometrial sloughing and an abrupt onset and end of menses (Altchek, 1977). Both menorrhagia and dysmenorrhea are thought to be related to the vascular effects of prostaglandin synthesized in the endometrium. In a study of prostaglandin content of menstrual fluid, Rees et al. (1984) documented higher levels of prostaglandin F_2 on day one of menses in patients with menorrhagia defined as blood loss of at least 80 ml.

As many as 80% of menstrual cycles are thought to be anovulatory in the first year after menarche (Gidwani, 1984); yet a regular pattern of bleeding often occurs (Altchek, 1977; Claessens and Cowell, 1981b). Ovulatory cycles occur in 32% of adolescents within 18 months after menarche, 46% between 19 and 30 months after menarche, and 61% at 31 months after menarche (Talbert et al., 1985). With pubertal maturation of the hypothalamic pituitary gonadal axis, negative feedback of estrogen on LH decreases and becomes positive feedback, leading to the midcycle ovulatory LH surge. Failure of the LH surge leads to chronic anovulation and tonic production of estrogen (Anderson et al., 1986). This continuous production of estrogen with endometrial stimulation unopposed by progesterone leads to endometrial proliferation and shedding with irregular, unexpected, and painless bleeding. The most characteristic pattern is 2–4 months of amenorrhea followed by heavy bleeding for 3–4 weeks (Altchek, 1977).

Although fewer than 5% of cases of dysfunctional bleeding in adolescents are due to an organic cause other than anovulation, the differential diagnosis is extensive (Gidwani, 1984). A high index of suspicion must be maintained that the bleeding represents a complication of pregnancy such as threatened, spontaneous, or incomplete abortion, or ectopic pregnancy (Altchek, 1977; Gidwani, 1984). In general, anovulatory bleeding tends to be painless, whereas a complication of pregnancy is more likely to produce painful bleeding; however, this symptom is not sufficiently reliable to negate the necessity of performing a pregnancy test.

One of the first steps in evaluating the patient is to determine that the bleeding is in fact uterine and not originating in the urinary tract, vagina, or bowel. Vaginal lacerations may be sustained during sexual assault, painful intercourse, or masturbation with foreign objects. Retained foreign bodies such as tampons, diaphragms, and contraceptive sponges may lead to vaginal bleeding often associated with a foul vaginal discharge (Anderson et al., 1986). Cervical friability or a cervical polyp may cause spotting or frank bleeding (Altchek, 1977). Clear cell adenocarcinoma of the vagina presents in the majority of cases with abnormal bleeding at an average age of 17.5 years (Claessens and Cowell, 1981b). The incidence of this malignancy is estimated at 0.14–1.4 cases/1,000 women exposed to diethylstilbesterol (DES) in utero (Gidwani, 1984). Bleeding may also occur with submucosal myomas, sarcoma botyroides, hemangiomas, and hormone-producing ovarian tumors, all of which are rare during adolescence (Altchek, 1977; Gidwani, 1984). Vaginitis, cervicitis, salpingitis, and endometriosis may occasionally present with abnormal bleeding (Anderson et al., 1986). A contraceptive history is essential, since both the oral contraceptive pill and intrauterine devices are commonly associated with irregular bleeding.

In a study of 59 adolescents requiring hospitalization with acute menorrhagia, Claessens and Cowell (1981a) found a 19% incidence of an underlying coagulation disorder, including four patients with idiopathic thrombocytopenic purpura, three with von Willebrand's disease, two with a qualitative platelet defect, and two with thrombocytopenia. A bleeding disorder was found in 45% of adolescents with menorrhagia presenting at menarche, 35% of those requiring transfusion while hospitalized, and 28% of those with severe menorrhagia defined by a hemoglobin of less than 10 g/100 ml. A family history of bleeding disorders should be obtained, and the patient should be questioned about easy bruising, epistaxis, or gingival bleeding. Laboratory evaluation for the possibility of a bleeding disorder should be obtained prior to transfusion or hormonal therapy and must include prothrombin time, partial test thromboplastin, platelet count, and bleeding time.

Hypothyroidism commonly leads to menorrhagia, whereas hyperthyroidism is often associated with amenorrhea. The hypothyroid patient with heavy bleeding may also present with fatigue, lethargy, constipation, dry skin, hair loss, and sluggish deep tendon reflexes on examination (Gidwani, 1984). Abnormal bleeding can be seen in Addison's disease and in diabetes mellitus (Altchek, 1977). Polycystic ovary syndrome most often presents with amenorrhea; however, one-third of patients present with menorrhagia usually following a prolonged period of amenorrhea due to unopposed estrogen effect (Gidwani, 1984). Hyperprolactinemia also characteristically presents with amenorrhea rather than DUB, but this diagnosis should always be considered in the presence of galactorrhea, which may be noted in hypothyroidism and pregnancy as well. Chronic illness, particularly renal and hepatic disease, may result in irregular bleeding (Altchek, 1977; Gidwani, 1984). Among the drugs associated with dysfunctional menses are narcotics, anticoagulants, anticholinergics, gonadal and adrenal steroids, monoamine oxidase inhibitors, and tranquilizers, which may affect the menstrual cycle through central neurotransmitters (Mishell, 1984; Anderson et al., 1986).

Management

Management of dysfunctional bleeding in the adolescent depends upon the degree of blood loss, frequency of bleeding, presence of anemia, and discomfort to the patient. A detailed menstrual history should be obtained along with a history of maternal DES exposure and a confidential sexual and contraceptive history. A general physical examination should be performed with particular attention to signs of chronic illness, petechiae or ecchymoses, hirsutism, thyroid enlargement, or galactorrhea. A complete pelvic exam should be performed, followed by the laboratory studies suggested in Table 8–8. Additional diagnostic studies, such as pelvic ultrasound, might be considered based upon presentation.

In contrast to adult women, dysfunctional bleeding in the adolescent, even if severe, can most often be managed medically without resorting to surgical dilatation and curettage (Altchek, 1977; Claessens and Cowell, 1981b; Gidwani, 1984). Intermittent heavy or prolonged bleeding unassociated with anemia can often be managed expectantly in the adolescent with health education, use of a menstrual calendar, and ferrous sulfate supplementation. Recent studies in adult women have suggested a role for prostaglandin synthetase inhibitors in reducing menstrual blood loss in patients with menorrhagia (Fraser et al., 1981; Fraser et al., 1983; Ylikorkala and Pekonen, 1986). Hemostasis during menses is the result of a delicate balance between platelet aggregation, fibrin formation, vasoconstriction, and tissue regeneration in the uterus versus prostaglandin-induced platelet inhibition, vasodilatation, and fibrinolysis (Gidwani, 1984). Since increased prostacyclin levels in the endometrium are known to interfere with platelet aggregation, an inhibitor should theoretically reduce blood loss (Mishell,

Table 8–8   Laboratory Evaluation of Dysfunctional Uterine Bleeding

Complete blood count

Coagulation profile
   Prothrombin time
   Partial test thromboplastin
   Platelet count
   Bleeding time

Thyroid studies
   Thyroxine (T4)
   T3 uptake
   Thyroid-stimulating hormone (TSH)

Pregnancy test—urine or serum HCG

Urinalysis

1984). Fraser et al. (1981) documented a reduction of 28% in mean blood loss with the use of mefenamic acid in a dosage of 500 mg three times a day from the onset to the end of menstruation. In a follow-up study of patients treated for over 1 year, the reduction in menstrual blood loss was maintained at 6–9 months and 12–15 months along with an increase in serum ferritin (Fraser et al., 1983). Gastrointestinal side effects were minimized by taking the drug with food. In a trial using naproxen in a dose of 500–1,000 mg a day for 5 days, menstrual blood loss was reduced by 36%, no side effects were reported, and enhanced iron stores resulted in increased hemoglobin (Ylikorkala and Pekonen, 1986). No studies have been reported to date on the use of prostaglandin synthetase inhibitors for menorrhagia in adolescents, and Food and Drug Administration (FDA) approval for this indication is pending. Aspirin is not effective for this indication and may actually increase uterine bleeding (Mishell, 1984).

For moderate nonemergent uterine bleeding, hormonal hemostasis may be achieved with a variety of outpatient regimens. Although the basic defect in anovulatory cycles is an absence of progesterone, progestins alone may not be sufficient, and some supplemental estrogen is usually needed to control bleeding. A progestin-dominant oral contraceptive pill such as Ovral (0.5 mg norgestrel with 0.05 mg ethinyl estradiol) or Norlestrin 2.5 (2.5 mg norethindrone acetate with 0.05 mg ethinyl estradiol) may be used (Altchek, 1977; Gidwani, 1984). Regimens include simply administering one tablet twice daily for 10 days, or rapid tapering, starting with one tablet every 4–6 hours for the 1st day, then one tablet three times a day for 2 days, and one tablet twice a day for 2 days, followed by one tablet daily for 20 days (Gidwani, 1984). In either regimen withdrawal bleeding is allowed to occur, and the patient is then cycled for 3 months with the same oral contraceptive pill. If contraception is not needed, this regimen can be discontinued after 3 months followed by a period of observation of 6–10 weeks. If normal cyclic menses do not resume, Provera (medroxyprogesterone acetate) may be administered on the first 5 days of every other month in a dose of 10 mg twice daily to induce withdrawal bleeding and prevent unopposed estrogen effect with the associated risk of endometrial hyperplasia and carcinoma (Alchek, 1977).

The adolescent with severe, life-threatening uterine bleeding should be hospitalized, rapidly evaluated for the possibility of a complication of pregnancy, and transfused as needed after obtaining appropriate laboratory studies. Premarin (conjugated estrogens) in a dose of 25 mg IV has been used to induce rapid cessation of uterine bleeding (Altchek, 1977). The dose may be repeated if needed in 3–6 hours, and a cyclic oral regimen including progestin should be initiated simultaneously. In a critique of this approach, Jones (1983) questioned the efficiency and efficacy of IV Premarin and advocated use of an antiprostaglandin as an alternative. Adolescents with bleeding of this severity should be followed concurrently with a gynecologist, since surgical dilatation and curettage may occasionally be needed. In both moderate and severe menorrhagia, ferrous sulfate supplementation should be initiated, and the use of a prostaglandin synthetase inhibitor such as mefenamic acid may be considered during subsequent menses. Management is summarized in Table 8–9. In patients with unstable hematologic diseases complicated by frequent menorrhagia, the use of Depo-Provera (depot medroxyprogesterone acetate), 150 mg by intramuscular injection every 3 months, may be considered as a means of inducing prolonged but reversible amenorrhea.

In a follow-up study of patients with dysfunctional bleeding, problems continued to be noted in 60% at 2 years, 50% at 4 years, and 30%–40% at 10 years

Table 8–9   Management of Dysfunctional Uterine Bleeding

Pelvic examination—confirm uterine source

Pregnancy testing

Hormonal hemostasis with multiple doses of a progestin-dominant oral contraceptive pill

Continue oral contraceptive pills for three or more menstrual cycles

Consider daily mefenamic acid or naproxen use during subsequent menses

Ferrous sulfate supplementation—monitor hemogram

Maintain menstrual calendar

following the initial episode. The prognosis was worse when menorrhagia occurred from the time of menarche (Southam and Richart, 1966).

Dysmenorrhea

> The dysmenorrhea which is so extremely common in young girls may be due to a variety of causes. Insufficient development of the uterus and a slight stenosis at the internal os are the causes in some cases; while chlorosis and insufficient bodily development, associated with mental overexertion, are responsible for others. (Winter G: *Textbook of Gynecological Diagnosis*. J.B. Lippincott, Philadelphia, 1909, p. 630)

Despite the introduction of safe, effective, short-term therapy for dysmenorrhea during the past decade, many young women continue to suffer from debilitating menstrual cramps. Among adolescent females, dysmenorrhea is the leading cause of short-term absence from school and work and results in 140 million lost hours each year. Klein and Litt (1981) analyzed data obtained from 1966 to 1970 in the National Health Examination Survey and found a 60% incidence of dysmenorrhea in a national probability sample of 12- to 17-year-old females. Dysmenorrhea was reported as mild by 49%, moderate by 37%, and severe by 14%. Prevalence was strongly correlated with biologic variables, including chronologic age, with dysmenorrhea reported by 39% of 12-year-olds and 72% of 17-year-olds; sexual maturity rating, with 38% at Tanner stage III and 66% at Tanner stage V; and gynecologic age, with 31% at a gynecologic age of 1 year and 78% at a gynecologic age of 5 years. They found no correlation with preparation for menarche or with race and only a mild correlation with increased socioeconomic status. The prevalence of dysmenorrhea was 56% in low socioeconomic groups and 63% in high socioeconomic groups. Black adolescents were nearly twice as likely to miss school due to dysmenorrhea, although the severity of their symptoms was no greater than in white adolescents. Overall, 14% of adolescent females reported missing school due to cramps, including 50% of those with severe dysmenorrhea and 17% of those with mild dysmenorrhea. Only 14.5% of adolescents with dysmenorrhea ever sought help from a physician, and among their parents, 30% were unaware of their daughter's symptoms. It should be noted that these data were obtained prior to the widespread use of prostaglandin synthetase inhibitors in the management of dysmenorrhea.

In a more recent study, Andersch and Milsom (1982) reported a 72% prevalence of dysmenorrhea in a random sample of 19-year-old women residing in Gothenburg, Sweden. Menstrual cramps were absent in 28%, mild in 34%, moderate in 23%, and severe in 15%. The severity of dysmenorrhea correlated with early menarche, increased duration and degree of menstrual flow, and history of dysmenorrhea in mother and sister. The prevalence and severity of dysmenorrhea was significantly lower in parous women but not in women with a history of therapeutic or spontaneous abortion. Absence from work or school for dysmenorrhea was reported by 51%, and 8% reported absence with every menstrual period. As in the previous study, the onset of dysmenorrhea was closely correlated with gynecologic age. Onset during the 1st year after menarche was reported by approximately 40%, during the 2nd year by 20%, during the 3rd year by 20%, and during the 4th through the 6th years by the remaining 20% of women surveyed.

In another Swedish study, Svanberg and Ulmsten (1981) administered a questionnaire to 502 adolescent females between the ages of 10 and 19 years and found a 43% incidence of dysmenorrhea overall. The percentage of adolescents reporting absence from school rose from 8.3% at 13 years to 18.2% at 17 years, and 8.3% of 17-year-olds reported staying in bed at least 1 day with severe dysmenorrhea. Approximately 25%–30% of adolescents reported use of analgesics or antispasmodic drugs for dysmenorrhea. The interval from menarche to the onset of dysmenorrhea was reported within the 1st year in 72%, within the 2nd year in 19%, within the 3rd year in 7%, and within the 4th year in the remaining 2% of all patients with dysmenorrhea. This was a recall study of adolescents wth a mean age of 15 years, thus accounting for lower percentages in comparison with the previous study of older adolescents.

Finally, in a survey of New England high school students, dysmenorrhea was reported by 60% and described as mild in 32%, moderate in 15%, and severe in 6% (Wilson et al., 1984).

Etiology

Lawlor and Davis (1981) tested the hypothesis that personality factors are related to the pain of dysmenorrhea. They studied 127 women aged 12–21 years of whom 75% reported dysmenorrhea. The personality profiles of women with dysmenorrhea did not differ significantly from those without pain. Nearly 40% of subjects with dysmenorrhea changed their activities due to pain, and these changes correlated with increased pain severity. There was no evidence that menstrual pain was used as a contrived excuse to miss school or work. Pain was unrelated to attitudinal variables, acceptance of the sex role, and social adjustment. The study concluded that primary dysmenorrhea is physiologically based, that terming the pain psychogenic is harmful to self-esteem, and that appropriate management includes education, reassurance, and specific medical therapy.

Nelson et al. (1984) applied the Menstrual Symptom Questionnaire in order to test the validity of the distinction between spasmodic and congestive dysmenorrhea. Spasmodic dysmenorrhea, equivalent to primary dysmenorrhea, is defined as acute spasmodic pain primarily in the lower abdomen, lower back, and thighs which occurs during the first day or two of menstrual flow and is often accompanied by diarrhea, nausea, and vomiting. Congestive dysmenorrhea is related to the premenstrual syndrome, occurs for several days prior to the onset of menstrual flow, and is characterized by dull aching pain and feelings of heaviness, muscle and joint stiffness, edema, constipation, depression, irritability, and lethargy. The study concluded that this distinction was weak and not very useful. No biochemical or hormonal factors currently distinguish these entities, and there are no differentially effective treatments. In practical terms, congestive dysmenorrhea may simply be a component of the premenstrual syndrome.

Primary dysmenorrhea refers to painful menstruation in the absence of significant pelvic pathology (Table 8–10). Symptoms often begin with the onset of ovulatory cycles approximately 6–12 months after menarche (Rosenwaks and Seegar-Jones, 1980). Sharp, spasmodic suprapubic abdominal pain with radiation to the lower back and anterior thighs may begin a few hours prior to onset of menses and persist for 1–3 days (Dawood, 1985). Pain may be accompanied by gastrointestinal and vascular symptoms including nausea, vomiting, diarrhea, headache, irritability, fatigue, and syncope (Gantt and McDonough, 1981). Nulliparous patients are most likely to be affected by primary dysmenorrhea which commonly improves after the first pregnancy. Structural changes in the uterus that result in a net increase in vascular supply during pregnancy persist postpartum and may be related to relief of pain (Dingfelder, 1981). Myometrial adrenergic nerves also disappear with pregnancy and only partially regenerate after delivery. Thus, altered neuromuscular activity may contribute to reduced menstrual pain (Andersch and Milsom, 1982).

Prostaglandins have been studied extensively during the past three decades and are clearly implicated in the etiology of dysmenorrhea. Prostaglandin synthesis in the uterus is thought to be regulated by progesterone. Anovulatory cycles are painless, since the progesterone level does not rise without a corpus luteum. Higher prostaglandin levels have been documented in the menstrual fluid in ovulatory as compared with anovulatory cycles (Ylikorkala and Dawood, 1978). Progesterone drops rapidly late in an ovulatory cycle if pregnancy has not occurred. This is followed by a dramatic increase in prostaglandin $F_{2\alpha}$ which leads to powerful labor-like uterine contractions, arteriolar constriction, ischemia, and sloughing of the endometrium (Rosenwaks and Seegar-Jones, 1980). In a study of the prostaglandin content of menstrual fluid, both prostaglandin $F_{2\alpha}$ and prostaglandin E_2 were increased with dysmenorrhea, irrespective of the volume of blood loss, and both prostaglandin levels were higher on day 1 than on day 2 of menses. The presence of pain was associated with an elevated ratio of prostaglandin $F_{2\alpha}$ over E_2 (Rees et al., 1984). Clinical symptoms correlate with the amount of prostaglandin released per unit time (Dawood, 1986).

Prostaglandins, which are thought to mediate myometrial activity, are synthesized locally in the endometrium under the control of the prostaglandin synthetase enzyme system in the microsomes. Prostaglandins are synthesized immediately prior to release and are not stored in tissues. Due to rapid metabolism, prostaglandin blood levels correlate poorly with symptoms; however, prostaglandin production in the secretory endometrium has been demonstrated to be up to seven times greater in women with dysmenorrhea as compared with controls (Ylikorakala and Dawood, 1978). This results in elevated myometrial resting tone, elevated active myometrial pressure, increased frequency of uterine contractions, and dysrhythmic contractions (Dawood,

Table 8–10   Characteristics of Primary Dysmenorrhea

Sharp, spasmodic, suprapubic pain

Radiation to lower back and anterior thighs

GI symptoms: nausea, vomiting, diarrhea

Vascular symptoms: headache, fatigue, irritability, syncope

Onset 6–12 months after menarche

More common in nulliparous females

Absence of pelvic pathology

1985, 1986). Prostaglandins may also sensitize nerve endings and stimulate smooth muscle contraction in the stomach, intestines, and blood vessels, thus accounting for the associated symptoms of nausea, vomiting, diarrhea, irritability, and headache. This hypothesis does not account for the small number of adolescents with primary dysmenorrhea who report onset of cramping with menarche or in the absence of ovulatory cycles (Alvin and Litt, 1982).

Management

Diagnosis of primary dysmenorrhea is confirmed by a typical history and normal pelvic or bimanual rectoabdominal examination. The adolescent should be reassured of the absence of pelvic pathology and the likelihood of normal fertility. Failure to respond to a therapeutic trial with either a combined oral contraceptive pill or a prostaglandin synthetase inhibitor should lead to a renewed search for pelvic pathology, including possible laparoscopy (Heinrichs and Adamson, 1980; Gantt and McDonough, 1981).

A low dose combined oral contraceptive pill is effective in approximately 95% of cases of primary dysmenorrhea by suppressing ovulation and growth of the endometrium where prostaglandin production takes place. Since the combined pill requires daily medication and is associated with mild side effects in the first few cycles of use, it should be prescribed only for young women who have chosen the pill as a method of contraception (Cholst and Carlon, 1987). Use of supplemental drug therapy is indicated only if the suppression of ovulation does not abolish symptoms.

Nonsteroidal antiinflammatory drugs (NSAIDs), which act as inhibitors of prostaglandin synthesis, have proven highly effective in the management of primary dysmenorrhea. Specific therapy is provided wth direct action upon the etiologic agent. Use is limited to symptomatic periods. Onset of symptomatic relief is prompt, and therapy is highly successful without undue side effects (Dingfelder, 1981). Prostaglandin synthetase inhibitors have been shown to diminish endometrial prostaglandin synthesis and thereby reduce uterine resting pressure as well as the force and frequency of contractions as measured by uterine manometry (Rosenwaks and Seegar-Jones, 1980). Dosage and frequency of administration of the most commonly employed medications are outlined in Table 8–11. Each of these drugs is likely to result in a dramatic response in approximately 70%–80% of patients treated.

Ibuprofen (Dawood, 1984) is available over-the-counter in a 200-mg dosage and may be a reasonable starting point for adolescents with mild symptoms. NSAIDs may be administered with impending menses or at the onset of bleeding and should be continued for 1–3 days as needed. Early treatment in order to prevent build up of prostaglandins is unnecessary, since metabolism is very rapid and use prior to menses might result in exposure to these agents early in pregnancy. The same class of drug has been employed in achieving pharmacologic closure of the patent ductus arteriosus in the preterm infant; however, effects on the fetus are unknown. NSAIDs are contraindi-

Table 8–11   Nonsteroidal Antiinflammatory Drugs for Dysmenorrhea

Drug	Dosage and frequency
Ibuprofen (Motrin)	400 mg QID
Mefenamic acid (Ponstel)	500 mg initially, then 250 mg TID-QID
Naproxen (Naprosyn)	250 mg BID
Naproxen sodium (Anaprox)	550 mg initially, then 275 mg TID-QID

cated in women with aspirin hypersensitivity, peptic ulcer disease, bleeding diathesis, and hepatic or renal disease. Side effects are infrequent but may include gastrointestinal symptoms, headache, dizziness, tinnitus, or rash. A potential beneficial side effect may be reduction in menstrual blood flow in some women (Ylikorkala and Dawood, 1978).

In a review of 51 outcome trials, Owen (1984) concluded that prostaglandin synthetase inhibitors are safe and effective in the management of primary dysmenorrhea and that pretreatment is unnecessary. Significant pain relief was noted in 72% of the patients studied, minimal or no relief in 18%, and a placebo response in 15%. Minimal side effects were reported except with indomethacin, which has been demonstrated to be less effective than ibuprofen in a comparative study. Mefenamic acid has the theoretical advantage of an additional direct effect but has proven no more effective than ibuprofen in a comparative trial.

Milsom and Andersch (1985) compared ibuprofen, 400 mg TID, with naproxen, 250 mg bid, in a study of women with severe dysmenorrhea. A significant reduction in the severity of pain was noted with both drugs; however, pain relief with ibuprofen was significantly greater than with naproxen. Moderate to complete relief of pain was reported in 50%–80% of patients, and there was no difference in the low incidence of side effects reported. Hanson (1982) compared ibuprofen, 400 mg every 4–8 hours with naproxen sodium, 500 mg initially followed by 275 mg every 4–8 hours, in women with severe dysmenorrhea. No statistically significant difference was noted in the analgesic effect of ibuprofen and naproxen. No significant side effects were reported with either drug. In one of the few studies limited to adolescents, DuRant et al. (1985) studied five treatment regimens with naproxen sodium and concluded that 550 mg initially followed by 275 mg every 6 hours was an optimal dose. In adolescents who did not respond to treatment, exploration of social, psychologic, and environmental stress was recommended to assess impact on compliance and response to therapy. In another study of adolescents, aspirin, 600 mg QID was prescribed 3 days prior to menses and resulted in significantly greater pain relief and less school absence when compared with placebo; however, only 48% of patients improved with aspirin, and six patients reported increased menstrual flow due to a presumed effect on platelets (Klein and Litt, 1981). Aspirin is a weak inhibitor of prostaglandin synthesis and is more likely to be associated with gastrointestinal distress and increased bleeding (Alvin and Litt, 1982). Although side effects with NSAIDs are uncommon, Halbert (1983) reported 12 adult women with reversible delay of menses on antiprostaglandin therapy for dysmenorrhea. Nine had been taking ibuprofen, three mefenamic acid, and six started treatment up to 7 days before expected onset of menses.

Pelvic Pain

Secondary dysmenorrhea refers to that associated with pelvic pathology (Table 8–12). Onset of dysmenorrhea at the time of menarche suggests anatomic obstruction to uterine or vaginal outflow. Chronicity of the pain throughout the menstrual cycle or lateralization of the pain strongly suggests a secondary cause. Diagnostic laparoscopy should be considered, especially in the presence of an abnormal pelvic examination (Gantt and McDonough, 1981).

In a study of 140 adolescents with chronic pelvic pain, Goldstein et al. (1980) found a cyclic relationship to menstrual periods in 30 of the 52 patients in whom the pain interfered with normal activities. Physical findings in these patients, who ranged in age from 10.5 to 19 years, included pelvic tenderness in 65%, cul-de-sac nodularity in 29%, a distinct mass in 19%, adnexal thickening in 17%, and fixed uterine retroversion

Table 8–12   Characteristics of Secondary Dysmenorrhea

Dull, diffuse pelvic pain

Chronic pain throughout menstrual cycle

Lateralization of pain

Onset at menarche or late in adolescence

Tenderness and/or nodularity on pelvic examination

Presence of pelvic pathology or IUD

in 12%. No specific physical abnormalities were noted in 23%. Laparoscopic findings revealed endometriosis in 47%, postoperative adhesions in 13%, uterine anomalies in 8%, pelvic inflammatory disease in 7%, hemoperitoneum in 4%, functional ovarian cysts in 4%, serositis in 3%, and normal laparoscopy in 14%. These findings indicate that endometriosis should be considered in an adolescent who reports cyclic pelvic pain associated with menses and whose pelvic examination reveals tenderness with or without nodularity. Secondary dysmenorrhea has also been associated with adenomyosis, endometrial polyps, and uterine fibroids (Gantt and McDonough, 1981). Although use of an intrauterine device (IUD) is not recommended in adolescents, this method of contraception is associated with a 5%–10% prevalence of dysmenorrhea due to increased prostaglandin release. Dysmenorrhea is less likely with a progesterone-containing IUD (Gantt and McDonough, 1981).

Ovulatory pain, termed mittelschmerz, is distinguished from dysmenorrhea by its midcycle timing and is estimated to affect 50% of all women at some time. An ultrasound study confirmed that pain occurred on the same side as follicular rupture in 86% of women with symptoms. The pain is acute and peristaltic and is thought to be a good indicator for the immediate prediction of ovulation. Etiology has been attributed to tubal, uterine, or cecal spasm, increased tension in the ovary or follicle, or peritoneal irritation by blood or fluid from the ruptured follicle (Marinho et al., 1982). In contrast, another study related the pain to the LH surge which precedes follicular rupture as determined by ultrasound (O'Herlihy et al., 1980). The pain is brief, self-limited, and often responds to the administration of oral analgesics.

Premenstrual Syndrome

> When symptoms of the approach of the menses are noted, such as flushes of heat, giddiness, pain in the back, and heaviness of the limbs, take two tablets of No. 11, four times a day until the menses appear. (Humphreys F: *Humphreys' Mentor*. Humphreys' Homeopathic Medicine Co, New York, 1941, p. 129)

In contrast to dysmenorrhea, current knowledge regarding premenstrual symptoms is limited by the absence of uniform diagnostic criteria and a lack of understanding of etiology, pathogenesis, and effective management. Premenstrual syndrome (PMS) is characterized by cyclically recurring symptoms during the luteal phase of the menstrual cycle (O'Brien, 1985; Boyle et al., 1987). Symptoms regress at onset or during menses, and a symptom-free week follows the menstrual period (Labrum, 1983; O'Brien, 1985). More formal diagnostic criteria proposed by the National Institutes of Mental Health include "marked change in intensity of symptoms measured on cycle days five to ten compared with premenstrual days twenty-two to twenty-eight and documentation of these changes for at least two consecutive cycles" (Freeman et al.,

1985). Problems with studies of premenstrual syndrome include an inexact definition of the disorder, lack of an objective measurable means of assessing the syndrome, complete reliance on patient report, inconsistent physiologic, biochemical, and endocrinologic changes, and treatment studies which lack placebo controls despite a demonstrated placebo effect of greater than 50%. O'Brien (1985) concludes that "much of the data is nearly meaningless."

Few studies have addressed this disorder in the adolescent age group. Since luteal phase deficiency is common in PMS (Hargrove and Abraham, 1983) and in adolescent menstrual cycles, one might expect an increased incidence of premenstrual symptoms compared with adults. In one outpatient gynecologic practice, 18% of 13- to 15-year-olds and 31% of 16- to 20-year-olds reported premenstrual symptoms (Norris, 1983). In a recent survey among high school students, premenstrual symptoms were reported in 63%, with bloating or weight gain in 42%, mood changes in 30%, and cramps in 19% (Wilson et al., 1984). Among college sophomores, 73% reported premenstrual symptoms, and 43% of those described the symptoms as moderate to severe (Rossignol, 1985).

Fisher et al. (1989) administered the Premenstrual Assessment Form, a 95-item questionnaire describing the severity of premenstrual changes in mood, behavior, and physical condition, to 207 adolescent females in suburban New York City. At least one premenstrual change was reported of minimal severity in 96%, moderate in 89%, severe in 59%, and extreme in 43% of subjects. In contrast with adult women, adolescents reported significantly more impulsive behavior and impairment in social function and significantly fewer water retention symptoms.

Symptoms may be classified as somatic, including weight gain, bloating, headache, and cramps, or emotional, such as mood swings, irritability, or depression. A list of commonly reported premenstrual symptoms is included by frequency and severity in Table 8–13.

Abraham (1983) has further divided premenstrual tension (PMT) into four subgroups. PMT-A, reported by 75% of women, includes anxiety, irritability, and tension. PMT-H, reported by 72%, includes water and salt retention, abdominal

Table 8–13   Reported Symptoms in Patients with Premenstrual Syndrome

	Mild to moderate (%)	Severe to disabling (%)
Mood swings	47	5
Irritability	44	12
Weight gain	40	6
Swelling	40	5
Tension	34	8
Skin disorders	32	7
Depression	30	7
Fatigue	29	4
Painful breasts	28	8
Headache	27	7
Anxiety	27	3
Cramps	25	6
Crying	20	5
Taking naps	17	1
Backache	17	5
Lowered work or school performance	12	3

Adapted from Woods et al., 1982.

bloating, mastalgia, and weight gain. PMT-C, reported by 35%, includes craving for sweets and increased appetite. PMT-D, reported by 37%, includes depression, withdrawal, insomnia, forgetfulness, and confusion. In an attempt to validate subgroups of PMS, Siegel et al. (1987) conducted factor analysis of symptoms in 156 women with PMS ranging in age from 18 to 48 years with a mean age of 33 years and determined that five distinct clinical clusters were apparent. Withdrawn mood accounted for 66% of the total variance, anxious and tense mood 13%, physical discomfort 9%, water retention 8%, and arousal 4%. These symptom clusters could be further combined into emotional and behavioral problems accounting for 79% of the overall variance, with physical symptoms accounting for 17%.

In a study using the Moos Menstrual Distress Questionnaire, age at menarche was not associated with any perimenstrual symptoms. Prevalence of symptoms decreased with increasing age, but symptoms increased with a longer menstrual cycle and longer menstrual flow (Woods et al., 1982). Friedman and Jaffe (1985) found no relation with age, race, sexual preference, pronounced athletic activity, marital status, or income, but noted that "occupational and educational achievement was associated with a significantly lower expression of complaints." In a study of premenstrual "bloatedness," Faratian et al. (1984) noted that although the perception of body size increased, there was no change in body weight or measured body dimensions, suggesting that fluid retention was not a common component of PMS. In an attempt to objectively measure functional ability in women with PMS, Posthuma et al. (1987) administered Part II of the Crawford Small Parts Dexterity Test, which requires manual dexterity in the form of bilateral coordination, balance, concentration, control, and perseverance as 36 small screws are turned into a board with a narrow-slotted screwdriver. In comparing the early follicular to late luteal phase, performance improved in asymptomatic women but worsened in women with PMS. In a study of adult women attending a specific clinic for PMS patients, the severity of symptoms was found to correlate positively with increasing dysmenorrhea and premenstrual spotting, suggesting possible progesterone deficiency. There was no correlation with cycle regularity, interval or duration of flow, amount of flow, and duration of cramps (Steege et al., 1985).

Rubinow and Schmidt (1987) recently addressed the difficulty in differentiating the affective and behavioral symptoms of premenstrual syndrome from psychiatric disorders. They concluded that disturbed menstrual function may lead to psychiatric morbidity, psychiatric illness may disrupt mentrual function or timing, and menstrual cycle-related events may modulate or exacerbate psychopathology or lead directly to the appearance of mood and behavior disorders.

Etiology

Among the early theories of PMS causation were estrogen excess and unopposed estrogen effect due to deficient progesterone production with an inadequate luteal phase (Reid and Yen, 1981). No consistent hormonal patterns have been found in investigating the syndrome, and response to hormonal therapy is equally inconsistent. Vitamin deficiency, particularly B_6 (pyridoxine), has been proposed as a major factor since B_6 acts as a coenzyme in the final step of dopamine and serotonin biosynthesis. Changing carbohydrate tolerance during the menstrual cycle has been studied, with many PMS symptoms attributed to reactive hypoglycemia, but timing of symptoms is inconsistent, and no relief is afforded by food intake. Sodium and fluid retention have been studied; however, there is no consistent pattern of premenstrual weight gain, no relation between the degree of fluid retention and severity of other symptoms, and no consistent effect of diuretic therapy (Reid and Yen, 1981). Other theories include an abnormal sensitivity to normal levels of prolactin and a functional deficiency of essential fatty acids due either to inadequate linoleic acid intake or absorption or to a failure of normal conversion of linoleic acid to γ-linolenic acid, a prostaglandin precursor (Horrobin, 1983).

Recent studies have focused on the role of neuropeptides in premenstrual symptoms. A central etiology for PMS is suggested by a report of five women who had persistent PMS symptoms after total hysterectomy and bilateral salpingo-oophorectomy (Labrum, 1983). These studies have focused on the role of α-melanocyte-stimulating hormone (MSH) and endorphins and their effects on dopamine and serotonin. Reid and Yen (1981) hypothesized that aberrant release of, or sensitivity to, α-MSH and β-endorphin during the luteal phase triggers a cascade of neuroendocrine changes that result in premenstrual symptoms. Fluctuations in brain serotonin levels could cause many of the affective changes described in PMS, since this neurotransmitter modulates brain centers controlling sleep, appetite, thirst, and sexual feelings (Labrum, 1983). A premenstrual fall in estrogen could result in decreasing serotonin levels and affective changes. Higher relative estrogen levels in the luteal phase of the cycle would lead to more pronounced withdrawal effects when estrogen levels decline (Labrum, 1983). Prostaglandin activity may also be inhibited by this mechanism (Reid and Yen, 1981).

Investigating the etiology of PMS symptoms, Rossignol (1985) determined the daily consumption of caffeine-containing beverages among college sophomores ranging in age from 18 to 21 years. Compared to women with no daily consumption of caffeine-containing beverages, the prevalence of moderate to severe PMS symptoms was increased 3-fold in women with a consumption of approximately two beverages a day and 7.5-fold in women with an average of six beverages a day. Sources of caffeine included cola in 49%, coffee in 32%, tea in 19%, and over-the-counter drugs in 1%.

Management

In evaluating therapeutic approaches to PMS, it should be noted that no single treatment has proven universally effective and that most treatment studies have been associated with a placebo response of greater than 50%.

In a survey of treatment modalities for PMS recommended by 503 practitioners, Lyon and Lyon (1984) reported that 70% employed progesterone, 63% dietary management, 60% multivitamins, 50% exercise, 23% stress management, anxiolytics, antidepressants, or diuretics, 16% prostaglandin inhibitors, 14% no treatment, and 6.4% bromocriptine. Most of these practitioners utilized multiple treatment options concurrently. In a two-phase study, Prior and Vigna (1987) concluded that exercise training in ovulatory sedentary women and intensified training in female athletes decreased mild premenstrual symptoms, including diminished fluid retention and breast symptoms, and improved mood. They attribute this improvement to the effect of exercise on neurotransmitters and endorphins.

Dietary changes and the use of specific multivitamin and mineral supplements have been extensively studied in the management of premenstrual symptoms, based upon laboratory evidence of significant deficiencies of vitamin B_6 and red blood cell magnesium in patients with PMS. Abraham and Rumley (1987) recommended dietary changes including decreased intake of refined sugar, increased intake of protein, vegetables, and fruits with a switch from meat to fish, and decreased intake of sodium coupled with supplements of pyridoxine, 100–400 mg daily, and calcium, 1–2 g daily. Stewart (1987) administered Optivite, a patented multivitamin multimineral supplement in a dosage of six tablets daily for 6 months and found that PMS symptoms were significantly improved by placebo in 55% and by the supplement in 71%. In a trial of α-tocopherol (vitamin E), 400 IU daily for three cycles, London et al. (1987) reported improvement in both physical and affective symptoms of PMS without side effects. Improvement was attributed either to modulation of prostaglandin production or effect on neurotransmitters; however, comparison of improvement with vitamin E versus placebo did not reach statistical significance. Hagen et al. (1985) compared pyridoxine, 100 mg daily, with placebo and found a 21% improvement in premenstrual symptoms with placebo and only a 4% improvement with pyridoxine therapy. Pyridoxine did cause a significant increase in blood magnesium, but there was no correlation with improvement in symptoms. Dalton (1985) has cautioned that vitamin B_6 therapy may not be innocuous. She measured serum vitamin B_6 levels in women taking supplementation for PMS. Sensory neuropathy was reported in 40% of women with levels above normal who were taking from 50 to 300 mg daily. When vitamin supplementation was discontinued, headache, fatigue, bloating, irritability, and neuropathy resolved. Dalton states that the daily requirement for pyridoxine is only 2–4 mg.

Mefenamic acid, an inhibitor of prostaglandin synthesis, has proven especially effective when PMS is associated with dysmenorrhea and/or menorrhagia. Mira et al. (1986) found mefenamic acid to be effective for fatigue, headache, mood swings, and general aches and pains but found no significant effect on breast or abdominal symptoms, change in appetite, or cyclic mood symptoms. Other studies with mefenamic acid have demonstrated substantial improvement or complete relief in 86% of patients with PMS symptoms (Budoff, 1983; O'Brien, 1985). Therapy has been initiated with onset of symptoms and has resulted in diminished tension, irritability, depression, pain, and headache but no changes in fluid retention or breast symptoms. In contrast, Budoff (1983) found diminished breast tenderness, abdominal bloating, and ankle swelling but no significant difference in tension, lethargy, or depression with mefenamic acid therapy.

Premenstrual symptoms have long been attributed to deficiencies in gonadal steroids leading to therapeutic trials with oral contraceptive pills and progesterone supplementation. Symptoms are reported to be 29% lower in users of the combined oral contraceptive pill and formulations with a greater progestin effect are thought to be more effective (O'Brien, 1985). When oral contraceptive therapy is initiated in patients with PMS, one-third are said to improve, one-third remain unchanged, and one-third become worse (Labrum, 1983). Progesterone is known to have a direct sedative effect on the central nervous system. Progesterone deficiency is associated with irritability, tension, anxiety, and aggressive behavior (O'Brien, 1985). This does not explain the absence of symptoms in the first half of the menstrual cycle when progesterone levels are normally low. Progesterone therapy is not approved by the FDA for PMS, and side effects include spotting, irregular cycles, and rashes (Norris, 1983). Progesterone may be administered by rectal or vaginal suppository, injection, or implant. Due to a short half-life and rapid liver metabolism, large doses are required for effective oral administration (Norris, 1983). However, bioavailability may be considerably enhanced by the use of oral micronized progesterone in a dosage of 300 mg daily (Chakmakjian and Zachariah, 1987).

In a review of diuretic therapy in PMS, Vellacott and O'Brien (1987) conclude that there is little consistent scientific evidence for weight gain or fluid retention with PMS but suggest that spironolactone therapy may have a role when bloating is the dominant symptom. Diuretics have been used primarily for complaints of bloating, weight gain, and abdominal distention. Danazol and bromocriptine have been used primarily for the management of severe breast symptoms. Watts et al. (1987) administered danazol in a daily dose of 100, 200, or 400 mg for 3 months and found improvement in breast pain, irritability, anxiety, and lethargy but no effect on bloating. Optimal dosage was determined to be 200 mg daily, since 400 mg inhibited the ovulatory gonadotropin surge and resulted in complete suppression of menstrual cycles. Bromocriptine promotes dopamine release which inhibits prolactin secretion and is also very useful in managing breast symptoms (Chakmakjian, 1983). Common side effects include fainting and nausea which may be avoided by administering the medication at night (O'Brien, 1985).

Muse et al. (1984) demonstrated relief of physical and behavioral premenstrual symptoms via the daily administration of a gonadotropin-releasing hormone agonist. This effect is rapidly reversible with no influence on subsequent cycles when therapy is discontinued, but prolonged suppression leads to amenorrhea with potential complications of hypoestrogenism. Finally, both clonidine and verapamil are currently being investigated as potentially useful agents in the management of premenstrual symptoms (Chihal, 1987).

Given this bewildering array of often conflicting data, a practical, common sense approach to premenstrual symptoms in the adolescent is proposed in Table 8–14 (Budoff, 1983; Chakmakjian, 1983; Labrum, 1983; O'Brien, 1985; Chihal, 1987).

Table 8–14   Guidelines for Management of Adolescent Premenstrual Syndrome

Confirm the cyclicity of symptoms through the use of a menstrual calendar. Symptoms should disappear with onset of menses and be followed by a symptom-free week.

Identify the symptoms of greatest concern and severity as reported by the patient.

Provide education and reassurance about current knowledge of premenstrual symptoms. Relieve fears about adverse reproductive outcome or cancer.

Maintain ideal body weight.

Encourage aerobic exercise.

Decrease or eliminate use of coffee, tea, cola, chocolate, and tobacco.

Encourage dietary change, including increased intake of protein, vegetables, fruits, fish. Increase calcium and decrease sodium intake. Consider pyridoxine in a dosage of 100 mg daily *or* from day 14 of cycle through onset of menses.

Consider a progestin-dominant oral contraceptive pill if needed for contraception and if PMS is associated with dysmenorrhea and/or menorrhagia.

Consider mefenamic acid, 500 mg TID from day 14 of the cycle through onset of menses, for headache, uterine pain, or bowel cramps.

Consider bromocriptine, 5 mg each night, from day 10 through 26 of the menstrual cycle *or* danazol, 200 mg daily, for severe breast pain or swelling.

Consider spironolactone, 50 mg daily, from day 14 of the cycle to onset of menses for patients with fluid retention documented by cyclic weight gain. Dietary sodium restriction should also be emphasized in this subgroup.

In patients with incapacitating premenstrual symptoms unresponsive to other modalities, long-term menstrual suppression with danazol, progesterone implants, or Depo- Provera (medroxyprogesterone acetate) might be considered.

References

Abraham GE: Nutritional factors in the etiology of the premenstrual tension syndromes. *J Reprod Med* 28:446–464, 1983.

Abraham GE, Rumley RE: Role of nutrition in managing the premenstrual tension syndromes. *J Reprod Med* 32:405–422, 1987.

Altchek A: Dysfunctional uterine bleeding in adolescence. *Clin Obstet Gynecol* 20:633–650, 1977.

Alvin PE, Litt IF: Current status of the etiology and management of dysmenorrhea in adolescence. *Pediatrics* 70:516–525, 1982.

Andersch B, Milsom I: An epidemiologic study of young women with dysmenorrhea. *Am J Obstet Gynecol* 144:655–660, 1982.

Anderson MM, Irwin CE, Snyder DL: Abnormal vaginal bleeding in adolescents. *Pediatr Ann* 15:697–707, 1986.

Bachmann GA, Kemmann E: Prevalence of oligomenorrhea and amenorrhea in a college population. *Am J Obstet Gynecol* 144:98–102, 1982.

Baker ER: Body weight and the initiation of puberty. *Clin Obstet Gynecol* 28:573–579, 1985.

Birnbaum MD, Rose LI: Late onset adrenocortical hydroxylase deficiencies associated with menstrual dysfunction. *Obstet Gynecol* 63:445–451, 1984.

Boyle CA, Berkowitz GS, Kelsey JL: Epidemiology of premenstrual symptoms. *Am J Public Health* 77:349–350, 1987.

Budoff PW: The use of prostaglandin inhibitors for the premenstrual syndrome. *J Reprod Med* 28:469–478, 1983.

Bullen BA, Skrinar GS, Beitins IZ, et al: Induction of menstrual disorder by strenuous exercise in untrained women. *N Engl J Med* 312:1349–1353, 1985.

Chakmakjian ZH: A critical assessment of therapy for the premenstrual tension syndrome. *J Reprod Med* 28:532–538, 1983.

Chakmakjian ZH, Zachariah NY: Bioavailability of progesterone with different modes of administration. *J Reprod Med* 32:443–448, 1987.

Chihal HJ: Indications for drug therapy in premenstrual syndrome patients. *J Reprod Med* 32:449–452, 1987.

Cholst IN, Carlon AT: Oral contraceptives and dysmenorrhea. *J Adolesc Health Care* 8:121–128, 1987.

Claessens EA, Cowell CA: Acute adolescent menorrhagia. *Am J Obstet Gynecol* 139:277–280, 1981a.

Claessens EA, Cowell CA: Dysfunctional uterine bleeding in the adolescent. *Pediatr Clin North Am* 28:369–378, 1981b.

Cox NH: Amenorrhoea during treatment with isotretinoin. *Br J Dermatol* 118:857–858, 1988.

Dalton K: Pyridoxine overdose in premenstrual syndrome. *Lancet* 1:1168–1169, 1985.

Dawood MY: Ibuprofen and dysmenorrhea. *Am J Med* 77:87–94, 1984.

Dawood MY: Dysmenorrhea. *J Reprod Med* 30:154–167, 1985.

Dawood MY: Current concepts in the etiology and treatment of primary dysmenorrhea. *Acta Obstet Gynecol Scand [Suppl]* 138:7–10, 1986.

Dingfelder JR: Primary dysmenorrhea treatment with prostaglandin inhibitors: A review. *Am J Obstet Gynecol* 140:874–879, 1981.

Drinkwater BL, Nilson K, Chestnut CH, et al: Bone mineral content of amenorrheic and eumenorrheic athletes. *N Engl J Med* 311:277–281, 1984.

DuRant RH, Jay MS, Shoffitt T, et al: Factors influencing adolescents' responses to regimens of naproxen for dysmenorrhea. *Am J Dis Child* 139:489–493, 1985.

Emans SJ, Grace E, Goldstein DP: Oligomenorrhea in adolescent girls. *J Pediatr* 97:815–819, 1980.

Faratian B, Gaspar A, O'Brien PMS, et al: Premenstrual syndrome: Weight, abdominal swelling, and perceived body image. *Am J Obstet Gynecol* 150:200–204, 1984.

Fears WB, Glass AR, Vigersky RA: Role of exercise in the pathogenesis of the amenorrhea associated with anorexia nervosa. *J Adolesc Health Care* 4:22–24, 1983.

Fisher M, Trieller K, Napolitano B: Premenstrual symptoms in adolescents. *J Adolesc Health Care* 10:369–375, 1989.

Flug D, Largo RH, Prader A: Symptoms related to menstruation in adolescent Swiss girls: A longitudinal study. *Ann Hum Biol* 12:161–168, 1985.

Fraser IS, McCarron G, Markham R: A preliminary study of factors influencing perception of menstrual blood loss volume. *Am J Obstet Gynecol* 149:788–793, 1984.

Fraser IS, McCarron G, Markham R, et al: Long-term treatment of menorrhagia with mefenamic acid. *Obstet Gynecol* 61:109–112, 1983.

Fraser IS, Pearse C, Shearman RP, et al: Efficacy of mefenamic acid in patients with a complaint of menorrhagia. *Obstet Gynecol* 58:543–551, 1981.

Freeman EW, Sondheimer S, Weinbaum PJ, et al: Evaluating premenstrual symptoms in medical practice. *Obstet Gynecol* 65:500–505, 1985.

Friedman D, Jaffe H: Influence of life-style on the premenstrual syndrome: Analysis of a questionnaire survey. *J Reprod Med* 30:715–719, 1985.

Frisch RE: Body fat, puberty and fertility. *Biol Rev* 59:161, 1984.

Frisch RE, Gotz-Welbergen AV, McArthur JW, et al: Delayed menarche and amenorrhea of college athletes in relation to age of onset of training. *JAMA* 246:1559–1563, 1981.

Frisch RE, McArthur JW: Menstrual cycles: Fatness as a determinant of minimum weight for height necessary for their maintenance or onset. *Science* 185:949–951, 1974.

Frisch RE, Wyshak G, Vincent L: Delayed menarche and amenorrhea in ballet dancers. *N Engl J Med* 303:17–19, 1980.

Gadpaille WJ, Sanborn CF, Wagner WW: Athletic amenorrhea, major affective disorders, and eating disorders. *Am J Psychiatry* 144:939–942, 1987.

Gantt PA, McDonough PG: Adolescent dysmenorrhea. *Pediatr Clin North Am* 28:389–395, 1981.

Gardner J: Adolescent menstrual characteristics as predictors of gynaecological health. *Ann Hum Biol* 10:31–40, 1983.

Gidwani GP: Vaginal bleeding in adolescents. *J Reprod Med* 29:417–420, 1984.

Goldstein DP, deCholnoky C, Emans SJ, et al: Laparoscopy in the diagnosis and management of pelvic pain in adolescents. *J Reprod Med* 24:251–256, 1980.

Granoff AB: Treatment of menstrual irregularities with dexamethasone in congenital adrenal hyperplasia. *J Adolesc Health Care* 2:23–27, 1981.

Hagen I, Nesheim BI, Tuntland T: No effect of vitamin B-6 against premenstrual tension. *Acta Obstet Gynecol Scand* 64:667–670, 1985.

Halbert DR: Menstrual delay and dysfunctional uterine bleeding associated with antiprostaglandin therapy for dysmenorrhea. *J Reprod Med* 28:592–594, 1983.

Hanson FW: Naproxen sodium, ibuprofen and a placebo in dysmenorrhea. *J Reprod Med* 27:423–427, 1982.

Hargrove JT, Abraham GE: The ubiquitousness of premenstrual tension in gynecologic practice. *J Reprod Med* 28:435–437, 1983.

Harkins JL, Gysler M, Cowell CA: Anatomical amenorrhea: The problems of congenital vaginal agenesis and its surgical correction. *Pediatr Clin North Am* 28:345–354, 1981.

Heinrichs WL, Adamson GD: A practical approach to the patient with dysmenorrhea. *J Reprod Med* 25:236–242, 1980.

Horrobin DF: The role of essential fatty acids and prostaglandins in the premenstrual syndrome. *J Reprod Med* 28:465–468, 1983.

Hughes EG, Garner PR: Primary amenorrhea associated with hyperprolactinemia: Four cases with normal sellar architecture and absence of galactorrhea. *Fertil Steril* 47:1031–1032, 1987.

Hull MGR, Bromham DR, Savage PE, et al: Post-pill amenorrhea: A causal study. *Fertil Steril* 36:472–476, 1981.

Jones G: Commentary on the use of intravenous Premarin in the treatment of dysfunctional uterine bleeding. *Obstet Gynecol Surv* 37:478–479, 1983.

Kase NG: The neuroendocrinology of amenorrhea. *J Reprod Med* 28:251–255, 1983.

Kemmann E, Pasquale SA, Skaf R: Amenorrhea associated with carotenemia. *JAMA* 249:926–929, 1983.

Klein JR, Litt IF: Epidemiology of adolescent dysmenorrhea. *Pediatrics* 68:661–664, 1981.

Klein JR, Litt IF, Rosenberg A, et al: The effect of aspirin on dysmenorrhea in adolescents. *J Pediatr* 98:987–990, 1981.

Koppelman MCS, Jaffe MJ, Rieth KG, et al: Hyperprolactinemia, amenorrhea, and galactorrhea: A retrospective assessment of twenty-five cases. *Ann Intern Med* 100:115–121, 1984.

Labrum AH: Hypothalamic, pineal and pituitary factors in the premenstrual syndrome. *J Reprod Med* 28:438–445, 1983.

Lawlor CL, Davis AM: Primary dysmenorrhea. Relationship to personality and attitudes in adolescent females. *J Adolesc Health Care* 1:208–212, 1981.

London RS, Murphy L, Kitlowski KE, et al: Efficacy of alpha-tocopherol in the treatment of the premenstrual syndrome. *J Reprod Med* 32:400–404, 1987.

Lyon KE, Lyon MA: The premenstrual syndrome: A survey of current treatment practices. *J Reprod Med* 29:705–711, 1984.

Mansfield MJ, Emans SJ: Adolescent menstrual irregularity. *J Reprod Med* 29:399–410, 1984.

Marinho AO, Sallam HN, Goessens L, et al: Ovulation side and occurrence of mittelschmerz in spontaneous and induced ovarian cycles. *Br Med J* 284:632, 1982.

Milsom I, Andersch B: Ibuprofen and naproxen-sodium in the treatment of primary dysmenorrhea: A double-blind cross-over study. *Int J Gynaecol Obstet* 23:305–310, 1985.

Mira M, McNeil D, Fraser IS, et al: Mefenamic acid in the treatment of premenstrual syndrome. *Obstet Gynecol* 68:395–398, 1986.

Mishell DR, ed: Menorrhagia: A symposium. *J Reprod Med* 29:763–782, 1984.

Muse KN, Cetel NS, Futterman LA, et al: The premenstrual syndrome: Effects of "medical ovariectomy." *N Engl J Med* 311:1345–1349, 1984.

Nelson RO, Sigmon S, Amodei N, et al: The Menstrual Symptom Questionnaire: The validity of the distinction between spasmodic and congestive dysmenorrhea. *Behav Res Ther* 22:611–614, 1984.

Norris RV: Progesterone for premenstrual tension. *J Reprod Med* 28:509–516, 1983.

O'Brien PMS: The premenstrual syndrome. A review. *J Reprod Med* 30:113–126, 1985.

O'Herlihy C, Robinson HP, Ch de Crespigny LJ. Mittleschmerz is a preovulatory symptom. *Br Med J* 280:986, 1980.

Ojofeitimi EO: Effect of duration and frequency of breast-feeding on postpartum amenorrhea. *Pediatrics* 69:164–168, 1982.

Owen PR: Prostaglandin synthetase inhibitors in the treatment of primary dysmenorrhea: Outcome trials reviewed. *Am J Obstet Gynecol* 148:96–103, 1984.

Posthuma BW, Bass MJ, Bull SB, et al: Detecting changes in functional ability in women with premenstrual syndrome. *Am J Obstet Gynecol* 156:275–278, 1987.

Prior JC, Vigna Y: Conditioning exercise and premenstrual symptoms. *J Reprod Med* 32:423–428, 1987.

Rees MCP, Anderson ABM, Demers LM, et al: Prostaglandins in menstrual fluid in menorrhagia and dysmenorrhoea. *Br J Obstet Gynecol* 91:673–680, 1984.

Reid RL, Yen SSC: Premenstrual syndrome. *Am J Obstet Gynecol* 139:85–104, 1981.

Reindollar RH, McDonough PG: Etiology and evaluation of delayed sexual development. *Pediatr Clin North Am* 28:267–286, 1981.

Reindollar RH, McDonough PG: Adolescent menstrual disorders. *Clin Obstet Gynecol* 26:690–701, 1983.

Rosenwaks Z, Seegar-Jones G: Menstrual pain: Its origin and pathogenesis. *J Reprod Med* 25:207–212, 1980.

Rossignol AM: Caffeine-containing beverages and premenstrual syndrome in young women. *Am J Public Health* 75:1335–1337, 1985.

Rubinow DR, Schmidt PJ: Mood disorders and the menstrual cycle. *J Reprod Med* 32:389–394, 1987.

Russell JB, Mitchell D, Musey PI, et al: The relationship of exercise to anovulatory cycles in female athletes: Hormonal and physical characteristics. *Obstet Gynecol* 63:452–456, 1984.

Sadeghi-Nejad A, Wolfsdorf JI, Biller BJ, et al: Hyperprolactinemia causing primary amenorrhea. *J Pediatr* 99:802–804, 1981.

Sanborn CF, Martin BJ, Wagner WW: Is athletic amenorrhea specific to runners? *Am J Obstet Gynecol* 143:859–861, 1982.

Sandler DP, Wilcox AJ, Horney LF: Age at menarche and subsequent reproductive events. *Am J Epidemiol* 119:765–774, 1984.

Schwartz B, Cumming DC, Riordan E, et al: Exercise-associated amenorrhea: A distinct entity. *Am J Obstet Gynecol* 141:662–670, 1981.

Shangold MM: Athletic amenorrhea. *Clin Obstet Gynecol* 28:664–669, 1985a.

Shangold MM: Causes, evaluation, and management of athletic oligo-/amenorrhea. *Med Clin North Am* 69:83–95, 1985b.

Siegberg R, Nilsson CG, Stenman UH, et al: Sex hormone profiles in oligomenorrheic adolescent girls and the effect of oral contraceptives. *Fertil Steril* 41:888–893, 1984.

Siegberg R, Nilsson CG, Stenman UH, et al: Endocrinologic features of oligomenorrheic adolescent girls. *Fertil Steril* 46:852–857, 1986.

Siegel JP, Myers BJ, Dineen MK: Premenstrual tension syndrome symptom clusters: Statistical evaluation of the subsyndromes. *J Reprod Med* 32:395–399, 1987.

Snow LF, Johnson SM: Modern day menstrual folklore. *JAMA* 237:2736–2739, 1977.

Soltan MH, Hancock KW: Outcome in patients with post-pill amenorrhoea. *Br J Obstet Gynaecol* 89:745–748, 1982.

Soules MR: Adolescent amenorrhea. *Pediatr Clin North Am* 34:1083–1103, 1987.

Southam AL, Richart RM: The prognosis for adolescents with menstrual abnormalities. *Am J Obstet Gynecol* 94:637–645, 1966.

Steege JF, Stout AL, Rupp SL: Relationship among premenstrual symptoms and menstrual cycle characteristics. *Obstet Gynecol* 65:398–402, 1985.

Stewart A: Clinical and biochemical effects of nutritional supplementation on the premenstrual syndrome. *J Reprod Med* 32:435–441, 1987.

Svanberg L, Ulmsten U: The incidence of primary dysmenorrhea in teenagers. *Arch Gynecol* 230:173–177, 1981.

Talbert LM, Hammond MF, Groff T, et al: Relationship of age and pubertal development to ovulation in adolescent girls. *Obstet Gynecol* 66:542–544, 1985.

Vellacott ID, O'Brien PMS: Effect of spironolactone on premenstrual syndrome symptoms. *J Reprod Med* 32:429–434, 1987.

Venturoli S, Porcu E, Fabbri R, et al: Postmenarchal evolution of endocrine pattern and ovarian aspects in adolescents with menstrual irregularities. *Fertil Steril* 48:78–85, 1987.

Warren MP, Brooks-Gunn J, Hamilton LH, et al: Scoliosis and fractures in young ballet dancers: Relation to delayed menarche and secondary amenorrhea. *N Engl J Med* 314:1348–1353, 1986.

Watts JF, Butt WR, Edwards RL: A clinical trial using danazol for the treatment of premenstrual tension. *Br J Obstet Gynaecol* 94:30–34, 1987.

Wentz AC: Body weight and amenorrhea. *Obstet Gynecol* 56:482–487, 1980.

Wilson C, Emans SJ, Mansfield J, et al: The relationships of calculated percent body fat, sports participation, age, and place of residence on menstrual patterns in healthy adolescent girls at an independent New England high school. *J Adolesc Health Care* 5:248–253, 1984.

Woods NF, Most A, Dery GK: Prevalence of perimenstrual symptoms. *Am J Public Health* 72:1257–1264, 1982.

Wyshak G, Frisch RE: Age of menarche. *N Engl J Med* 307:753–754, 1982a.

Wyshak G, Frisch RE: Evidence for a secular trend in age of menarche. *N Engl J Med* 306:1033–1035, 1982b.

Ylikorkala O, Dawood MY: New concepts in dysmenorrhea. *Am J Obstet Gynecol* 130:833–847, 1978.

Ylikorkala O, Pekonen F: Naproxen reduces idiopathic but not fibromyoma-induced menor-rhagia. *Obstet Gynecol* 68:10–12, 1986.

9

Evaluation and Management of Abdominal and Pelvic Pain

Jerold C. Woodhead, Douglas W. Laube, Kevin M. Wood, Lynn C. Richman, Susan R. Johnson, Vera Loening-Baucke, and Wilbur L. Smith

An adolescent girl with abdominal pain causes anxiety at home and in the physician's office. Whether the pain is acute, recurrent, or chronic, adolescents and their parents may have great concern about the existence of a serious disease. The physician faces the tasks of diagnosis, explanation, and management. Explanation is often the most difficult task of all, especially if organic illness cannot account for the pain experienced by the adolescent. Thorough knowledge of pubertal development greatly aids evaluation of abdominal pain because it allows more complete consideration of possible organic causes and provides the physician with an understanding of the psychoemotional causes or consequences of pain.

Pain is always subjective. The response to a painful stimulus depends upon complex interactions among biologic, psychologic, and social factors which, together, define a unique reactivity to pain for any individual (McGrath and Unruh, 1987a; Ross and Ross, 1988). Engel (1977) first proposed the "Biopsychosocial" model of illness, and many have used it as a basis for exploration of specific symptoms such as pain. The International Association for the Study of Pain (Merskey et al., 1979) defines pain as "an unpleasant sensory and emotional experience associated with actual or potential damage or described in terms of such damage." According to this definition, pain experience depends upon tissue damage and previous direct, personal exposure to pain or observation of the experience that others have with pain. Wall (1979) defines pain as a socially conditioned phenomenon affected by events distinct from the apparent noxious stimulus such as distracting stimuli, past events which color experience, and culturally learned reactions. Wall further observes that pain is "never neutral . . . [it is] packaged along with an emotional response of dislike, fear, anxiety or depression." Anxiety about the past and the present combines with fear of future consequences in painful situations, and both fear and anxiety are determined by an individual's personality, experience, knowledge, information, religion, and trust. Wall concludes his monograph with the comment that pain is not a "simple sensory experience signalling the existence of damaged tissue. The presence and intensity of pain is too poorly related to the degree of damage to be considered such a messenger . . . pain signals the existence of a body state where recovery and recuperation should be initiated."

In general, acute pain accompanies conditions that may produce physical damage and, hence, requires rapid evaluation and management. Complaint of pain over longer periods of time may reflect a chronic or a recurrent process, either of which may have both organic and psychologic components. Evaluation of chronic or recurrent pain will be time-consuming, may be extremely frustrating for physicians, adolescents, and parents, and necessitates a deliberate, thoughtful approach and a willingness to consider causes other than organic disease.

In the pages that follow, we shall focus on those aspects of adolescence that affect the presentation of abdominal pain and that set adolescent girls apart from children and adults. Because pubertal development results in marked physiologic and psychologic changes over a short time period, and because these changes introduce new considerations into the differential diagnosis of abdominal pain, we will address physiologic and psychologic aspects of abdominal pain extensively. Maturation of reproductive organs represents the major physiologic change of puberty in girls (Moscicki and Shafer, 1986); gynecologic causes of abdominal pain are among the "new" diagnoses which must be considered. Gynecologic, nongynecologic, and psychologic causes of pain will be covered, as will their interactions. Acute and recurrent abdominal pain will receive separate consideration.

Adolescent Development and Abdominal Pain

Beginning with the onset of puberty, girls begin to experience abdominal pain which may differ in its cause from that common to pubertal boys and prepubertal children of both sexes because of the maturation of the female reproductive organs. Thorough understanding of the physical growth (Daniel, 1985), the cognitive development (Blum and Stark, 1985), the psychosocial correlates (Kreipe and McAnarney, 1985) of adolescence, and the complexities of female adolescent reproductive development (Moscicki and Shafer, 1986) assists the physician who must evaluate a teenage girl with abdominal pain. Orr (1986) discusses in great detail the relationships that exist among stress, psychosomatic illness, and adolescence. Frey (1985) reviews adolescence and the family.

Many physicians fail to appreciate fully the unique relationship between an adolescent and her physician. Neither the adult-physician model nor the child-physician model suffices for the interaction between teen and doctor, although both provide important lessons. The complexities of adolescent growth and development (in all spheres) and the asynchrony of progress among the different aspects of growth make the adolescent an often confusing amalgam of child, adult, and something that is neither child nor adult.

Silber (1986) discusses the ways that the physician and the adolescent contribute to the success or failure of the clinical interaction. The physician may contribute to poor communication and resultant misdiagnosis because of unconscious biases or reactions to adolescents. If a physician does not have clinical expertise in the medical care of adolescents, errors in judgment and less than optimal medical care will result. The physician may also assume a parental role, with potentially damaging outcomes to the clinical encounter.

The adolescent, on the other hand, may bring to the clinical encounter her own biases and stereotypes as well as the inconsistencies and partial knowledge that characterize many phases of adolescent psychoemotional growth. She may assign to the physician the role of a parent figure, either positively or negatively.

To further complicate matters, parents, who have a legitimate interest in the health of their adolescent children, may place unrealistic demands on physicians with regard to the evaluation of symptoms. They may ally with or be hostile to the physician (openly or covertly). They may assume that the physician's primary responsibility is to them, when in reality it is to the adolescent. Parents may be unable or unwilling to accept a diagnosis that attributes pain to something other than disease or physical abnormalities. They may deny the effects of family dysfunction or may conceal incestual or abusive situations.

Silber (1986) suggests that optimal medical care of adolescents requires exploration of two key issues by the physician: 1) How does the adolescent make the physician feel? and 2) What is the effect of these feelings on the physician's clinical performance? Implicit in his suggestion is the necessity that physicians who treat adolescents have knowledge about the processes of physical and psychoemotional development and the ways this development affects individuals, families, and the doctor-patient relationship. Physicians must also be skilled in the clinical assessment of adolescents. Honesty, openness, and the willingness to listen to the adolescent help to promote successful medical care.

Abdominal Pain

Abdominal pain (McGrath and Unruh, 1987b) may originate from an intraabdominal organ (visceral pain) or from the parietal peritoneum (parietal pain). Pain also may be referred to the abdomen from extraabdominal sites or from the abdomen to sites distant. Referred pain is identified in areas which have the same sensory innervation as an organ affected by a noxious stimulus. Way (1983) discusses the types and origins of abdominal pain in detail. A basic understanding of abdominal pain presentation greatly enhances the clinician's diagnostic approach.

The intraabdominal and pelvic organs do not have pain receptors, as such. Instead, pain is detected by free nerve endings located in the walls of hollow organs, the capsules of solid organs, and in muscle, the mesentery, the parietal peritoneum, and the posterior peritoneum. The visceral peritoneum and greater omentum are insensitive to pain. Many stimuli, such as cutting, tearing, or crushing, which produce pain elsewhere in the body, do not cause pain in intraabdominal or pelvic organs. Processes that produce stretching or tension of the wall or capsule of an organ result in pain. The rate at which the stretching occurs is important: A slow process will not cause pain, whereas a rapid process will. Infiltration of the wall of an organ by a malignancy does not cause pain unless obstruction or ischemia result. Other stimuli that cause pain include inflammation, hemorrhage, and involvement of sensory nerves by neoplasms (Way, 1983).

Classification of Pain

The time-honored classification of abdominal pain into organic or functional etiologic groups has been modified by Barr (1983, 1987). According to Barr, abdominal pain may be organic, dysfunctional or psychogenic in origin.

Organic Pain   Organic pain originates from a disease process or a noxious stimulus in an organ system and responds to specific surgical or medical therapy. Such pain is most often acute in onset, although it may be chronic or recurrent.

Dysfunctional Pain   Dysfunctional pain tends to be recurrent and occurs as the result of normal, rather than pathologic, intraabdominal processes. Dysfunctional pain prompts medical attention because it interferes with everyday activities. The source of dysfunctional pain may be identifiable, such as dysmenorrhea or lactose intolerance, or nonspecific, without apparent mechanism. Barr observes that nonspecific abdominal pain tends to be persistent in adolescents (Barr, 1987).

Psychogenic Pain   Psychogenic pain has no apparent intraabdominal origin. Instead, it occurs as a behavioral response in situations where secondary gain results or is associated with a variety of psychogenic events, including acute or chronic stress or psychiatric syndromes. Diagnosis of psychogenic pain must be based on positive evidence of a relationship between pain and behavior; this diagnosis should not be one of "exclusion." Parental alcoholism and learning disabilities are examples of stressors which may provoke psychogenic pain in an adolescent. However, the concurrence of abdominal pain and stress in an adolescent does not necessarily mean that the stress is causal. Levine and Rappaport (1984) point out that stress is far more common than abdominal pain and that there is "no rigorous evidence for a direct *causal* linkage between stress and pain [emphasis added]." In addition, Levine and Rappaport observe that Barr's model describes the *types* of abdominal pain but does not address the *reasons* that one individual experiences pain while another does not when exposed to the same noxious stimulus.

The model for recurrent abdominal pain described by Levine and Rappaport (1984) ascribes pain experience to the convergence of multiple predisposing factors which create the symptom and modulate its impact and severity. Their model not only addresses the occurrence of pain in an individual but also explains the absence of pain or the ability to tolerate it in another individual exposed to the same stimulus. The factors that influence pain experience include:

1. Somatic predisposition, dysfunction, or disorder (i.e., disease)
2. Life-style and habit
3. Milieu and critical events
4. Temperament and learned-response patterns.

Each factor has an influence on the other factors and contributes directly and indirectly to the symptom of pain experienced by an individual. No single factor necessarily has more importance than any other.

Evaluation of Abdominal Pain

A physician's approach to an adolescent with abdominal pain, whether acute, chronic, or recurrent, will follow the "classic" sequence in most instances: history, physical examination, and judiciously chosen laboratory tests and imaging studies.

History

The history provides the key information on which the initial decisions about the diagnostic evaluation are based, even in the most acute situations. An accurate, detailed description of the nature of the pain, its severity, location, and timing, and any changes that have occurred over time, is well worth the effort spent to obtain it. Information about pubertal development, menstrual history, sexual activity, and associated fever, vomiting, diarrhea, constipation, voiding symptoms, or other systemic signs and symptoms will direct attention to specific diagnostic areas. Spiro (1970) notes the particular value of the past medical record and a review of the patient's previous experience with pain, either direct, such as trauma, or indirect, such as observation of a parent with ulcer pain. He further comments that knowledge of the patient's reaction style, as influenced by culture, family, and personality, assists in interpretation and management of abdominal pain.

The history will provide the physician with information to test against physiology, pathologic processes, anatomy, and disease entities. It will focus the differential diagnosis and direct the physical examination and choice of tests. In acute pain situations the working diagnosis may include disease processes that demand urgent intervention to prevent tissue damage. In nonacute situations the patient's symptom complex and results of the evaluation may not correspond to an identifiable disease process and, hence, not dictate rapid intervention; a more deliberate approach may be indicated.

Timing   Details of the time course of abdominal pain, especially its onset, provide information vital to early decision making (Way, 1983). Surgical problems have a high association with pain that has rapid onset; with a more gradual onset of pain, the differential diagnosis becomes more complex, and the likelihood of a surgically remediable etiology decreases.

Abrupt onset   The most rapid onset of pain occurs with intraabdominal catastrophic events such as ruptured ectopic pregnancy, vascular accident, or perforated ulcer, but abdominal pain referred from outside of the abdominal cavity, such as a spontaneous pneumothorax in an asthmatic, may also occur abruptly. The onset of such pain may be reported as instantaneous and may also be associated with shock. Rapid surgical consultation and intervention, if indicated, are mandatory. Blunt abdominal trauma with visceral rupture (spleen, liver, kidney) or hemorrhage into a solid organ or the bowel wall presents with abrupt onset of pain, although delayed symptoms may occur.

Rapid onset   When onset of pain can be identified as having occurred over a period of an hour or less, the list of possible causes increases. Small intestinal obstruction, torted or strangulated viscus, biliary or ureteral colic, peptic ulcer, staphylococcal food poisoning, and ectopic pregnancy are among the diagnoses relevant to adolescents.

Gradual onset   A more gradual onset of pain over a 12- to 24-hour period typically accompanies processes such as acute appendicitis, bowel obstruction, acute abdominal sickle cell crisis, diabetic ketoacidosis, regional enteritis, ulcerative colitis, constipation, and urinary tract infection. Blunt trauma to the abdomen occasionally may cause injury which becomes apparent 12–24 hours later with the onset of abdominal pain or with a change in the character of pain.

Recurrent pain   If pain is recurrent, times when pain occurs and times when it does not occur may offer clues to diagnosis, as do the severity of the recurrent pain, changes in pain presentation, and the appearance of new symptoms. Recurrent pain may be tolerated until an especially severe episode prompts medical attention to rule out a "surgical abdomen." On the other hand, acute pain without a definable cause frequently heralds subsequent development of recurrent abdominal pain.

Other aspects of timing   Other important aspects of pain timing include the frequency with which pain episodes occur, the duration of each episode, and the association of pain with activity, position, bowel movement, urination, or meals. Abdominal pain that begins shortly after an individual begins to eat a meal suggests constipation, since the gastrocolic reflex triggers increased rectosigmoid motility with resultant pain. Pain from peptic ulcer, gallbladder, pancreas, or small bowel typically occurs later in relation to meals. Nausea, vomiting, diarrhea, or anorexia may accompany abdominal pain, and, although none is specific for a surgically remediable process, vomiting usually occurs late in appendicitis and early in gastroenteritis.

Location   A noxious stimulus in a hollow or solid intraabdominal organ produces pain which is identified near the midline. There is a great deal of overlap and poor localization of pain from intraabdominal organs because innervation of most viscera comes from multiple dermatones. Pain localizes to the midline because most intraabdominal organs receive sensory fibers from both sides of the spinal cord. Visceral pain afferent fibers travel with both sympathetic and parasympathetic nerves, although the majority of pain afferents for the gastrointestinal and urinary tracts and the ovaries and distal fallopian tubes accompany the sympathetic fibers; pain afferents from the remainder of the reproductive organs travel primarily with the parasympathetic fibers of the pelvic nerve but also have a sympathetic component (Way, 1983; Bonica, 1967).

Pain with origin in the liver, stomach, and upper small intestine is experienced most often in the epigastric region. Pain originating in the bowel, from the ileum to the splenic flexure, is usually felt in the midabdomen. Pain from the remainder of the large bowel, the kidneys, the bladder, and the gynecologic organs is most often felt in the lower abdomen. Pain with origins in the body of the uterus is experienced in the lower abdomen, while pain arising in the lower uterine segment and cervix is felt in the lumbosacral area. Pain from the fallopian tubes and ovaries may be experienced in the anterior thigh as well as the lower abdomen.

In general, peritoneal irritation localizes to the area of inflammation with hyperesthesia of the overlying skin. Folkman (1979) observes that by the time pain has shifted in character from visceral to peritoneal, a fluid is responsible for transmission of the pain; only an inflamed gallbladder or liver touch the peritoneum and produce peritoneal pain. Large accumulations of blood or infectious exudate within the peritoneal cavity cause pain which is referred to the shoulder if subdiaphragmatic irritation occurs. Inflammatory involvement of the liver capsule causes right upper quadrant pain. Table 9–1 lists various fluids which may contaminate the peritoneal cavity and the pain associated with each.

Character   Hollow organs such as the bowel, ureters, fallopian tubes, uterus, and cervix respond to acute dilatation and inflammation with crampy or colicky pain which occurs intermittently and frequently causes a dull, aching sensation in between acute flare-ups. In contrast, solid organs such as the ovaries, liver, spleen, and kidneys respond to inflammation or abrupt distention of the capsule with continuous, severely throbbing pain which has occasional sharp exacerbations. Peritoneal irritation from infection or large blood accumulation (for example, from a ruptured ectopic pregnancy or endometrioma) generally causes intense, dull, constant throbbing pain made worse by movement or cough. Pain of peritoneal irritation is more steady, intense, and localized than visceral pain (Way, 1983).

Table 9–1   Pain Associated with Intraperitoneal Fluid

Fluid	Degree of pain	Comment
Ascites	0	If uninfected
Bile	4+	Continuous
Blood	2+	Few hours duration
		Pain remits when active bleeding stops
Chyle	0	—
Feces	3+	Continuous
Hydrochloric acid	3–4+	Unremitting
Inflammatory fluid or pus	3+	—
Pancreatic enzymes	3–4+	Continuous
Urine	2–3+	If infected or concentrated

Modified from Folkman, 1979.

Associated Signs and Symptoms   Abdominal pain of organic etiology rarely presents alone. Associated signs and symptoms most often point to an organ system or disease process. Pain originating from the bowel, for example, may have associated abdominal distention, constipation/obstipation, diarrhea, vomiting, gastrointestinal bleeding, or a palpable mass. Urinary tract disorders might have fever, dysuria, proteinuria, hematuria, or flank tenderness in addition to pain. Pain that originates in the reproductive organs can mimic both gastrointestinal and urinary diseases but also may have features specific to the reproductive tract, such as vaginal or cervical discharge, pain or mass on pelvic examination, or positive pregnancy test. Pallor may signal gastrointestinal bleeding. Weight loss accompanies chronic giardiasis and inflammatory bowel diseases. The list of associated signs and symptoms is extensive, and each patient presents the physician with a diagnostic challenge.

Physical Examination

Information obtained from the history will usually prompt a thorough, detailed physical examination, but on occasion may quickly focus the physical examination to a specific area of concern. Pelvic examination must be considered part of the evaluation of abdominal pain in adolescent females and is considered in a separate chapter. Textbooks of physical examination, such as *Major's Physical Diagnosis* (Delp and Manning, 1981), discuss the approach to the abdominal examination in detail and appropriately note that physical examination uncommonly identifies problems not elicited by the history.

Characteristic pain patterns, such as the progression of acute appendicitis, the discomfort of Mittelschmerz, or the association of pain with infrequent bowel movements will guide the physical examination. Less characteristic pain patterns, however, will require a more general physical examination and careful consideration of the relationship between history and physical findings. The physician must take care to avoid making judgments based on hurried or cursory consideration of the patient's pain history.

Observation   The physical examination should begin with the least invasive maneuver: observation. How ill does the patient appear, and what is her level of consciousness? How much pain does she appear to have? Does the patient's pain description correspond with observations of the patient's appearance and interaction?

Does she lie still on the examining table, does she writhe in discomfort, or does she sit in apparent comfort? Can the patient walk, stand, sit, and get herself onto and off of the examining table? Does movement or position appear to produce or exacerbate pain? Does the patient have respiratory distress, cough, rash, or abdominal distention, or does she have evident features of an acute or chronic illness which has abdominal pain as part of the symptom complex? These are but some of the observations that an astute physician will make during the initial evaluation of abdominal pain. These observations, coupled with the subjective history and the objective data from vital signs, will reduce the differential diagnostic possibilities, direct the physical examination, and, perhaps most importantly, help establish the seriousness of the complaint and the urgency with which it should be approached.

Auscultation, Percussion, and Palpation   The physical examination maneuvers of auscultation to evaluate bowel sounds, followed by percussion and, finally, palpation become increasingly more invasive, and, thus, more likely to evoke pain or localize it and to provide precise diagnostic information. Sensitivity to a patient's discomfort and awareness of her anxiety and apprehensiveness will improve the success of abdominal examination and should help the physician distinguish between voluntary rigidity of abdominal muscles and involuntary guarding. Such attention to the patient will also allow the physician to offer encouragement and reassurance, which may improve patient cooperation. Abdominal masses may be missed, even when large, if the physician does not carefully search for an enlarged organ, such as spleen or kidney, or does not suspect a condition, such as pregnancy, and thus overlooks the enlarged uterus. A thorough evaluation of abdominal pain includes examination of the chest, lungs, pelvic contents, and rectum, in addition to palpation of the abdomen.

Laboratory

Selected laboratory tests chosen carefully to fit the clinical situation complement the history and physical examination. Urinalysis and urine culture, most importantly, provide information about infectious and inflammatory processes in the urinary tract. In addition, hematuria may be detected with renal trauma, hydronephrosis, urinary stones, glomerulonephritis, and sickle cell disease. Either urine or serum human chorionic gonadotropin assay should be done to test for the possibility of pregnancy.

Fever usually prompts a complete blood count with differential white blood cell count. Although nonspecific, elevated WBC with immature forms (''left shift'') suggests infection or an inflammatory process such as Crohn disease or ulcerative colitis. An elevated erythrocyte sedimentation rate often accompanies inflammatory bowel disease. Anemia may be identified if vaginal or gastrointestinal bleeding is part of the clinical presentation or in a patient with an ''abdominal crisis'' caused by homozygous sickle cell anemia. The peripheral blood smear will demonstrate the characteristic red cell morphology of sickle cell anemia and the fragmented erythrocytes of hemolytic uremic syndrome.

Test for occult blood in stool obtained during rectal exam should be routine. Stool culture or evaluation for ova and parasites may prove useful in selected cases. Culture of vaginal discharge is always indicated. Serum electrolytes, glucose, creatinine, and urea nitrogen aid in the evaluation of abdominal pain when the differential diagnosis includes diabetic ketoacidosis, renal disease, anorexia nervosa, or other processes which cause metabolic disturbances. Liver function tests obviously have a place in evaluation of suspected liver disease.

Imaging Evaluation

The relatively high incidence of abdominal discomfort in adolescent females is accompanied by a low prevalence of correctable pathological disorders. This supports a minimalist approach toward the imaging evaluation of these patients. The ideal examination for such patients would be noninvasive, not involve the use of significant ionizing radiation, and have relatively few false negatives (i.e., have high sensitivity). Ultrasound fulfills the above criteria and, appropriately, has become the primary screening device for abdominal and pelvic discomfort in preteen and teenage females.

Ultrasound   Ultrasound imaging usually employs a 3.5 MHz transducer. Transabdominal imaging requires a full bladder as an acoustical window. A brief period of fasting (usually about 4 hours) and the urgency of a full bladder are the only discomforts of the procedure. Transvaginal scanning may have even better sensitivity than the transabdominal approach but is not appropriate for most young adolescents because of transducer size. Older, sexually active adolescents are the best candidates for transvaginal ultrasonography.

Evaluation of pelvic structures requires knowledge of the patient's menstrual history. The size and shape of the uterus and adnexa and the appearance of the ovaries vary with the stage of pubertal development, the phase of the current menstrual cycle, the periodicity or regularity of menses, and pregnancy (Ritchie, 1986; Filly, 1987). Both uterine and ovarian volume rapidly increase at the onset of puberty and reach adult size by the time of menarche (Orsini et al., 1984). Ultrasound can distinguish the anatomic characteristics of the uterine contents during the various phases of the menstrual cycle, which assists evaluation of menstrual irregularity.

Pregnancy   Intrauterine pregnancy is the most common primary uterine disorder seen in pubescent females. Haller et al. (1978) reviewed 350 females under age 15 who underwent pelvic ultrasound and found that 60% were pregnant. Ultrasound detects intrauterine pregnancy with great accuracy beyond eight weeks of gestation. Earlier in gestation, human chorionic gonadotropin assay greatly assists interpretation of the ultrasound image. The distinction between ectopic pregnancy and very early intrauterine pregnancy requires correlation of the ultrasound image with human chorionic gonadotropin levels, history, and physical examination.

Structural abnormalities   Vaginal duplication and hydrometrocolpos are the most common structural vaginal abnormalities which cause discomfort. The latter is easily detected with ultrasound. Occasionally, urinary tract abnormalities, such as an ectopic ureterocele, will be visualized on sonography of the vagina (McCarthy and Taylor, 1983). If a vaginal abnormality is identified, the kidneys should also be evaluated, as there is an established relationship between renal abnormalities and vaginal malformations.

Ovarian disorders   The ovaries show the widest range of variation in size and response to hormonal stimulation of any of the pelvic organs (Fig. 9–1). Flagrant ovarian polycystic disease is easily diagnosed. However, the Stein-Leventhal form of polycystic ovarian disease is often difficult to distinguish from the normal appearance of the ovary with developing follicles. Interpretation of subtle changes in ovarian pathology, particularly those related to follicles and cystic ovarian disease, requires close correlation with the phases of the menstrual cycle (Yeh et al., 1987).

True tumors of the ovary occur uncommonly in teenagers. Ovarian teratoma (Fig. 9–2) is the most common of these lesions and often exhibits a characteristic, highly echogenic appearance because of the presence of calcium. Ultrasound also aids

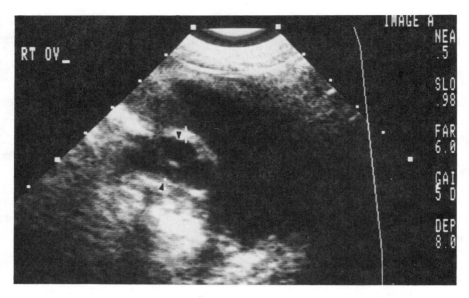

9–1   Ultrasound demonstrated multiple ovarian cysts probably representing polycystic ovarian disease.

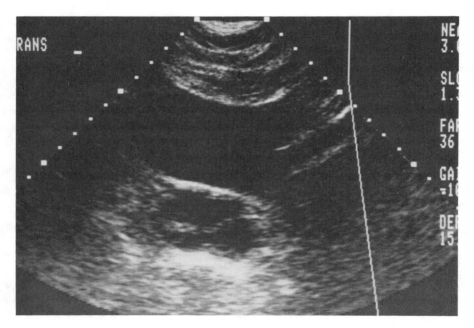

9–2   Ultrasound identified a cystadenoma of the left ovary, a benign ovarian tumor.

evaluation of ovarian torsion, whether acute with abrupt onset of severe pain, or chronic, with recurrent episodes of abdominal pain (Fig. 9–3). In chronic torsion the ovary is often hemorrhagic and appears solid on ultrasound, causing confusion with a true ovarian tumor.

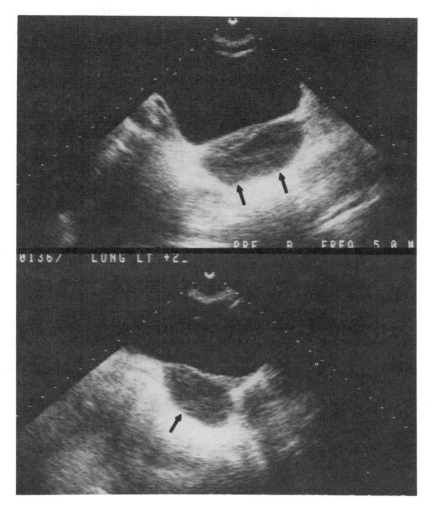

9–3 Ultrasound documented a mixed density predominantly solid L ovarian mass. At surgery this was chronic torsion of the left ovary.

Inflammatory processes All of the pelvic and abdominal organs can be involved with inflammatory disease or other processes that cause pain. Ultrasound can identify pelvic inflammatory disease, appendicitis, acute urinary tract obstruction, pancreatitis, cholecystitis, cholelithiasis, and regional enteritis, although another imaging modality may be required to improve the specificity of the diagnosis. Ultrasound in pelvic inflammatory disease classically identifies a mixed-density cystic and solid adnexal mass; occasionally, free fluid can be identified in the cul-de-sac. Differentiation of PID from appendicitis with ultrasound is possible if the cecum and normal appendix can be identified. Occasionally, however, the cecum and appendix may not be involved in the inflammatory process, or the appendix may not be visualized, which makes differentiation between PID, Crohn disease, and appendicitis difficult. An edematous gallbladder or absent gallbladder on ultrasound suggest cholelithiasis or cholecystitis. In acute pancreatitis the organ is enlarged and hypoechogenic. Renal and ureteral abnormalities appear readily on ultrasound images.

Other Imaging Techniques   Other useful imaging techniques include plain radiographs, contrast studies of the gastrointestinal and urinary tracts, computed tomography, and magnetic resonance imaging. Plain radiographs demonstrate bowel obstruction, perforation, radioopaque stones, such as appendicoliths or renal calculi, and the stool impactions found in constipated patients. Contrast studies aid in the diagnosis of inflammatory bowel disease, ulcers, structural bowel abnormalities, and hydroureteronephrosis. In addition, barium enema improves diagnostic accuracy in appendicitis (Lewin et al., 1978), although presence of an appendicolith on plain radiograph obviates the need for the contrast study.

Abdominal and pelvic CT is easily performed but should be reserved as a secondary imaging technique because of cost and ionizing radiation. Siegel et al. (1981) reported that CT provided supplementary diagnostic information in about 30% of pediatric patients with pelvic disorders and improved anatomic localization in about 60%. Acute abdominal trauma represents the major indication for CT evaluation (Berger and Kuhn, 1981; Kuhn, 1985). Its value lies in its ability to evaluate multiple organs, to detect accurately small amounts of intraperitoneal fluid or air, to visualize boney structures, and to assess vascular integrity of abdominal and pelvic organs when contrast is used. Magnetic resonance imaging will probably replace CT for many evaluations in the future, but MRI techniques are currently in early stages of development (Hricak, 1986).

Recommendations   Overall, ultrasound is the best initial choice for the screening evaluation of an adolescent with abdominal or pelvic pain. It allows evaluation of multiple organs with minimal discomfort and risk and detects abnormalities with a high degree of sensitivity. Although a normal ultrasound does not completely exclude organic pathology, it greatly reduces the likelihood that a definable lesion will be found. If the ultrasound is normal but symptoms persist, or if the ultrasound is clearly abnormal, consultation with the radiologist will determine further imaging needs and strategy.

Acute Abdominal Pain

Acute abdominal pain presents most commonly in the second decade of life and may be more common in females than in males (Edwards et al., 1985; Schuster, 1986a; Thomson, 1986). Certain causes of acute abdominal pain have a definite sex predilection in adolescents, with urinary tract infection and cholelithiasis much more common in girls, and appendicitis and trauma more common in boys. Obviously, abdominal pain which originates in the female reproductive tract presents a special case.

Surveys (Jones, 1969; de Dombal, 1979; Drake, 1980; Crossley, 1982) of patients of all ages, both male and female, admitted to hospital because of acute abdominal pain consistently identify acute appendicitis as the single most common diagnosis, but medical or gynecologic diagnoses are more common overall than appendicitis. These surveys also report spontaneous resolution of acute abdominal pain in 30%–40% of patients. Approximately 50% of patients hospitalized for acute abdominal pain have a discharge diagnosis of "nonspecific" pain. Diagnosis is more difficult in women than in men, and for the group aged 1–20 years there is a 30% rate of diagnostic error. Only a small number of patients with complaint of acute abdominal pain eventually prove to have the need for surgical exploration. Careful evaluation and observation allows timely selection of those patients in need of urgent surgery and reduces the number of patients operated on. Early detection of acute surgical conditions is clearly important to reduce to the absolute minimum the morbidity and mortality that accompanies such conditions.

Faced with an acutely ill teenage girl who complains of abdominal pain, the first task is to identify the need for surgical intervention. There is no clinical presentation, set of laboratory test results, or imaging procedure that uniquely identifies every process that causes acute abdominal pain, although certain historical and clinical features have a high likelihood of association with surgically remediable processes. Physicians must rely on experience and knowledge of pathophysiology to interpret history, physical findings, and test results and to generate a focused differential diagnosis. Careful assessment of the onset of abdominal pain (especially timing), the location, character, and severity of pain, plus any associated signs and symptoms provide the information necessary for the early stages of the evaluation process (Liebman and Thaler, 1978; Way, 1983).

Recurrent Abdominal Pain

Although acute abdominal pain prompts great anxiety among physicians, patients, and parents, recurrent abdominal pain is much more frequently encountered in day to day practice. Its prevalence, furthermore, means that recurrent pain has a much greater impact on the lives of adolescents (and their families) than does acute pain. Approximately 10%–18% of children from late elementary school through high school will experience recurrent episodes of abdominal pain over periods longer than three months (Pringle et al., 1966; Oster, 1972; Apley and Hale, 1973; Miller et al., 1974; Apley, 1975; Parcel et al., 1977). Apley and Naish (1958) found that girls were more commonly affected with recurrent abdominal pain than boys and that 9 years was the age of peak onset for girls. Galler et al. (1980) reported unpublished observations which identified a peak of recurrent abdominal pain in early adolescence. Demographic data have consistently documented an overrepresentation of female adolescents in the population with recurrent abdominal pain (Engel, 1959; Oster, 1972; Parcel et al., 1977; Starfield et al., 1980; Adelman and Metcalf, 1983); similar female overrepresentation exists in the population of young adults referred for evaluation of recurrent abdominal pain (Adelman and Metcalf, 1983). Most reviews of recurrent abdominal pain in children from Western Europe and the United States report a low prevalence of organic illness (Apley, 1975; Christensen and Mortenson, 1975; Berger et al., 1977).

The approach to the adolescent with recurrent abdominal pain demands patience, thoroughness, and willingness to explain details of the diagnostic process to the patient and her parents (Barr, 1983; Levine and Rappaport, 1984; Coleman and Levine, 1986). Unless the pain presents acutely, the diagnosis does not have to be made in one office visit. History and physical examination will provide the information necessary to exclude processes which require rapid surgical referral. Pain localized to areas other than the midline has a higher likelihood of an organic etiology, as does pain described precisely and consistently (Spiro, 1970).

All physicians have experienced the intense desire on the part of many parents to identify an easily treatable cause for the pain which affects their children, despite the low prevalence of disease among sufferers of recurrent pain. Demands for complex, costly, often invasive evaluations, and unwillingness to accept a diagnosis made without these tests, make the physician's role difficult and frustrating. All too often physicians "set themselves up" for such an interaction by failure to explain adequately the results of historical and physical findings and their relationship or lack of relationship with the presenting symptom. Furthermore, the common medical practice of "ruling out" diseases, even when rare or unlikely, sends a message to patients that only physical illness can cause abdominal pain, with the resultant demand that all possible causes be investigated. Popular media support the exclusionary approach by their reports of sensational diagnoses made after long, extensive (and expensive) investigations. Parental dissatisfaction or anxiety leads to doctor shopping, as well as self-referral to nontraditional, unorthodox, or potentially harmful providers of "health care." An analagous physician response to insecurity or frustration results in referral to numerous medical specialists and may lead to a series of interconsultant referrals. Parental or physician referral to other health care providers frequently causes the primary physician to lose contact with the patient.

Selected Causes of Nongynecologic Abdominal Pain

Gastrointestinal Disorders

Acute Appendicitis   Adolescents have the highest rate of acute appendicitis (Schrock, 1983; Smith, 1985; Strahlman, 1987). The average age of occurrence is 11 years, and more than half of all cases occur between age 10 and 19 (Folkman, 1979). The complication rate (Savrin and Clatworthy, 1979) remains persistently high because at least half of all patients have referral for surgical care only after perforation has occurred and peritonitis has developed. Perforation is most common in the very young and the elderly, but approximately one-third of adolescents have a perforated appendix at the time of initial diagnosis. Parents contribute to delayed diagnosis in approximately one-half of cases because they fail to recognize the severity of their child's illness. Physicians contribute to diagnostic delay in the other half by failure to recognize the signs of the "acute surgical abdomen." Most patients seek medical attention only after the pain has localized in the right lower quadrant, 12 or more hours after onset. The appendix perforates approximately 36 hours after the onset of pain. Diagnostic difficulty arises if the appendix lies retrocecally, because pain may remain periumbilical for days without shift to the right lower quadrant, even if perforation occurs.

    Differential diagnosis   Differentiation between acute appendicitis and other acute abdominal complaints may present a difficult diagnostic problem (Gilmore et al., 1975; Liebman and Thaler, 1978; Way, 1983). In adolescent girls particular attention must be paid to the possibility of urinary tract infection, pregnancy (especially ectopic pregnancy), and acute gynecologic infections. Acute gastroenteritis and mesenteric adenitis also complicate the diagnostic process. This is especially true for the gastroenteritis caused by *Yersinia*. Numerous other problems may mimic acute appendicitis, including peptic ulcer disease, sickle cell crisis, inflammatory bowel disease, dysfunctional gynecologic pain, and pneumonia, when pain is referred to the abdomen.

    In particular, pelvic inflammatory disease and appendicitis may have similar features. Bongard et al. (1985) prospectively studied a group of women with acute abdominal pain and identified features of history, clinical course, and pelvic/abdominal examination which allowed them to distinguish PID from appendicitis. Nausea and vomiting accompanied PID in only one-half of cases, contrasted with their occurrence in almost all cases of appendicitis. Symptom duration was greater than 48 hours for

PID compared with less than 24 hours for appendicitis. History of unusual vaginal bleeding and previous episodes of sexually transmitted disease occurred more commonly with PID than with acute appendicitis. When adnexal tenderness accompanied appendicitis, it occurred most often on the right side. More commonly, adnexal tenderness did not occur in appendicitis. PID most commonly had bilateral adnexal tenderness on pelvic examination. Both appendicitis and PID occurred throughout the menstrual cycle.

History　An episode of appendicitis begins with nonspecific symptoms that may include decreased appetite and general malaise, but pain and fever are the most consistent historical features. Pain begins as a colicky periumbilical discomfort which intensifies and becomes more of a steady pain over several hours. Fever characteristically follows the onset of pain and remains low grade until perforation occurs. Vomiting, when it occurs, follows the onset of pain. After the periumbilical pain reaches a peak, right lower quadrant pain develops as inflammatory fluid causes irritation of the parietal peritoneum adjacent to the inflamed appendix. Movement, cough, and straining at bowel movement aggravate the pain once it has shifted into the right lower quadrant, an important clue to the presence of peritoneal irritation. Most patients vomit at some time during the course of acute appendicitis, and anorexia often occurs in the absence of vomiting. Fever tends to be low grade in nonperforated appendicitis; a high fever or associated shaking chills suggest perforation of the appendix or another diagnosis. Patients may complain of constipation, "gas," or diarrhea.

Physical examination　Observation provides some of the best clues to the stage of appendicitis. If evaluated very early in the course of acute appendicitis, a patient may not appear especially uncomfortable and may not demonstrate the clues which suggest peritoneal irritation. With the passage of time, generally a few hours at most, more classic features of appendicitis will develop and allow surgical consultation and preparation for surgery. On the other hand, a girl who lies still and resists any motion is likely to have peritoneal inflammation and may have a perforated appendix; emergency surgical intervention is needed.

Before peritoneal irritation begins, pain is localized by the patient to the periumbilical area. Later in the course of appendicitis, most teenagers localize abdominal pain by pointing with one finger to a spot in the right lower quadrant. Auscultation reveals diminished bowel sounds in most cases, but they may be normal or hyperactive. Percussion produces discomfort in the right lower quadrant, even when the percussion is done at a site distant. Gentle palpation of the abdomen will reveal muscle rigidity, which indicates involuntary guarding, but no muscle tenderness. The skin of the right lower quadrant may be extremely sensitive to touch (hyperesthesia). Deeper palpation should begin as far away as possible from the site of maximal pain and progress towards that area.

Laboratory studies　White blood cell count with differential and urinalysis may provide clues to the presence of appendicitis, but only an appendicolith identified by plain x-ray of the abdomen consistently supports the diagnosis of appendicitis. Unfortunately, appendicoliths are not always visible. Barium enema improves diagnostic accuracy (Lewin et al., 1978). Ultrasound offers the least invasive screening evaluation.

Gastroenteritis　Most often viral in etiology and of short duration, gastroenteritis may occasionally result from bacterial infection and have a protracted course and serious consequences (Sack and Barker, 1986; Wyatt and Kapikian, 1987). The list of bacterial and viral pathogens is extensive (Pickering and Cleary, 1987; Bishop and Ulshen, 1988; Hamilton, 1988). Pain alone, without other gastrointestinal or systemic signs and symptoms, is uncommon in gastroenteritis.

Viral gastroenteritis   Rotavirus and the Norwalk agent are the most common viral causes of gastroenteritis. Both cause abdominal cramps, nausea, vomiting, diarrhea, and fever, although infection with the Norwalk agent causes more severe symptoms (Pickering and Cleary, 1987).

Salmonella   Gastroenteritis caused by *Salmonella* occurs in epidemics and usually affects infants and young children, although any age patient may be affected. Headache, chills, and abdominal pain are the initial symptoms, followed by fever, nausea, vomiting, and diarrhea. The organism is isolated from stool; blood cultures remain negative, in contrast to the septicemic form of *Salmonella* infection (Brandborg, 1978; Hornick, 1987a). Antibiotic treatment of the acute gastroenteritis is not indicated for most patients (Pickering, 1983).

Shigella   Bloody diarrhea, abdominal cramps, and fever characterize *Shigella* gastroenteritis. The illness is most severe in infants and young children, although adolescents may develop *Shigella* gastroenteritis. Culture of stool identifies the organism (Hornick, 1987b). Because ampicillin resistance has been reported with increased frequency, trimethoprim/sulfamethoxazole may be the treatment of choice (Pickering, 1983).

Traveller's diarrhea   Enteropathogenic *Escherichia coli* causes this form of gastroenteritis which typically has prominent abdominal cramps associated with profuse watery diarrhea but without systemic toxicity (Keusch, 1987a). History of travel to areas with poor sanitation points to this diagnosis. The organism and the enterotoxin can be identified in stool. Symptomatic and supportive therapy suffices during the several days of illness. Prevention is the best "therapy," but antibiotic prophylaxis with trimethoprim/sulfamethoxazole or doxycycline will greatly reduce risk of acquisition of the organism. Bismuth subsalicylate (Pepto Bismol®) also reduces risk of traveller's diarrhea (DuPont, 1985) but must be used with caution because of the association of Reye syndrome with salicylates.

Enteroinvasive E. coli   This organism usually causes moderate to severe illness with prominent fever, abdominal cramps, and watery diarrhea (Keusch, 1987b). Unlike *Shigella* enteritis, grossly bloody and mucus-containing stools are not common with enteroinvasive *E. coli* diarrhea. The route of infection has not been identified for most cases but is occasionally food-borne. Diagnostic approach includes stool culture which will be negative for gastrointestinal pathogens. A stool smear will show numerous leukocytes. Identification of the causative strain of *E. coli* is usually difficult.

Staphylococcal food poisoning   Ingestion of preformed toxin from food contaminated with *Staphylococcus aureus* results in rapid onset of cramping gastrointestinal pain and profuse vomiting and diarrhea. Systemic shock may develop (Eisenberg, 1985; Pickering and Cleary, 1987).

Yersinia and Campylobacter   In recent years, *Yersinia enterocoliticus* and *Campylobacter pylori* have been identified as relatively common causes of gastroenteritis. *Yersinia* (Weinstein, 1987), in particular, may mimic acute appendicitis because of its tendency to cause mesenteric adenitis. In addition, infection with this organism may produce small bowel lesions that mimic those of Crohn disease. Available data do not support the need for antibiotic treatment of *Yersinia* gastroenteritis (Pickering, 1983).

Infection with *Campylobacter* has burning midepigastric pain as a major symptom. This organism frequently produces gastric and duodenal ulcers. Over 60% of adults with preexisting peptic ulcer disease have *Campylobacter* isolated from biopsies of antral mucosa. This gastroenteritis usually does not need antibiotic therapy. When clinically indicated, erythromycin is the drug of choice (Pickering, 1983).

Aeromonas   A more uncommon cause of gastroenteritis, but one associated with abdominal cramps, *Aeromonas hydrophila* has been identified in adolescents and adults. Stool culture isolates this bacterial species. Treatment with trimethoprim/ sulfamethoxazole may be effective, but detailed guidelines for treatment have yet to be developed (Pickering and Cleary, 1987; Bishop and Ulshen, 1988).

Giardia lamblia   Gastroenteritis caused by *Giardia* infestation may have associated abdominal pain which is more often recurrent than truly acute. *Giardia* infestation is characterized by abdominal distention, passage of flatus and, often, weight loss caused by malabsorption (Pickering and Cleary, 1987).

Constipation   Constipation (stool retention) frequently causes abdominal pain in the teenager (Loening-Baucke, 1987). Unfortunately, many teenagers and their parents are not aware of the presence of constipation. Therefore, the physician has to consider constipation as a cause of abdominal pain, ask appropriate questions, and not exclude it simply because the patient gives a history of daily bowel movements. Appropriate abdominal and rectal examination are mandatory before constipation can be excluded as a cause of pain.

History   Acute, recurrent, or chronic abdominal pain may be reported by teenagers who have constipation. Some teenagers will have severe attacks of abdominal pain daily before each bowel movement or for several days before a large bowel movement. Others suffer from vague chronic abdominal pains or may have the onset of abdominal pain with meals, possibly related to the gastrocolic reflex. The relationship of pain to bowel movements varies among different patients but is usually quite consistent for an individual.

A careful history of bowel movement interval, size, and consistency usually reveals underlying constipation. Some teenagers have daily bowel movements but apparently do not evacuate completely, as evidenced by history of periodic passage of very large amounts of stool, once every 3 to 30 days. Occasionally the interval between huge bowel movements is longer. Most parents have not observed the stooling pattern of their teenagers, but, if asked, will remember stools which clogged the toilet. Some patients may not have signs of overt constipation at the time of abdominal pain, but the past history reveals enema treatment, laxative treatment, fecal soiling, or constipation with or without abdominal pain. Fecal soiling may be present and occur occasionally, once a day, or many times a day, but few teenagers or parents relate the soiling to constipation, and many are too embarrassed to disclose this information, except when asked about it directly.

One fourth of constipated teenagers experience daytime urinary incontinence. Typically, the daytime incontinence consists of small leaks once or many times daily. Nighttime enuresis is present in one-fourth of patients. Thirteen percent give a history of previous urinary tract infection (Loening-Baucke, 1987).

Rare organic causes for constipation include disorders of the spinal cord, cerebral palsy, hypotonia, hypothyroidism, cystic fibrosis, and Hirschsprung disease. Constipation may also be due to dietary factors or drugs like methylphenidate, imipramine, and phenytoin.

Physical examination   The physical examination can provide definite support for the diagnosis of constipation. A large abdominal mass may extend throughout the entire colon but more commonly is felt in the midline suprapubic area. Sometimes the mass fills the left lower quadrant or the right lower quadrant. The absence of an abdominal fecal mass does not rule out constipation as a cause of pain, however.

Rectal examination must be performed on every patient. Inspection of the anal opening may show protruding fecal material. Sometimes an anterior location of the anus is recognized. Often the rectum is packed with stool either of hard consistency, or, more commonly, the outside of the fecal impaction feels like clay and the core of the impaction is rock hard. Sometimes the retained stool is soft or loose. It is mandatory to ask when the last bowel movement occurred. A recent bowel movement may have emptied the rectum but not the sigmoid and descending colon.

Laboratory and radiographic evaluation   A supine abdominal roentgenogram carefully evaluated for colonic and rectal stool is helpful if stool retention is suspected but not detected on abdominal or rectal examination. All girls should have urinalysis and urine culture to screen for the presence of urinary tract infection. Blood or radiologic studies (other than plain abdominal film) are rarely necessary. A barium enema is seldom necessary.

Management Plan   The majority of teenagers with constipation will benefit from a precise, well organized plan designed to clear fecal impaction, prevent future impaction, and promote regular bowel habits. Although abdominal pain may have begun only recently, constipation frequently has persisted over many months or many years. Long-term treatment for months or even years may be necessary.

Management of constipation requires removal of impacted stool and prevention of recurrent impactions. Enemas are used for disimpaction, followed by daily laxatives to promote regular bowel habits and prevent abdominal pain. Support and encouragement with telephone consultations greatly enhance compliance and treatment outcome and allow assessment of laxative effectiveness and relief from abdominal pain. Reevaluation should be scheduled in one month to review symptoms and compliance and to repeat abdominal and rectal examinations. The patient is seen again approximately 3 months later to evaluate whether the laxative could be slowly discontinued or whether it is necessary to increase the dose to prevent recurrence of constipation and abdominal pain.

Enemas   Initial disimpaction should always be accomplished in the physician's office, most often with an adult sized hypertonic phosphate enema (4½ oz). In most teenagers, one to two enemas will result in good bowel cleanout, but occasionally, in severely impacted patients, a mixture of 50% milk and 50% molasses may be needed for disimpaction, using a volume tolerated by the patient, up to 1,000 ml each time, until disimpacted.

Laxatives   Daily defecation is maintained by daily administration of laxatives, such as milk of magnesia, beginning on the evening following the disimpaction. In severe constipation with rock hard stools, the starting dosage of milk of magnesia is approximately 2 cc/kg body weight per day given with the evening meal. In teenagers who have fecal retention of mostly soft-formed stools, usually 1 cc/kg body weight daily is adequate. Laxative dose should be individualized after the initial starting dose and adjusted to induce 1–2 bowel movements per day. Bowel movements should be loose enough to ensure complete emptying of the lower bowel every day. Milk of magnesia is available in liquid or tablet form. The liquid may be mixed with lemon juice, chocolate syrup, or other flavoring agents to make a more palatable mixture. Milk of magnesia concentrate reduces the volume necessary for each dose by approximately two-thirds. If the teenager refuses milk of magnesia, mineral oil may be substituted in approximately the same dose as the milk of magnesia. Another laxative, Chronulac®, contains lactulose, galactose, lactose, and other nonabsorbed sugars. The usual dose is from 15 to 60 ml daily.

Teenagers may also choose to use 10-mg bisacodyl suppositories rather than daily oral laxatives. If suppositories are chosen, one should be inserted into the rectum once daily at a regular time. Bisacodyl stimulates large bowel peristalsis. It is effective within 15–60 minutes.

Whether oral laxatives or rectal suppositories are chosen, therapy should continue on a daily basis for a minimum of 2 months. This allows improvement of rectosigmoid muscle tone and, thus, enhances the ability of the teenager to recognize distention of the bowel by a fecal bolus. The actual choice of medication is not as important as the teenager's compliance with the treatment regimen.

Toilet use   The constipated bowel needs to be retrained. This means encouraging the teenager to sit on the toilet for up to 5 minutes three times a day, following meals. The gastrocolic reflex, which goes into effect shortly after a meal, should be used to advantage. The teenager needs to keep a daily record of bowel movements, abdominal pain episodes, and laxative use. This allows the physician to evaluate the effectiveness of the laxative prescription and to make the necessary adjustments when abdominal pain ceases and bowel function has improved. Occasionally, mild constipation will improve during a 1-month trial of more frequent and timed toilet sitting, without need for laxatives.

High fiber diet   All constipated teenagers and their families should receive information about high fiber diet. They should be given verbal and written instructions about the value of fruits, vegetables, bran, natural cereals, and whole grains. Bulk laxatives containing dietary fiber from the husk psyllium seed are useful for teenagers who are unable or unwilling to increase the fiber content of their diet (Burkitt and Meisner, 1979; Committee on Nutrition, 1981; Yang and Banwell, 1986).

Outcome   Most teenagers with abdominal pain caused by constipation are compliant with treatment and experience relief from abdominal pain. We evaluated our teenagers with abdominal pain and constipation 12 months after the initial visit. Almost half (48%) had recovered from constipation, abdominal pain, and fecal soiling, and were off laxatives; 39% still used laxatives to prevent constipation and abdominal pain; and 11% had discontinued laxatives but still experienced constipation and abdominal pain.

The Irritable Bowel Syndrome   The most common gastrointestinal problem identified in adults is the irritable bowel syndrome which consists of abdominal pain, altered bowel habits (alternating constipation and diarrhea), and absence of detectable organic pathology (Schuster, 1986b; Silverberg, 1983). Existence of this syndrome in children with recurrent abdominal pain has been controversial, but Silverberg and Daum (1979) described its characteristic features in a large group of children and adolescents. Children tend to complain of recurrent abdominal pain or have nonspecific diarrhea, while adolescents have a clinical presentation identical to the adult syndrome. Schuster (1986b) identified the onset of the adult form of irritable bowel syndrome in late adolescence and noted a female predominance. The syndrome appears to reflect exaggerated intestinal motility with excessively strong, spastic contractions of either the segmenting type, which promote constipation, or the propulsive type, which cause diarrhea. Symptoms are usually intermittent, and there may be symptom-free periods, days to weeks in duration. Location and nature of pain tend to be consistent for any one patient, but pain descriptions may vary from patient to patient. Cramping lower abdominal pain is most common. Pain may remit temporarily after bowel movement. Bowel habits also tend to remain consistent for each patient, with variability among different patients. Pellet stools and narrow, formed stools alternate with loose, diarrheal stools accompanied by flatus and mucus. Epigastric discomfort, "heartburn," and nausea may accompany altered bowel habits in 25%–50% of patients. Anxiety, depression, and somatization are characteristic psychological findings in adults with the irritable bowel syndrome (Whitehead and Schuster, 1979). Pain does not wake the patient from sleep. Gastrointestinal bleeding and weight loss are *not* part of the syndrome. The most effective therapy addresses disordered bowel habits and encourages the patient to prevent pain by avoidance of constipation and diarrhea. A treatment plan similar to that discussed in the section on constipation with special attention to increased dietary fiber is most likely to establish regular bowel habits in patients with constipation-prone irritable bowel syndrome. Attention to the emotional component of this syndrome is important. Careful discussion of the absence of disease may greatly reduce anxiety. Medications such as antispasmodics have not proven helpful for most patients.

Inflammatory Bowel Disease   Ulcerative colitis and Crohn disease have abdominal pain as a prominent symptom (Ament, 1975; Burbige et al., 1975; Farmer, 1980; Messer and Keating, 1980; Daum and Aigues, 1983; Kirschner, 1988). Pain tends to be recurrent or chronic but may present acutely, along with fever and leukocytosis, and mimic appendicitis. Pain occurs more commonly in Crohn disease than in ulcerative colitis. Diarrhea and bloody stools also occur with both processes, but most often with ulcerative colitis. Retardation of physical growth and pubertal development, weight loss, low grade fever, malaise anorexia, arthralgias, arthritis, skin rashes (including erythema nodosum, pyoderma granulosum, and papulonecrotic lesions), digital clubbing, or aphthous lesions in the mouth may accompany or precede development of gastrointestinal symptoms. Adolescents with perianal lesions are much more likely to have Crohn disease than ulcerative colitis. Renal complications of Crohn disease include hydronephrosis, from obstruction of the ureter by an inflammatory mass (Present et al., 1969), and nephrolithiasis (Chadwick et al., 1973). Renal stones may also develop in ulcerative colitis (Bennett and Hughes, 1972; Chadwick et al., 1973). Crohn disease occasionally may present with abdominal pain and chronic constipation, along with other extraintestinal manifestations, such as retarded pubertal development. Diagnosis of inflammatory bowel disease first depends on its inclusion in the differential diagnosis of abdominal pain. Radiologic contrast studies, sigmoidoscopy, and colonoscopy, with mucosal biopsy, confirm the diagnosis. Treatment is well described in recent reviews (Gryboski, 1981; Messer and Keating, 1980; Kirschner, 1988).

Peptic Ulcer Disease   Adolescents with duodenal or gastric ulcers may have symptoms which fit the adult pattern of peptic ulcer disease: pain 1 to 3 hours after meals, nocturnal pain, recurrent vomiting, relief of pain with food or antacids, and symptom-free periods (Robb et al., 1972; Nord, 1983). However, atypical symptoms are especially common in young adolescents and may delay diagnosis (Bendig, 1985). Complaint of abdominal pain may focus on the midepigastric area, but in some adolescents pain may be poorly localized and vaguely described. Timing of pain is quite variable and ranges from intermittent to continuous; the relationship between pain and meals has similar variability. Painless bleeding may signal the presence of peptic ulcer in a previously asymptomatic patient (Tam et al., 1986). The likelihood that peptic ulcer disease is the cause of an adolescent's abdominal pain increases with a personal history of recurrent vomiting, gastrointestinal bleeding, or nocturnal pain, or a history of ulcer disease in parents or siblings.

Physical examination may identify tenderness in the midepigastric area and guaiac-positive stools, or it may be unremarkable except for nonspecific discomfort with abdominal palpation. High clinical suspicion of peptic ulcer disease should lead to more definitive evaluation. Endoscopy has replaced barium contrast studies as the method of choice for diagnosis of duodenal or peptic ulcer disease because of its greater sensitivity and specificity (Bendig, 1985).

Goals of treatment include relief of symptoms, ulcer healing, and prevention of recurrence and complications. Antacids and the H-2 receptor antagonists, cimetidine and ranitidine, offer the most predictable and consistent therapeutic results. Antacids, preferably liquid, taken between meals and at bedtime, buffer gastric activity and relieve pain. If pain is severe, more frequent dosing may help reduce symptoms. Cimetidine, 5–10 mg/kg/dose, QID, or ranitidine, 1.5–1.9 mg/kg/dose, BID, both inhibit gastric acid secretion. Side effects are minimal. Dietary changes and anticholinergics have little to offer for most adolescents with peptic ulcer disease. Rare complications, such as perforation, obstruction, uncontrollable bleeding, or intractable symptoms, may require surgical therapy. With medical therapy recurrence rate is high (Puri et al., 1978).

Bowel Obstruction   Mechanical obstruction of the bowel, paralytic ileus, or pseudoobstruction cause abdominal pain with associated vomiting, abdominal distention, and obstipation. Patients complain of paroxysmal cramping pain. The interval between painful episodes may be as short as 4–5 minutes with proximal bowel obstruction. Pain-free intervals are longer with more distal lesions. The majority of mechanical obstruction in adolescents occurs with intrinsic bowel disease (such as Crohn disease), as a result of adhesions from prior surgery or pelvic inflammatory disease, or because of intussusception associated with a Meckel diverticulum. Rarely, a congenital anomaly of midgut malrotation may present in adolescence with pain and obstruction (Brandt et al., 1985). Constipation causes mechanical bowel obstruction, although not usually complete obstruction. Paralytic ileus accompanies peritonitis, hypokalemia (e.g., anorexia nervosa), drugs, and surgery. Idiopathic intestinal pseudoobstruction is a syndrome in which functional obstruction with signs and symptoms indistinguishable from those produced by mechanical obstruction occur as a result of abnormal bowel and sphincter muscle activity (Stanghellini et al., 1987). Evaluation of presumed bowel obstruction must identify those patients who require surgical therapy to prevent strangulation and ischemia of bowel.

Eating Disorders   Diagnostic criteria for anorexia nervosa (Feighner et al., 1972) and bulimia (American Psychiatric Association, 1980) do not include abdominal pain, yet patients with both syndromes may complain of either acute or recurrent abdominal pain. The metabolic and physical consequences of repeated vomiting may cause ileus, gastritis, esophagitis, Mallory-Weiss tears of gastric and esophageal mucosa, and peptic ulcerations. Gastric distention during refeeding of an anorectic patient may also cause pain. The bulimic adolescent may have abdominal discomfort after binge eating, just before self-induced vomiting.

Abdominal Trauma   Trauma from vehicular accidents and falls may produce abdominal injury and resultant pain. Physical abuse is another important cause of abdominal trauma. Abdominal pain that follows trauma most commonly reflects blunt injury to the spleen, kidney, liver, or bowel. Pancreatic trauma occurs relatively uncommonly. In only 5%–15% of cases of trauma does a penetrating injury occur. Liver and bowel most often incur injury from penetrating trauma (Ramenofsky, 1987). Jewett et al. (1988) review a consequence of blunt abdominal trauma that may cause diagnostic confusion and delay: intramural hematoma of the duodenum. This uncommon injury presents with abdominal pain and vomiting and may not come to medical attention for more than 24 hours after the traumatic event. Ramenofsky (1987) describes an approach to the acutely injured child or adolescent. Computed tomography has proved to be the best imaging modality (Berger and Kuhn, 1981; Kuhn, 1985).

Renal/Urinary Tract Causes of Pain

Urinary Tract Infection   Infection of the urinary tract produces acute or recurrent abdominal pain throughout childhood and adolescence, interferes with activities, and may have serious long-term sequelae (Kunin, 1979). With infection localized to the bladder and urethra, adolescent girls typically give a history of dysuria, frequency, urgency, and lower midline abdominal pain. They may also notice foul smelling or bloody urine. Fever may be absent or minimal. The association of voiding symptoms with high fever, chills, and flank pain suggests pyelonephritis. *E. coli* causes approximately 80% of urinary tract infections, but other organisms, including *Klebsiella* species, *Proteus* species, and enterococci, may cause infection. Another cause of voiding symptoms and lower abdominal discomfort is the dysuria-pyuria syndrome, described in adult women who have persistent voiding symptoms but negative or "nonsignificant" urine cultures (Komaroff, 1984). This syndrome probably occurs in adolescents. *Staphylococcus saprophyticus* and *Chlamydia trachomatis* have been identified as common causes of the dysuria-pyuria syndrome.

Diagnosis of urinary tract infection relies on urine cultures which will detect >50,000 colony-forming units per ml except in the dysuria-pyuria syndrome when colony counts less than 10,000 per ml are common. Detection of pyuria, hematuria, or proteinuria on urinalysis aids in the diagnosis of infection but is not specific for infection.

Treatment with antibiotics for 10–14 days has been the standard (Kunin, 1979) until recently, when short course regimens have been advocated for adult women. Moffatt and co-workers (1988) reviewed all of the studies of short course therapy in children and adolescents and found all to be methodologically flawed. Examinations of studies which support the efficacy of short course therapy for adults with urinary tract infection have identified similar methodologic flaws (Fihn and Stamm, 1985; Philbrick and Bracikowski, 1985). Until better studies demonstrate efficacy of short course therapy for children and adolescents, standard 10-day antibiotic therapy remains the treatment of choice.

Henoch-Schoenlein Purpura   This vasculitis is also known as anaphylactoid purpura and primarily affects the young child, but adolescents and adults may also develop HSP. Abdominal pain, purpura, joint pain, and glomerulonephritis are the major features of this syndrome. Gastrointestinal and renal complications appear to occur more frequently in adolescents and adults than in children as do recurrent episodes of symptomatic HSP (Allen et al., 1960; Ballard et al., 1970; Meadow et al., 1972; Kobayashi et al., 1977).

Diagnosis of HSP is based on the clinical features. Gastrointestinal, joint, skin, or renal aspects of the syndrome may occur alone or in combination. The most common gastrointestinal complaint is cramping pain. Ileus occurs frequently, and intussusception may occasionally develop. The purpuric rash characteristically appears on dependent areas, especially legs and buttocks. The nonrenal symptomatology may fluctuate for a period up to several weeks before resolution. In general, hematuria follows the other clinical features of this syndrome, but it may be the presenting complaint. Approximately 80% of patients develop hematuria within 1 month after onset of other manifestations. Hematuria may persist for several months but usually resolves without residual renal damage.

Treatment of Henoch-Schoenlein purpura is largely symptomatic, although steroid therapy has been advocated for patients with severe abdominal pain (Allen et al., 1960). Glasier et al. (1981) noted that abdominal pain was self-limited, and Rosenblum and Winter (1987) found no difference in duration or complication rate among patients with Henoch-Schoenlein purpura treated or not treated with steroids. They questioned the value of steroids in this syndrome and suggested a prospective, controlled study to address the issue.

Urinary Tract Stones Acute ureteral obstruction that occurs with passage of renal stones produces severe colic, with pain located in the flank and radiating to the groin. Urinary stones occur more commonly in adults (Burton and Smolev, 1986) than children and adolescents (Stapleton, 1986). Approximately 70% of stones in the pediatric population are comprised of calcium oxalate and have a tendency to present as asymptomatic hematuria (Stapleton, 1986). Urinalysis has an important role in evaluation of suspected urinary stones, as does renal excretion of calcium, oxalate, uric acid, and cystine.

Congenital Abnormalities Congenital urinary tract obstruction or hydronephrosis caused by vesicoureteral reflex may occasionally be undetected until adolescence (Dunn et al., 1978). Abdominal discomfort, recurrent urinary tract infections, an indistinct abdominal mass which represents the enlarged ureter and kidney, and inability to concentrate the urine all point to the need for urinary tract imaging. History of enuresis often suggests lack of urine-concentrating ability.

Hemolytic-Uremic Syndrome (HUS) HUS may present with abdominal pain and bloody diarrhea. Elevated serum creatinine and urea nitrogen, and evidence of hemolysis, such as schistocytes, helmet cells, and anemia, confirm the diagnosis (Berman, 1972; Kaplan and Proesmans, 1987).

Acute Renal Vein Thrombosis Adolescent girls with sudden onset of flank and back pain may have acute renal vein thrombosis. In adults, renal vein thrombosis occurs as a primary renal disease or with thromboembolic disease, pregnancy, lymphoma, and retroperitoneal tumors. Patients may vomit but typically do not have evidence of urinary tract infection. Urinalysis reveals microscopic hematuria and proteinuria. Pain progresses under observation, and edema may develop if urinary protein loss continues. Function of the affected kidney declines, and serum creatinine rises. Intravenous pyelography shows delayed nephrogram of the kidney, nonvisualization of the collecting system, and renal enlargement. Arteriography and venography confirm the diagnosis. Therapy may include anticoagulation because of concern about clot propagation and pulmonary embolus (Kettwich et al., 1980).

Hepatitis

Inflammatory diseases of the liver may have abdominal pain as one of the prominent symptoms. Viral hepatitis is the most common inflammatory liver disease and may present acutely or may be asymptomatic (Krugman, 1985). An acute "flu-like illness" more commonly accompanies hepatitis A than the other forms, but the different forms of viral hepatitis, including hepatitis A, hepatitis B, non-A, non-B hepatitis, and hepatitis D (delta), have clinical presentations which may be indistinguishable. Serologic evaluation must be used to differentiate between these forms of infection (Krugman, 1985; Aach, 1987a). In symptomatic patients, malaise, fatigue, fever, anorexia and weight loss frequently precede jaundice and midepigastric or right upper quadrant abdominal discomfort. The liver may be enlarged and tender. Other associated signs and symptoms include urticaria or other rashes, arthralgias and arthritis, lymphadenopathy, sore throat, diarrhea, and cough. Dark urine and acholic stools accompany icteric hepatitis. Anicteric hepatitis may be 2–6 times more frequent than the icteric form, especially in children and young adolescents. Symptomatic hepatitis occurs more frequently in adolescents and young adults than in children. Hepatitis A resolves completely in almost all patients at all ages, but both hepatitis B and non-A, non-B hepatitis may progress to chronic hepatitis or a carrier state (Berman et al., 1979).

History provides important information for differentiation among the types of hepatitis. Hepatitis A occurs most commonly in crowded, unsanitary environments. Rate of infection is three-fold higher among families in the lowest socioeconomic classes than among the middle and upper classes (Szmuness et al., 1976). Epidemics of hepatitis A have followed contamination of a variety of foods by the virus. If family members of a patient with hepatitis A do not receive prophylactic immune globulin, spread of the disease within the family is likely. Intravenous drug abusers, sexual partners of individuals known to have hepatitis B, and patients with sexually transmitted diseases have increased risk for acquisition of hepatitis B. Hepatitis D occurs in the presence of hepatitis B virus and causes both acute and chronic hepatitis. Non-A, non-B hepatitis accounts for approximately 90% of posttransfusion hepatitis. This form of hepatitis is diagnosed by exclusion of infection with hepatitis A, B, or D and the other forms of viral hepatitis, including Epstein Barr virus and cytomegalovirus (Krugman, 1985; Aach, 1987a). Pre- and postexposure protection against viral hepatitis are discussed in a recent publication from the Centers for Disease Control (ACIP, 1985).

Cholecystitis

Abdominal pain associated with gallbladder inflammation may occur in adolescent girls, although less commonly than in older women. Female predominance of gallbladder disease becomes apparent in early adolescence and eventually reaches the 3:1 to 4:1 female to male ratio noted in adults (Aach, 1987b). Obesity (Bennion and Grundy, 1975), oral contraceptive agents (Bennion et al., 1976), and Crohn disease (Pellerin et al., 1975) predispose to production of lithogenic bile with resultant stone formation. Patients with homozygous sickle cell disease have high prevalence of bilirubin gallstones (Barrett-Connor, 1968); cholesterol stones account for the majority of calculi in patients without hemolytic processes. Gallstone disease may mimic an acute abdominal crisis in patients with sickle cell anemia (Ariyan et al., 1976). Cholecystitis may be identified with or without gallstones, although the latter is more often seen in infants and young children (Ternberg and Keating, 1975). Obstruction of the duct or bile stasis typically precedes development of acute gallbladder infection.

Abdominal pain of acute onset, characterized as severe and unremitting and localized in the midepigastrium or right upper quadrant, signals acute cholecystitis. Pain may radiate to the right shoulder or back, but it may also be periumbilical and confounded with the pain of early appendicitis. Body temperature typically is not markedly elevated. Jaundice may occur in a small percentage of patients with acute attacks of pain. Tenderness to palpation of the right upper quadrant and, occasionally, guarding and rebound tenderness are the most common physical findings. Unfortunately, recurrent attacks of less severe pain in the upper abdomen may be indistinguishable from recurrent pain of various etiologies; unless gallbladder disease is considered in the differential diagnosis it may be undetected for long periods. Diagnosis is most easily made with ultrasound imaging (Greenberg et al., 1980).

Pancreatitis

Pancreatitis occurs uncommonly (Lerner and Lebenthal, 1986), usually after trauma or as a result of infection, drugs, or hereditary processes. A cause of severe, unremitting abdominal pain, pancreatitis most commonly enters the differential diagnosis after blunt abdominal trauma or when a patient has perplexing recurrent abdominal pain. Young adolescents may not provide the "classic" description of intense, continuous, knife-like pain which radiates to the back (Eichelberger et al., 1982). Pain is midepigastric, made worse with eating, and has associated fever, nausea, and vomiting. Pain does not resolve after vomiting. A patient with pancreatitis generally appears ill and has a slightly distended, tender abdomen. Shock may develop rapidly on occasion. If hemorrhagic pancreatitis occurs there may be a bluish discoloration in the periumbilical area (Cullen sign) or in the flanks (Grey-Turner sign). Diagnosis must have laboratory support, specifically, elevated serum amylase and lipase (Adams et al., 1968; Moosa, 1984).

Pneumonia

Lower lobe pneumonia may present with fever and abdominal pain. Pain may be located anywhere in the abdomen, although there is a tendency for pain to be maximal in the upper quadrant on the side of the infiltrate. Abdominal pain may draw attention from the lungs as a source of fever. This occurs especially in the occasional patient with minimal pulmonary findings. Fever is usually higher than that typically seen with acute appendicitis. Leukocytosis with a prominent "left shift" in the differential white blood cell count often accompanies pneumonia. Abdominal pain does not localize with time to the right lower quadrant. The patient may splint her abdomen on the side of the infiltrate. The pneumonia may be apparent on x-rays of the abdomen but is often overlooked.

Gynecologic Pain

History and physical findings may be similar for gynecologic and nongynecologic causes of pain, which makes differentiation difficult. Tenderness to abdominal palpation or rectal examination, rebound tenderness, and altered bowel sounds accompany both gastrointestinal and gynecologic causes of acute abdominal pain. History of vaginal bleeding or altered menses point to the pelvic organs as the source of pain, as does an abnormality identified on pelvic examination. Certain conditions occur commonly in adolescent girls, including pregnancy-related phenomena such as spontaneous abortion or ectopic pregnancy, disorders of the uterus and cervix, such as acute cervicitis and endometritis, and disorders of the adnexa, such as salpingitis, tuboovarian abscess, torsion, rupture of a functional ovarian cyst, and endometriosis. In addition, primary dysmenorrhea occurs commonly in adolescents and may present as acute or recurrent pain.

Acute Pelvic Pain in Adolescents

Table 9–2 lists common pelvic disorders that may present with acute findings. An attempt is made to correlate specific findings with each diagnosis. Although the summaries are not intended to provide a comprehensive review of each disorder, the clinical findings can be used by the clinician to pursue specific entities in more detail. Table 9–3 lists the same disorders and summarizes laboratory findings that are consistent with each diagnosis.

  Acute disorders of gynecologic origin may present as pelvic or lower abdominal pain and may mimic disease in the genitourinary tract, gastrointestinal tract, and musculoskeletal system. In a pubertal adolescent with abdominal pain of sudden onset, physical examination of the abdomen may demonstrate tenderness to palpation, rebound tenderness, and, occasionally, diminished or absent bowel sounds. Common gynecologic disorders which cause acute abdominal pain include salpingitis, tuboovarian abscess, ectopic pregnancy, and ruptured ovarian cysts (which occasionally include those related to endometriosis). Patients with acute salpingitis generally appear to be less ill than patients with appendicitis but usually have higher fever.

Pregnancy-Related Causes of Acute Pain

Spontaneous Abortion Spontaneous abortion is the most common cause for acute lower abdominal pain in sexually active women, including adolescents. This pain is generally characterized as acute in onset, colicky, and located in the lower midline. Pain results from the progressive softening and dilatation of the internal os of the cervix and usually occurs in association with varying degrees of vaginal bleeding. The bleeding might be quite profuse for a short period of time as the conceptus is passed spontaneously from the uterus. An adolescent whose abdominal/pelvic pain is pregnancy-related usually gives a history of missed menstrual periods, sexual activity, and complaints such as anorexia, vomiting, urinary frequency, or breast tenderness or fullness.

  Most spontaneous abortions occur within the first 6–8 weeks of amenorrhea and are usually complete, without the need of surgical or medical treatment. A spontaneous abortion later than 8 weeks after cessation of menses or with prolonged acute bleeding (more than 8 hours), or thought to be incomplete for any reason, mandates complete evacuation of the conceptus by suction curettage. The primary care clinician who has had experience with uterine evacuation by suction curettage may perform this procedure in the office quite easily with analgesia and local anesthesia. Lack of experience with this technique mandates quick referral of a patient who is experiencing incomplete spontaneous abortion for completion of the process. Remember to obtain blood type and Rh so that patients (approximately 15%) who are Rh-negative may receive Rh immunoglobulin to minimize the chances of isoimmunization.

Ectopic Pregnancy Ectopic pregnancy often has associated acute unilateral lower quadrant pain characterized as continuous but crampy. It is associated with menstrual

Table 9–2   An Approach to the Sexually Active Adolescent with Acute Abdominal/Pelvic Pain

Acute disorders	Pain	Fever	Abnormal bleeding	Vaginal discharge	GI symptoms	Rebound tenderness	Adnexal mass	Adnexal tenderness
1. Mucopurulent cervicitis	Low suprapubic +	Low grade	Postcoital	Slight increase yellow/green	None	None	None	None; cervical motion, ++
2. Salpingitis/PID	Low abdomen ++	Low grade to marked	About 1/3 have irregular bleeding	Slight increase	Mild anorexia	None to marked	Bilateral tenderness; thickening or masses	Marked
3. Cystitis	Low suprapubic ++	Low grade to absent	None	None	None	None	None	None
4. Appendicitis	RLQ - mild to marked	Low grade	None	None	Anorexia; may have nausea vomiting	Mild to marked RLQ	Fullness in RLQ on rectal	Right-sided tenderness
5. Ectopic pregnancy	Mild to marked	May have transient, lowgrade in 20%	Usually	None	None	Mild to marked unilateral	Fullness or mass unilateral	Marked
6. Ruptured cyst	Mild to marked	None	Often none but may have delayed menses	None	None	None to marked	Usually mass or fullness	Marked
7. Adnexal torsion	Mild to marked	Low grade to none	Unusual	None	None	Mild to marked	Usually palpable	Unilateral marked
8. Spontaneous abortion	Colicky; mild to marked low midline	None	Always; often marked	None	Anorexia with pregnancy	None	Unusual	Unusual
9. Primary dysmenorrhea	Colicky with menses	None	Menses usually normal flow	None	May have nausea and vomiting with menses	None	None	None
10. Endometriosis	Usually with menses	None	Usually not; 30% have premenstrual spotting	None	May have nausea and vomiting with menses	Usually none	Usually not; may have small adnexal irregularities	Usually

Table 9–3   Laboratory Assessment of the Sexually Active Adolescent with Acute Abdominal/Pelvic Pain

Acute disorders	CBC with diff.; sed. rate	Cervix culture for STD	Urine analysis or culture	Ultrasound pelvic	Pregnancy test	Wet prep vag. discharge
1. Mucopurulent cervicitis	Not usually helpful	Mandatory for G.C.; *Chlamydia*	+/−	Not helpful	Not helpful	Mandatory
2. Salpingitis/PID	Inflammatory changes 75%	Mandatory for GC; chlamydia	+/−	Usually not helpful	Yes; to help rule out ectopic	May help if + for mucopurulent discharge
3. Cystitis	Usually not helpful	Probably should screen	Mandatory	Not helpful	Not helpful	Mandatory to R/O vaginitis
4. Appendicitis	Mandatory	May help to R/O salpingitis	Not usually helpful	May help if + gas in appendix	May help to R/O ectopic	Not usually helpful
5. Ectopic pregnancy	Mandatory to check for anemia	May help to R/O salpingitis	Not usually helpful	May help to see gestational sac	Mandatory	Not usually helpful
6. Ruptured cyst	Check for anemia if indicated	Screening if indicated	Not usually helpful	May help define presence of cyst	May help in diff., dx, ectopic	Not usually helpful
7. Adnexal torsion	May help to diff. from appendicitis	Screening if indicated	Not usually helpful	May document presence of mass	May help in diff., dx, ectopic	Not usually helpful
8. Spontaneous abortion	May help to document anemia	Not helpful	Not helpful	May show presence of gestational sac	Mandatory	Not helpful
9. Primary dysmenorrhea	Not helpful	Screening if necessary	Not helpful	Not helpful	Not helpful	Not helpful
10. Endometriosis	Not usually helpful	Screening if indicated	Not helpful	May show ovarian involvement	Not usually helpful	Not helpful

aberrations, including a missed period and some degree of vaginal bleeding in most cases. The vaginal bleeding may occur at the onset of pain or before the onset of pain and frequently represents both the passage of necrotic intrauterine decidual tissue as well as retrograde blood flow from the hemorrhagic fallopian tube into the peritoneal cavity. Other findings associated with ectopic pregnancy are transient low grade fever and elevation in white blood cell count, especially if there has been significant intraperitoneal hemorrhage. It is important to remember these points because the differential diagnosis of ectopic pregnancy includes acute pelvic infection and/or appendicitis. Pregnancy testing with either urine or serum human chorionic gonadotropin (HCG) assay is mandatory in all adolescent girls with acute lower abdominal pain and/or vaginal bleeding. HCG assays detect virtually all early pregnancies, including ectopic pregnancy. The clinician who provides medical care to adolescents needs to maintain an awareness of ectopic pregnancy so that early referral for appropriate surgical treatment is not delayed (Coupet, 1989).

Disorders of the Cervix

Both acute and chronic uterine and cervical infection may cause pain characterized as a dull, aching, lower midline abdominal discomfort. Pain from the lower uterine segment or endocervical canal may be referred to the low back or lumbosacral region.

Acute Cervicitis   Acute cervicitis is most commonly caused by either *Neisseria gonorrhoeae* (Asgeirssen and Weintzen, 1986; Wilfert and Gutman, 1987) or *C. trachomatis* (Figelman, 1986; Wilfert and Gutman, 1987). Usually, patients present with cervical or vaginal discharge, low grade fever, and slight leukocytosis. Definitive diagnosis requires culture of the discharge. Pelvic examination reveals a moderate to marked degree of cervical tenderness, especially with lateral motion of the cervix. Acute cervicitis may occur in the absence of obvious upper tract inflammatory disease. Cervicitis caused by *N. gonorrhoeae* and *Chlamydia* is sexually transmitted. The male partner should be identified and receive antibiotic treatment identical to that provided to his sexual partner.

    Gonorrheal cervicitis   The treatment of choice for culture-proven acute *N. gonorrhoeae* cervicitis is 4.8 million units of intramuscular procaine penicillin G administered approximately ½ hour after 1 g of oral probenecid. For patients allergic to penicillin, tetracycline or doxycycline may be used. Tetracycline dose is 500 mg orally, four times a day for 7 days; doxycycline dose is 100 mg twice daily for 7 days. Other agents which may be used include amoxicillin, 3 g, or ampicillin, 3.5 g, orally as a single dose approximately ½ hour after 1 g of oral probenecid, or ceftriaxone, 250 mg intramuscularly as a single dose (Wilfert and Gutman, 1987).

    Chlamydial cervicitis   *C. trachomatis* is the most common cause of acute mucopurulent cervicitis in most women. Two simple, definitive, objective clinical findings establish this diagnosis: 1) yellow mucopurulent material obtained from the cervix on a white swab and 2) the presence of 10 or more polymorphonuclear leukocytes per high-powered microscopic field on gram stain of the material obtained from the endocervix. Treatment for *Chlamydia* cervicitis is oral tetracycline, 500 mg four times a day for 7 days, or doxycycline, 100 mg twice daily for 7 days. If the patient is allergic to tetracycline, erythromycin, 500 mg four times a day for 7 days, is acceptable. Another alternative is trimethoprim, 160 mg, plus sulfamethoxazole, 800 mg, twice daily for 10 days (Figelman, 1986; Wilfert and Gutman, 1987).

Disorders of the Adnexa

The pain response to inflammatory and reactive disorders of the adnexa differs somewhat from that of uterine and cervical disorders. Patients with a diffuse inflammatory process of the fallopian tubes and/or ovaries will have moderate to severe acute lower back or pelvic pain with bilateral pain to palpation of the abdomen and involuntary guarding and rebound tenderness. Pelvic examination reveals bilateral adnexal tenderness, adnexal thickening, or frank adnexal enlargement. The degree of pain and the physical findings will vary, depending on the duration of illness, the organism, whether the process represents a primary or a recurrent infection, and the adequacy of prior treatment in recurrent cases.

Pelvic Inflammatory Disease   Pelvic inflammatory disease (PID) is an acute, intrinsic (or primary) gynecologic infectious process (Freij, 1986; Wilfert and Gutman, 1987). The term most commonly refers to inflammation in the upper genital tract, including the endometrium, the fallopian tubes, the ovaries, the uterine wall, the broad ligaments, and the pelvic peritoneum. Risk factors for PID include sexual activity, multiple sexual partners, age below 25 years, presence of an intrauterine device, previous PID or lower genital tract infection with *Chlamydia* or *N. gonorrhoeae*, and uterine instrumentation. When possible, upper tract genital infections should be labeled with specific terms, such as acute salpingitis (Shafer et al., 1982), acute salpingooophoritis, and acute parametritis, although severe cases may involve all of these structures as part of the same inflammatory process.

Acute pelvic inflammatory disease is usually a polymicrobial infection caused by organisms which ascend from the vagina and cervix along the mucosa of the endometrium to infect the mucosa of the fallopian tube. Bacteria cultured directly from tubal fluid commonly include endogenous aerobic and anaerobic bacteria, as well as *C. trachomatis* and *N. gonorrhoeae*.

With a fulminant infectious process, pus spills into the lower abdominal cavity and may migrate along the right paracolic gutter to the liver. Fifteen to 20% of patients will have right upper quadrant pain and/or tenderness caused by pericapsular inflammation of the liver. Thus, right upper quadrant pain occurs in patients with primary pelvic infections as well as with gastrointestinal, liver, or gallbladder disease.

The present epidemic of sexually transmitted diseases and corresponding pelvic inflammatory processes is a major public health concern (Washington et al., 1986). PID is a generic term which does not necessarily implicate a sexually transmitted process, although the majority of intrinsic upper tract genital infections *are* sexually transmitted and extremely rare in women who are not sexually active. Pelvic inflammatory disease is the most common serious infection in women age 16–25. The morbidity produced by it exceeds that produced by all other infections in this age group. Washington and co-workers (1986) reported 42,000 new cases of acute pelvic infection, which required hospitalization, and another 158,000 cases of early pelvic infection, which were treated as outpatients, in girls age 15–19. Approximately 85% of these cases were spontaneous infections in sexually active adolescents; the remainder followed procedures that broke the cervical mucus barrier and allowed the vaginal flora the opportunity to colonize the upper genital tract.

Chlamydia   Special attention should be paid to a sexually active teenager who has more than one sexual partner. She is at high risk for infection by *C. trachomatis*. Young women who have colonization of the cervix by *Chlamydia* have a higher incidence of upper tract genital infection than do older women. Between 10% and 30% of women with cervical cultures positive for *Chlamydia* also have positive upper tract or peritoneal cultures. From 20% to 40% of sexually active women have antibodies against *C. trachomatis*; and between 10% and 30% of women with acute pelvic inflammatory disease documented by laparoscopy have evidence of acute chlamydial infection by serial antibody testing even in the absence of positive cultures (Eschenbach, 1985).

Chlamydia may produce a subacute infection with an insidious onset. After infecting the upper tract, including fallopian tubes, the *Chlamydia* organism may remain in the fallopian tubes for a number of months after initial colonization. This is in contrast to *Gonococcus* which remains in the fallopian tube a few days, at the most. Experimental evidence indicates that *Chlamydia* may cause disruption of the tubal mucosa by an immunopathologic mechanism rather than by direct cellular toxicity as is the case with *N. gonorrhoeae* (Eschenbach, 1985). The clinical course of *Chlamydia* is often indolent to the extent that these patients may be confused with patients who have other forms of chronic pelvic pain and, therefore, may be inappropriately treated or not treated at all. In the adolescent with unexplained pelvic pain, examination of the endocervical mucus as well as endocervical cultures for *Chlamydia* should be done. The amount of tubal destruction from these infections is frequently disproportionate to the severity of the symptoms that the patients may have.

Diagnosis   A clinical diagnosis of acute pelvic inflammatory disease is difficult at best. The differential diagnosis includes lower genital tract pelvic infection, ectopic pregnancy, torsion or rupture of an adnexal mass, acute appendicitis, and endometriosis. Before development of laparoscopy, the diagnosis of acute pelvic inflammatory disease was based on the triad of fever, elevated erythrocyte sedimentation rate, and adnexal tenderness or mass. Jacobsen (1980) has shown that only 17% of laparoscopically confirmed cases of acute PID have this classic triad. Therefore, reliance on even stringent clinical criteria causes the majority of these cases to be overlooked and, thus, untreated. More liberal use of diagnostic laparoscopy would allow identification of such cases, but, in practice, the majority of women with acute pelvic inflammatory disease do not undergo laparoscopy because of the expense, inconvenience, and invasiveness of the procedure. Recently, uniform clinical and laboratory criteria have been developed by the Obstetric and Gynecologic Infectious Disease Society, adapted from the work of Hager et al. (1983) (Table 9–4). The use of

Table 9–4   Clinical Criteria for the Diagnosis of Pelvic Inflammatory Disease

Essential criteria (all 3)
  Lower abdominal tenderness (direct and rebound)
  Cervical and uterine motion tenderness
  Adnexal tenderness

Additional criteria (one or more)
  Rectal temperature $>38°C$
  Peripheral white blood cell count $>10,000/mm^3$
  Erythrocyte sedimentation rate >15 mm/hour
  Peritoneal fluid obtained by culdocentesis containing white blood cells and bacteria
  An inflammatory mass detected by bimanual examination or ultrasonography
  Presence of *C. trachomatis* (direct immunofluorescence test) or gram-negative intracellular
    diplococci suggestive of *N. gonorrhoeae* (gram-stain) in endocervical specimens

Adapted from Hager et al., 1983.

strict criteria, in conjunction with clinical experience and common sense, will allow early identification of the majority of patients with PID so that treatment may begin early enough to guarantee successful outcome.

General clinical guidelines for the diagnosis of PID include:

1. Pain in the lower abdomen is by far the most frequent symptom of acute pelvic infection. More than 90% of women present with diffuse, bilateral lower abdominal pain, usually described as constant and dull. Generally the pain is of a relatively short duration, lasting less than 7 days. If the pain has been present more than 3 weeks, it is unlikely that the patient has acute pelvic inflammatory disease.
2. Approximately three quarters of patients with acute pelvic inflammatory disease have an associated endocervical infection with co-existent purulent discharge.
3. Abnormal vaginal bleeding is noted in slightly less than half of patients.
4. Approximately 10% of women with acute pelvic inflammatory disease develop symptoms of perihepatic inflammation, the Fitz-Hugh-Curtis syndrome. This condition is often mistaken for either lower lobe pneumonia or acute cholecystitis. These patients have right upper quadrant pain, pleuritic pain, and tenderness in the right upper quadrant to palpation.

Treatment   An adolescent with acute pelvic inflammatory disease may be treated either as an outpatient (Table 9–5) or an inpatient (Table 9–6) (Centers for Disease Control, 1985). When considering patients for hospitalization, certain criteria can be followed reliably (Table 9–7). The guidelines for outpatient treatment are tailored to a mildly ill patient with positive abdominal and/or adnexal findings who does not meet the criteria for hospitalization. The routine investigation should include cultures for *C. trachomatis* and *N. gonorrhoeae*. The primary care clinician who sees adolescent patients is encouraged to obtain gynecologic consultation in cases where hospitalization and inpatient treatment are thought to be necessary.

Sequelae   The most serious sequelae of acute pelvic inflammatory disease involve the morbidity and mortality associated with rupture of tuboovarian abscesses, ruptured ectopic pregnancy, and subsequent infertility. However, the adolescent care

Table 9–5   Outpatient Therapy of Acute Pelvic Inflammatory Disease

Initial Therapy		
Antibiotic	Single Dose	Route
Ampicillin[a]	3.5 g	p.o.
Amoxicillin[a]	3.0 g	p.o.
Penicillin G[a], procaine	4.8 million units	IM
Cefoxitin[a]	2 g	IM
Ceftriaxone	250 mg	IM

Followed by			
Antibiotic	Dose	Route	Frequency	Duration
Doxycycline	100 mg	p.o.	BID	10–14 days
Tetracycline[b]	500 mg	p.o.	QID	10–14 days

From Centers for Disease Control, 1985.

[a]Give probenecid 1 g p.o. 30 minutes before antibiotics.

[b]Tetracycline has lower activity against certain anaerobes *and* requires more frequent administration than doxycycline. Both factors make tetracycline potentially less effective in treatment of pelvic inflammatory disease.

Table 9–6   Inpatient Therapy for Acute Pelvic Inflammatory Disease

Regimen A

Doxycycline, 100 mg intravenously twice daily, plus cefoxitin, 2 g intravenously four times daily. Continue intravenous drugs for at least 4 days and at least 48 hours after the patient's condition improves. Then continue doxycycline, 100 mg by mouth twice per day, to complete 10–14 days total therapy.

Regimen B

Clindamycin, 600 mg intravenously four times daily, plus gentamicin, 2 mg/kg intravenously followed by 1.5 mg/kg three times daily in patients with normal renal function. Continue intravenous drugs for at least 4 days and at least 48 hours after the patient's condition improves. Then continue clindamycin, 450 mg by mouth four times daily to complete 10–14 days total therapy.

Centers for Disease Control, 1985.

Table 9–7   Indications for Hospitalization of Patients with Pelvic Inflammatory Disease

Nulliparity
Presence of tuboovarian complex or abscess
Gastrointestinal symptoms
Peritonitis in upper quadrants
Presence of an intrauterine device
History of operative or diagnostic procedures
Inadequate response to outpatient therapy

clinician should understand that chronic pelvic pain commonly develops following acute pelvic inflammatory disease. The risk is four times greater for PID patients than for control subjects. Overall, approximately 20% of all women with prior acute pelvic infections will develop chronic pelvic pain (Stenchever, 1987). This observation is important to keep in mind for clinicians who expect to maintain long-term contact with their adolescent patients.

Functional Ovarian Cysts   Functional ovarian cysts commonly cause acute abdominal pain in the adolescent age group. Rupture of an ovarian cyst may cause sudden onset of pain in the lower abdominal quadrant on the side of the involved ovary. Diagnosis and management are facilitated by knowledge of the normal menstrual cycle and its ovarian changes (Moscicki and Shafer, 1986). All too often, a diagnosis of "ovarian cysts" leads to inappropriate imaging of pelvic structures with subsequent referral for unnecessary surgery. *It should be remembered that all young ovulatory women have ovarian cysts*, which are usually follicle cysts.

Mittelschmerz   Midcycle ovulatory pain, or Mittelschmerz, is a reproducible monthly discomfort of varying intensity at or about the time of ovulation. It infrequently causes pain severe enough to be incapacitating but may be interpreted by the adolescent as a serious problem. The pain of Mittelschmerz is generally short lived, lasting anywhere from a few hours to perhaps a day. Most often Mittelschmerz does not cause long-term sequelae. Occasionally, a corpus luteum cyst will be symptomatic through the remainder of the menstrual cycle until the next menses ensues.

Follicle cysts   The most common form of ovarian cyst is the follicle cyst which has an average diameter of approximately 2 cm. Follicle cysts are not neoplastic and are incapable of autonomous growth. They represent a temporary variation of a normal process (Fig. 9–4). The majority of follicle cysts are asymptomatic and are discovered only during routine pelvic examination. The pain experienced with an occasional

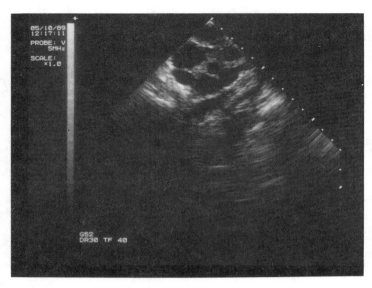

9–4   An ovary with numerous follicular cysts.

symptomatic follicle cyst is usually transient; only rarely does significant intraperitoneal bleeding occur which requires definitive treatment. In general, surgical excision of functional ovarian cysts is contraindicated. Occasionally patients with follicle cysts may experience intermittent menstrual irregularities because of the large amount of estrogen secreted into the cyst fluid. The typical picture of a patient with intermittent recurrent follicle cysts is that of a regular menstrual cycle with a prolonged intermenstrual interval followed by occasional episodes of heavier menstrual bleeding.

Initial management for an isolated episode of pain associated with follicle cysts is to observe and reexamine the patient during a subsequent menstrual cycle. For the occasional patient in whom pain recurs, oral contraceptives may provide adequate temporary relief by suppression of follicular activity through gonadotropin suppression. This may be done for intervals as short as four to six weeks, but more commonly treatment for six or more oral contraceptive cycles is recommended in an effort to render the ovaries temporarily quiescent.

Corpus luteum cysts   A less common but potentially more serious variant of functional cysts occurs with abnormalities of the corpus luteum. When ovulation takes place at midcycle, the corpus luteum forms as the hormone-producing organelle that supports the endometrium in the second half of the menstrual cycle (Fig. 9–5). Most corpus luteum cysts are asymptomatic, but occasionally a cyst will rupture and cause intraperitoneal hemorrhage. Hallatt et al. (1984) observed that sudden, severe lower abdominal pain was the prominent symptom in all patients with hemoperitoneum caused by a ruptured corpus luteum cyst. The majority of the patients surveyed were in the luteal phase of the menstrual cycle and not pregnant. Approximately one-third of women noted unilateral lower quadrant cramping and lower abdominal pain for 1–2 weeks before overt rupture of the corpus luteum cyst. For reasons unknown, the right ovary was the source of hemorrhage in two-thirds of the cases.

The differential diagnosis of young women with acute lower abdominal pain and suspected ruptured corpus luteum cyst includes ectopic pregnancy. Therefore, these patients should have urine or serum assays for human chorionic gonadotropin

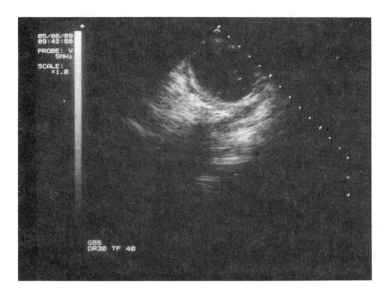

9–5 A typical corpus luteum cyst. It has a size of approximately 4½ × 3 cm, contains a thickened wall at one pole which represents hypertrophic, luteinized elements derived from the ovarian follicle, and may have small amounts of blood represented by the white flecks seen inside the cyst.

(HCG) to help exclude ectopic pregnancy. Intraperitoneal bleeding of a magnitude to cause signs of an acute surgical abdomen or of hypovolemia will require surgical intervention. However, the majority of patients will not need surgery, since bleeding from a corpus luteum cyst is usually of small amount and short duration.

Torsion of the Adnexa Adnexal torsion occurs rarely but can cause sudden onset of moderate to severe abdominal pain. The history reveals sudden pain without signs or symptoms of infection. Peritoneal signs are limited to the quadrant involved. Pelvic examination will reveal an exquisitely tender adnexa usually associated with a tense cystic enlargement. Pain may be referred to the ipsilateral anterior and anterior-medial thigh. In addition to pain, nausea and vomiting occur in approximately two-thirds of patients. This symptom complex sometimes leads to a preoperative diagnosis of acute appendicitis, especially if the torsion occurs on the right ovary. The most common etiology of adnexal torsion is ovarian enlargement, with true neoplasms (usually benign) present in approximately 60% of these patients.

Other Pelvic Causes of Pain

Dysmenorrhea The term dysmenorrhea, literally "difficult monthly flow," commonly refers to painful menstruation. This is one of the most frequently encountered pain-related gynecologic disorders (ACOG, 1983). Primary dysmenorrhea, characteristic of adolescence, generally has no associated pelvic pathology, whereas secondary dysmenorrhea involves an older group of patients and typically results from a pathological process in the pelvis. Dysmenorrhea causes absenteeism from school and work more often than any other problem among young women, with estimates of more than 140 million working hours lost annually.

The etiology of primary dysmenorrhea is generally attributed to the presence of uterine prostaglandins (ACOG, 1983) which give rise to pain through two mechanisms:

1. The uterotonic or spasmodic activity of the uterine musculature
2. Hypersensitization to the effect of chemical and physical stimuli on pain nerve terminals by cyclic endoperoxides and prostaglandin E_2

Diagnosis   Primary dysmenorrhea can be diagnosed in most cases by characteristic clinical features. It occurs almost invariably with ovulatory cycles and usually appears within 12 months after menarche. The pain starts a few hours before or just after the onset of menstrual flow and lasts 48–72 hours. Pain is cramping, spasmodic, or labor-like, localized in the lower midline, and radiates to the back and inner thighs. Some patients occasionally complain of a pelvic ache or the sensation of pelvic pressure. Pelvic examination, including rectovaginal examination, is normal. Adolescents with dysmenorrhea may have other associated symptoms which include nausea and vomiting (89%), fatigue (85%), diarrhea (60%), lower back ache (60%), and headache (45%).

Treatment   Either oral contraceptives or inhibitors of prostaglandin synthetase activity may be used to treat dysmenorrhea. Oral contraceptives effectively treat primary dysmenorrhea while affording contraception. Combination pills reduce prostaglandin levels in menstrual fluid with subsequent reduction in menstrual fluid volume and suppression of endometrial proliferation. In addition, contraceptives suppress ovulation, resulting in an altered endocrine environment. More than 90% of patients can be relieved of primary dysmenorrhea using oral contraceptives.

Patients who do not wish or need contraception may use prostaglandin synthetase inhibitors. Prostaglandin synthetase inhibitors effectively block dysmenorrhea when taken on the first 2–3 days of each menstrual cycle. These agents work through a variety of mechanisms, but in general, they inhibit cyclic endoperoxide synthesis and inhibit the prostaglandin synthetase enzyme system (ACOG, 1983). A variety of medications, including aspirin, effectively treat primary dysmenorrhea if given appropriately. Table 9–8 outlines the more commonly used prostaglandin synthetase inhibitors and their dosages. With these rapidly absorbed prostaglandin inhibitors, treatment before the onset of pain is not necessary. Advise patients to begin treatment at the very

Table 9–8   Treatment of Dysmenorrhea with Prostaglandin Synthetase Inhibitors

Drug	Dose	Route	Frequency	Comment
Aspirin	325–650 mg	p.o.	q4h	May need around-the-clock dosing
Ibuprofen (Motrin)	400 mg	p.o.	q6h	—
Mefenamic acid (Ponstel)	500 mg	p.o.	Initial dose q6h	—
	250 mg	p.o.		
Naproxen (Naprosyn)	500 mg	p.o.	Initial dose q6–8h	Maximum daily dose 1250 mg
	250 mg	p.o.		(5 tablets)
Naproxen sodium[a] (Anaprox)	550 mg	p.o.	Initial dose q6–8h	Maximum daily dose 1375 mg
	275 mg	p.o.		(5 tablets)

[a]Naproxen sodium has more rapid onset of action (30 minutes) than the other medications.

outset of symptoms or when menstrual flow begins, whichever comes first. Contraindications to the use of prostaglandin inhibitors include the presence of gastrointestinal ulcers, bleeding disorders, and hypersensitivity to aspirin or similar agents.

Endometriosis   Endometriosis occurs uncommonly in adolescents but should remain a consideration for patients with a history of progressive dysmenorrhea and pelvic pain. It is especially difficult to differentiate endometriosis from primary dysmenorrhea in adolescents. The pain of endometriosis varies from a mild discomfort associated only with menstruation to marked abdominal pain with peritoneal signs related to the rupture of endometriomas. Chronic pelvic pain occurs in about 20% of patients with endometriosis. Young women who do not respond to treatment for primary dysmenorrhea may have endometriosis. Diagnosis requires laparoscopy. Unusual symptomatic variants may cause diagnostic confusion. Occasional patients have otherwise unexplainable cyclic dysuria or other voiding symptoms, while others may have symptoms primarily related to difficult stool evacuation and/or dyschezia at the time of menstruation.

Chronic Pelvic Pain in Adolescents

The term "chronic pelvic pain" describes pelvic discomfort present for at least six months for which no etiology has been discovered, despite repeated clinical evaluations. The clinical distinction between pelvic and abdominal pain is often arbitrary, and causes of chronic pelvic pain (Pearce et al., 1982; Slocumb, 1984) should be considered in the differential diagnosis of any menstruating teenager who complains of lower abdominal pain. Often, a characteristic history accompanied by specific findings on pelvic examination will suggest a diagnosis.

Table 9–9 summarizes the clinical approach to the sexually active adolescent with chronic abdominal/pelvic pain. Findings are categorized by diagnosis. Table 9–10 summarizes laboratory findings which are consistent with the diagnoses in chronic pelvic pain patients.

Differential Diagnosis

Functional Ovarian Cysts   Although sporadic functional ovarian cysts occur commonly, a small number of young women will develop recurrent symptomatic cysts that present a difficult management problem. Classically, these women experience intermittent episodes of pain lasting for several days or weeks, and pelvic examination identifies the presence of a unilateral cystic mass. Chronic ovulation suppression with oral contraceptives usually prevents recurrence of symptomatic cysts. Surgery should be reserved for patients who fail to respond to medical management.

Endometriosis   Endometriosis may be found in as many as 15%–20% of adolescents with unexplained chronic pelvic pain. Often, adolescents do not have the classic findings of dysmenorrhea, dyspareunia, and infertility. Suggestive findings on pelvic examination include uterosacral ligament nodularity, fixed uterine retroversion, and/or ovarian cysts. The diagnosis may require laparoscopy.

Chronic Endometritis   Chronic endometritis, also known as nonpuerperal endometritis (NPE), generally causes low, midline, dull aching pain which may or may not

Table 9–9   An Approach to the Sexually Active Adolescent with Chronic or Recurrent Abdominal/Pelvic Pain

Chronic disorders	Pain	Fever	Abnormal bleeding	Vaginal discharge	GI symptoms	Rebound tenderness	Adnexal mass	Adnexal tenderness
1. Constipation	RLQ—may be colicky	None	None	None	May have infrequent BM dyschesia	None	May have large amount of stool LLQ	Mild; RLQ or LLQ
2. Recurrent PID	Mild to marked	Low grade to none	About 1/3 have irregular bleeding	Slight increase to none	Usually not	Usually not	Bilateral thickening or small masses	Mild to marked bilaterally
3. Emotional/functional	Mild to moderate	None	May have anovulatory pattern	None	Often have constipation or diarrhea	None	None	None
4. Ovulation	Midcycle, mild to moderate	None	May have midcycle spotting 20%	None	None	None	May have small unilateral fullness or cyst	Mild to moderate
5. Chronic endometritis	Mild, low midline or suprapubic	Low grade to none	Usually >75%	May have associated mucopurulent discharge 20%	None	None	None	May have mild

Table 9–10 Laboratory Assessment of the Sexually Active Adolescent with Chronic or Recurrent Abdominal/Pelvic Pain

Chronic disorders	CBC with diff.; sed. rate	Cervix culture for STD	Urine analysis or culture	Ultrasound pelvic	Pregnancy test	Wet prep vag. discharge
1. Constipation	Not helpful	Screening if indicated	Not helpful	May show stool and R/O adnexal mass	Not helpful	Not helpful
2. Recurrent PID	May show low grade changes	Mandatory	May help R/O UTI	May show adnexal complex	Screening if indicated to R/O ectopic	May show mucopurulent cervicitis
3. Emotional/functional	Not helpful	Screening if indicated	Screening if indicated	Not helpful	Not helpful	Not helpful
4. Ovulation	Not helpful	Screening if indicated	Screening if indicated	May show functional cyst	Screening if indicated	May show ovulatory mucus
5. Chronic endometritis	May show low grade inflammatory changes	Mandatory	Helpful to R/O UTI	Not helpful	Not helpful	Mandatory

be referred to the low back or inner groin area, depending on whether or not inflammation extends into the endocervical canal. NPE may occur in 40%–50% of women who have had mucopurulent cervicitis caused by either *C. trachomatis* or *N. gonorrhoeae*. Chronic endometritis most commonly presents as lower abdominal pain with intermenstrual spotting or bleeding, although some women only complain of dull, constant, lower midline abdominal pain. Many young women with this entity are asymptomatic. Treatment can be based on history of pain and spotting, especially if there is an associated mucopurulent cervical discharge. To prove the diagnosis of NPE, endometrial biopsy and culture are necessary, although these tests are not always practical. The treatment of chronic endometritis is oral tetracycline 2 g/day or doxycycline 100 mg twice daily for 10 days. Other antibiotic alternatives are similar to those listed for the treatment of acute cervicitis.

Pelvic Inflammatory Disease   The prevalence of pelvic inflammatory disease is unfortunately increasing among adolescents. Chronic pelvic pain may result from the residual damage to fallopian tubes caused by multiple episodes of acute infection, but, with the exception of rare infections with the tubercle bacillus or *Actinomyces*, pelvic infections are *not chronic*. There is little or no place for the term ''chronic pelvic inflammatory disease.'' The chronic symptoms that result from acute infection are caused by bacteriologically sterile processes, such as adhesions and hydrosalpinx. The resulting pain is often described as a dull, aching sensation punctuated by episodes of sharp pain precipitated by movement or intercourse. Secondary dysmenorrhea may sometimes accompany this disorder.

Adhesions   Adhesions resulting from previous surgeries or other abdominal infections (most commonly appendicitis) may also contribute to chronic abdominal pain, although the idea that adhesions cause pain has been questioned. Chan and Wood (1985) reported that lysis of adhesions in a group of 43 women with both infertility and chronic pelvic pain resulted in pain relief for 65% lasting from 1–5 years following surgery. On the other hand, many asymptomatic women have extensive adhesions identified at surgery performed for other reasons (Rapkin, 1986). As a general rule, chronic pain should be ascribed to adhesions only when they are extensive and/or dense.

Sexual Abuse   Sexual abuse appears to be common in this group of patients. Harrop-Griffiths et al. (1988) found a history of childhood sexual abuse in 64% of a group of adult women with chronic pelvic pain compared with 23.3% in a pain-free control group. This pattern of abuse often carries over into adult relationships; in the Harrop-Griffiths study 48% of the women with chronic pain also reported experiencing sexual abuse as an adult in contrast to only 16% of the controls.

Psychoemotional   Adult women with chronic pelvic pain commonly have a chaotic social history. Although often married, their relationships are frequently unstable. Many studies have attempted to define psychologic characteristics associated with chronic pelvic pain, but few have been well designed. Renaer et al. (1979) compared women with chronic pain to women with acute pain and found few measurable psychologic differences. Women with chronic pain are often anxious, depressed, and frustrated with the inability of health care providers to solve their problem (Rapkin and Kames, 1987). Psychoemotional problems may result from chronic or recurrent pain or may be part of the cause.

Evaluation

History   The historical evaluation of chronic pelvic pain should focus on the menstrual history, events associated with exacerbation or improvement in the pain, and previous surgical procedures. Women who have organic disorders most often provide a clear and precise description of their pain with respect to location and timing; those with chronic pain of unknown etiology often provide a vague description with many different descriptors. Such vague pain might be described as a dull, aching sensation with occasional fleeting sharp exacerbations; the pain occurs daily and changes location from time to time.

History should focus on sexual activity, with particular attention to contraceptive use, symptoms of sexually transmitted disease, and abuse or incest. The adolescent may be reluctant to provide this information unless the history is taken in the absence of the parent and with assurances of confidentiality. Many adolescents will not volunteer information about sexual activity or abuse because they believe that the physician can identify both simply by doing a physical examination (Cavanaugh, 1987). The clinician, therefore, should clearly state that it is not always possible to determine sexual activity and abuse by the examination and should ask direct questions about them.

Additionally, other stressors should be sought, including family problems, difficulties at school, and problems dealing with peer pressure. The psychosocial history may be emotionally difficult for the adolescent to provide, and several visits may be required before she feels comfortable enough to discuss some issues.

Physical Examination   A thorough general physical examination should pay particular attention to the abdominal and pelvic examination. There should be no reluctance to perform a pelvic examination even in very young adolescents. A variety of speculum sizes is available, and the smallest speculum that will provide adequate visualization should be used. Occasionally it may be impossible to perform a speculum or bimanual examination because of patient discomfort. However, a rectal abdominal exam can usually provide sufficient information to make a provisional diagnosis.

Laboratory and Imaging Tests   Women with chronic pelvic pain are often subjected to multiple diagnostic tests, including ultrasound, intravenous pyelogram, barium enema, cystoscopy, and sigmoidoscopy. Unless symptoms or physical findings suggest specific disorders of the urinary or gastrointestinal tract, these studies almost always provide negative results (Johnson and Laube, 1986).

Laparoscopy   Diagnostic laparoscopy provides the most consistently useful information. Between 15% and 50% of adult women with chronic pain have abnormal laparoscopic findings, including endometriosis, significant adhesions, or tubal damage. The few studies of diagnostic laparoscopic in teenagers with chronic pain have identified findings similar to those in adult women (Kleinhaus et al., 1977; Goldstein et al., 1979).

Summary   In summary, the evaluation of chronic pelvic pain begins with a careful history and physical exam. Normal pelvic examination, presence of pain for several months, and pain-related dysfunction support the need for diagnostic laparoscopy. Other diagnostic tests have value only if warranted by specific symptoms and signs.

Management

Management depends upon the specific diagnosis. Minimal endometriosis in the teenager most often responds to oral contraceptives. Extensive endometriosis may require conservative surgical therapy. Management of pelvic adhesions is more controversial. Division of adhesions through the laparoscope should be done if possible. However, extensive damage from pelvic inflammatory disease will require surgical therapy which should be as conservative as possible. Even if the fallopian tubes appear to be extensively damaged, the availability of newer reproductive technologies demands preservation of the uterus and ovaries in cases in which preservation of fertility is desired. The occasional patient who experiences intermittent episodes of pain because of recurrent, functional cysts is best managed with oral contraceptive suppression. Surgical intervention should be minimized, since adhesion formation may become a significant iatrogenic problem.

Patients who have no identifiable organic cause for pain present difficult management problems. Empirical use of antidepressant therapy in chronic pain syndrome cannot be recommended for adolescents. In the absence of demonstrable depressive symptoms, such therapy will have little effect. Referral for psychologic or psychiatric evaluation may be necessary.

Some have suggested that performance of a negative diagnostic laparoscopy will result in improvement in the pain because of the reassurance provided by the negative exam. Although this hypothesis has not been sufficiently studied, it is consistent with our clinical impression that some women do benefit from a negative laparoscopy. These women may have been concerned about cancer or a problem affecting reproduction, and when they learn that their pelvic organs are normal, their pain improves.

However, many young women with chronic pain continue to be symptomatic after negative laparoscopy. We believe that the best strategy in this group of patients includes the following:

1. Avoid unnecessary diagnostic tests and, instead, rely on history and physical examination when recurrent episodes of pain occur.
2. Plan to see the patient on a scheduled basis. This provides reassurance to the patient that her pain is being taken seriously and begins to modify her pain-associated behavior.
3. Help the patient understand that your goal is to help her deal with the pain, rather than to find a "cure."
4. Use a nondirective counseling approach which focuses on the patient's worries and problems in any area of her life (Pearce et al., 1982).
5. When appropriate, make referral for evaluation of psychosocial problems (Harrop-Griffiths et al., 1988).

Psychogenic Abdominal Pain

This section outlines and discusses an approach to psychogenic recurrent abdominal pain (McGrath and Unruh, 1987c) that may be used to clarify diagnostic issues and thereby enhance the practitioner's ability to affect behavioral change. Aspects of the clinical interview, descriptions and uses of several personality and behavioral measures, differential diagnosis, and specific treatment concerns are discussed.

Clinical Interview Techniques

After an appropriate evaluation finds no disease process or physiologic and/or structural reasons for abdominal pain, assessment of psychologic factors assumes the highest importance if the symptom complex persists (Barr, 1983; Barr and Feuerstein, 1983). Occasionally, symptoms cease when the patient (and her parents) are reassured that no serious disease exists; more commonly pain continues. Throughout the investigation, it is important to stress that physical complaints and related symptoms are real, not "made up" or "in the patient's head." In addition, symptoms themselves often create stress between and within family members, which clouds and complicates the diagnostic picture.

The use of the clinical interview as a tool in the differential diagnosis of recurrent abdominal pain is central to the accurate assessment of psychosomatic factors and treatment of this disorder. Separate interviews with the adolescent and her parents plus observation of parent/child interactions during a joint interview will provide the foundation for the initial evaluation of psychosomatic issues and will assist in the decision to refer the patient for a formal psychologic assessment.

Having developed one or more hypotheses that possibly explain the complaints of abdominal pain, information gathered during an interview with the adolescent should serve to support, refute, or perhaps generate new hypotheses. While it is true that critical life setbacks (e.g., parents' divorce, death of family member) may account for transient or initial somatic complaints in some patients, the vast majority of recurrent abdominal complaints are thought to be the result of an interaction between environmental stressors (including both daily and critical life events), preexisting somatic susceptibilities, and the adolescent's repertoire of emotional/behavioral strategies used to cope with these stressful events.

Parental Interview   The parental interview focuses on the teen's symptom complex within the framework of a carefully elicited history of birth, growth and development, illnesses and hospitalizations, family illnesses and structure, and parental perception of the patient's behavior patterns, school performance, and peer relations. Birth events, developmental delays, or frequent medical crises which have necessitated hospitalizations or frequent visits to the physician's office may promote feelings of helplessness in the patient as well as an attitude of overprotectiveness in one or both parents. Similarly, medical or behavioral problems in family members may provide behavioral models from which the patient may learn to gain acceptance, approval, or attention. The extent to which the patient's current behavior reflects her past behavior in similar situations might reveal a pattern of somatization as a reaction to stress in the home or at school. Limited cognitive ability or poor academic achievement increase the likelihood that physical complaints may serve as a way to avoid homework, tests, or even a competitive classroom atmosphere. Parental perceptions of the patient's peer relationships will provide clues about her social acceptance as well as the extent to which she may seek peer approval, yield to peer pressure, and perhaps reject social conventionality. Abdominal pain which elicits parental response may allow the adolescent to exercise power and control over her parents and thus serve as a way to demonstrate personal independence.

Patient Interview   The interview with the teenager (Table 9–11) also focuses on the symptom complex but with emphasis on her perception of the pain and its relation to past and current medical, social, family, and personal experiences.

Table 9–11   The Interview of an Adolescent with Recurrent Abdominal Pain

School
1. Academic performance level
2. Self-perception versus school records
3. Career aspirations

Peer relations
1. Social structure of peer group
2. Behaviors of peer group
3. Drug and/or alcohol use by peer group
4. Sexual activity

Family interactions
1. Day-to-day communication
2. Sources of conflict within family
3. Sibling behavior
4. Marital harmony
5. Financial stress

School   This should be one of the primary topics of the interview with the adolescent, since the majority of daily primary and secondary reinforcers which shape emotional and behavioral responses to life events occur within the school setting. Questions about academic performance, peer relationships (i.e., level of participation and acceptance), and career aspirations are important for comparisons with parental perceptions and with objective information from school. An attempt should be made to assess the frequency and intensity of any academic and/or social failure, as viewed by the adolescent, and more importantly, how that adolescent deals with these setbacks.

Peers   Discussion of peer relationships (especially outside of school) may provide information about the importance of peer activities, the social structure of the peer group, requirements for membership and acceptance in the group, and expectations for behavior. Sexual activity and involvement with drugs or alcohol are likely to take place within the peer group. Much of this information may have been elicited during the "medical" evaluation, but greater detail or new material may surface with repeated discussion. When approached tactfully, sympathetically, and with guaranteed confidentiality, candid discussions of such issues can occur. In such an environment, the practitioner may be viewed as a nonjudgmental source of useful and reliable information. Additionally, these discussions may dispel myths related to pregnancy, venereal disease, and the casual use of "recreational" drugs.

Family   Interactions among family members, from the adolescent's perspective, represent the third area of emphasis in the patient interview. Specific questions about family dysfunction, including day-to-day relations between the patient and her parents, sources of conflict, parental and sibling alcohol or substance abuse, physical and/or sexual abuse, antisocial or illegal behavior, parental marital stability, and financial stress may uncover information of importance to the diagnosis or management of the symptom complex. Many of these issues may not be covered in a "medical" interview or may not be volunteered unless the clinician specifically explains their importance to the evaluation.

Objective Assessment of Behavior

While critically useful information can and should be gathered during the clinical interview, additional supportive data can be obtained with the use of one or more available objective tests (Risser et al., 1987) purported to measure emotional/personality dimensions, behavioral problems, and academic achievement. These tests have great utility in the practice of adolescent medicine. They do not require the input of a psychologist. All are self-administered, except for the WRAT-R, and all are easily scored.

Specific Objective Tests

SCL-90-R (Derogatis, 1977)   This is a 90-item self-report symptom checklist designed to reflect psychologic symptom patterns of psychiatric and medical patients. There are nine primary symptom dimensions (Somatization, Obsessive-Compulsive, Interpersonal Sensitivity, Depression, Anxiety, Hostility, Phobic Anxiety, Paranoid Ideation, Psychoticism) and three global indices (Global Severity Index, Positive Symptom Total, Positive Symptom Distress Index) of distress. Administrative instructions take approximately 2 minutes, while the test itself is typically completed in 15 minutes. Results yield a multidimensional symptom profile within which scores on particular symptom dimensions may be interpreted. Separate norms for male and female adolescents have been developed.

The State-Trait Anxiety Inventory (STAI) (Speilberger et al., 1969)   The STAI is a brief questionnaire designed to reflect the degree and nature of the patient's anxiety. Results may suggest that a patient's anxiety level is either a relatively permanent personality dimension (trait) or the result of situational stress (state). This particular test has been shown to differentiate subgroups of patients with nonorganic abdominal pain.

The Revised Behavior Problem Checklist (RBPC) (Quay and Peterson, 1983)   The RBPC is the revised form of a widely used, well researched behavior rating scale. It contains 89 items that yield four major factors labeled Conduct Disorder, Socialized Aggression, Attention-Immaturity, and Anxiety-Withdrawal. Numerous studies have lent support for the basic validity of the RBPC and for the ability of the scales to discriminate deviant groups and to detect changes purportedly due to treatment.

The Wide Range Achievement Test-Revised (WRAT-R) (Jastak and Wilkinson, 1984)   The WRAT-R is simple in its design, administration, and scoring. It provides grade equivalents and standard scores on measures of Reading (word recognition), Spelling, and computational Arithmetic skills. Normative data are provided from ages 5 to 75 years. The Reading and Spelling portions can be administered in approximately 15 minutes, while the Arithmetic portion can be self-administered in 10 minutes.

Data Integration

Interviews and one or more of the standardized assessment measures will provide the practitioner with the information necessary to determine the need for further evaluation and treatment by a mental health professional (Risser et al., 1987). Diagnosis of a psychoemotional basis for abdominal pain requires positive psychologic findings. Caution must be shown not to assume emotional problems because organic etiology cannot be identified. In general, abdominal pain complaints may be the result of a number of multifaceted and integrated factors. Questions designed to assess the presence or absence of environmental stressors, preexisting somatic susceptibilities, and the patient's repertoire of emotional/behavioral strategies to cope with stress should be the primary focus of the separate interviews with parents and patients. Information and impressions gathered from these interviews, when combined with results from self-administered measures of behavior, emotional/personality dimensions, and/or achievement can serve to enhance the practitioner's ability to diagnose and treat effectively patients with abdominal pain complaints.

Differential Diagnosis

Differential diagnosis of nonorganic abdominal complaints includes three major categories of behavioral responses: depression, anxiety/insecurity, or anger (Table 9–12). Development of appropriate treatment plans depends on this categorization and also on the distinction between chronic and acute symptoms.

Depression   Depression may be either a chronic behavioral pattern or an acute reaction to antecedent events (e.g., divorce of parents, death of loved one, school failure) which often are readily apparent but which need not immediately precede the somatic complaint. Careful questioning often reveals such events. Chronic depressive reactions typically are stereotyped behavioral responses which vary little with time or changing situations and often have no apparent connection to a specific situation. Acute depressive episodes differ from chronic patterns because the behavioral response is specific to the precipitating event.

Anxiety/Insecurity   The second major response category, anxiety/insecurity, essentially involves an exaggerated emotional reaction to situational events based on an illogical or irrational fear of failure or rejection. The somatic complaints typically help the adolescent avoid or delay an action that might lead to an undesired failure (e.g., school exam) and the rejection that accompanies failure (i.e., loss of love or acceptance by significant others such as parents and peer groups). Children and adolescents commonly use somatic complaints to gain attention, sympathy, or to feel liked and accepted by others. Sufficient reinforcement (e.g., attention, sympathy, avoidance of responsibilities) increases the likelihood that an individual may develop and use a sick role for secondary gain. The sick role will be reinforced as long as the social stigmas associated with being sick are overcompensated by the benefits gained, and desirable

Table 9–12   Differential Diagnosis of Behavioral Responses in Nonorganic Abdominal Complaints

I.	Depression	
	1.	Acute reaction (divorce, death, school failure, loss of boyfriend, etc.)
	2.	Chronic behavioral pattern (no apparent precipitating event)
II.	Anxiety/insecurity	
	1.	Avoidance due to fear of failure (school work, social activities, etc.)
	2.	Rejection fears (loss of love from parents or peers)
	3.	Attention/sympathy seeking (use sick role for secondary gain)
III.	Anger	
	1.	Complaint is manipulative of others
	2.	Passive-aggressive expression of anger
	3.	Expression of striving for more independence

activities are not significantly reduced. When evaluating somatic complaints, the physician should attempt to determine whether the family and the patient's immediate social systems support and encourage such behavior. Overprotective family environments or those which encourage family unity at the expense of individuality are particularly likely to promote "sick role" behavior in family members.

Anger   A third major response category, anger, is less common than either the depression or anxiety/insecurity categories but, nevertheless, provides another reasonable explanation for abdominal complaints in children and adolescents. The primary assumption is that the somatic complaints are manipulative and are used to demonstrate anger and personal independence, or to exert control over others. Manipulative and/or passive-aggressive tendencies may be apparent from the patient's behavior history. Somatic complaints used as passive-aggressive expressions of anger are clearly more subtle and sophisticated than temper tantrums used by young children. Thus, adolescents are more likely to use somatic complaints for this purpose. Within this context, the "sickness" of the patient may be used to inconvenience or perhaps to control the parent. Another less hostile interpretation for the somatic complaints is that they reflect the adolescent's striving for personal independence. By choosing when and where to be sick, the adolescent feels she is exercising considerable control and autonomy.

Treatment Considerations

Even though somatic and behavioral events occur simultaneously, a causal relationship does not necessarily exist. Identification of a psychologic problem in a female adolescent with recurrent abdominal pain does not imply that the abdominal complaints necessarily have a psychologic basis. Therefore, thorough medical evaluation should be completed to the extent appropriate for historical and physical findings regardless of psychologic indicators. Barr (1983) and Coleman and Levine (1986) present practical approaches to recurrent abdominal pain which emphasize attention to psychoemotional issues.

Recurrent abdominal pain itself may precipitate psychologic stress, since the pain may create feelings of lethargy or dysphoria. Thus, establishment of relationships between abdominal pain and psychologic stress helps in the differential diagnosis only when there exists more than simultaneous occurrence. Behavioral manipulation of the symptom may facilitate ongoing diagnosis and treatment decisions.

Symptom removal has several components. Elimination of the reinforcement or alteration of the precipitating events may allow extinction or removal of the symptom. While this may be the total treatment needed, prudence suggests caution before attempts to remove symptoms by elimination of reinforcements or alteration of precipitating events. The value of the symptom to the patient and the consequences of symptom removal must be evaluated. For example, if the symptom of abdominal pain serves as a defense against underlying depression, simple symptom removal may unmask depression and increase the potential of suicide for some adolescents unless this possibility has been anticipated and appropriate management planned for.

Behavioral Analysis of Recurrent Abdominal Pain   The following model presents three levels of behavioral analysis of patients with recurrent abdominal pain (Table 9–13). In general, the more complex the psychoemotional issues, the more likely the need for referral to a mental health professional.

Table 9–13   Levels of Behavioral Analysis and Treatment

Level I: Somatic symptom only behaviorally based
  1.   Symptom maintained by either a or b or both
      a.   Positive reinforcement
      b.   Avoidance of negative consequences
  2.   No primary anxiety
  3.   No major psychological conflict
Treatment of level I
  Discuss absence of disease
  Explain relationship of complaint to behavior of others
  Counsel others to cease reinforcement of complaint

Level II: Somatic symptom behaviorally based, but accompanied by interpersonal conflict
  1.   Symptom is a defense against either a or b or both
      a.   Anxiety
      b.   Interpersonal conflict (not readily apparent)
  2.   A primary anxiety or source of conflict exists
Treatment of level II
  Symptom removal alone may be harmful
  Remove symptom as in level I while exploring source of anxiety or conflict
  Provide counseling for anxiety or conflict

Level III: Somatic symptom with underlying emotionally damaging circumstances
  1.   Symptom is a defense against emotional disaster
  2.   A primary depression exists
Treatment of level III
  Do *not* remove symptom
  Refer for extensive personality evaluation and counseling by a trained mental health expert

Level I: Somatic symptom—Behaviorally based only   At the simplest level, the symptom of abdominal pain may exist and be maintained purely on the basis of positive behavioral reinforcement or avoidance of negative consequences. In this case, the adolescent will demonstrate no major anxiety or psychologic conflict. An example would be a patient whose abdominal pain generates overly solicitous behaviors from others in the environment, especially parents or peers. Another example could be an abdominal complaint to avoid difficult circumstances. The symptom thus would be frequently reinforced by the reactions of people important to the patient.

Symptom removal requires a thorough discussion of the absence of disease and dysfunctional causes of pain and an explanation of the way parental or peer behavior promotes and reinforces pain. Cessation of reinforcement usually promotes pain resolution. While many cases appear to be at this simple level, the clinician should carefully analyze possible anxiety-based psychologic factors and depressive components in the patient before proceeding with symptom removal.

Case example: Susan was a 14-year-old ninth grader who had begun to complain of abdominal pain following her first semester in high school. Although her grades were generally acceptable (e.g., mostly B's), they represented a drop from the A's she received in earlier grades. Her peer and family relationships were reported to be adequate. However, with the increasing frequency of her abdominal complaints, her attendance at school had begun to suffer, and she was no longer willing to participate in favored extracurricular activities. The parents requested a medical evaluation. Her history of birth, growth and development, and illness/hospitalization was noncontributory. A thorough physical examination found no disease process or physiologic and/or structural causes for the abdominal pain.

During separate interviews with Susan and her parents, it became apparent that both she and her parents were disappointed in her recent school performance, particularly in light of her previous "straight A" academic record in earlier grades. It was further acknowledged that an older sister received straight A's and was in the high school "honors program." Results from standardized symptom checklist and achievement tests suggested that she was mildly dysphoric, but not significantly depressed, and she showed social withdrawal. She demonstrated above grade-level development scores in reading, spelling, and math. Susan's physical complaints were the result of an exaggerated situational emotional response to her lowered grade point average (i.e., fear and anxiety associated with the "possible" rejection by and disappointment of her parents).

Treatment consisted of a discussion of the absence of disease and dysfunctional causes of the pain with Susan and her parents. The discussion also included an attempt to develop an awareness of how unrealistic expectations can undermine both performance and motivation to perform. Parents were encouraged to place less emphasis on Susan's grades and to praise and reinforce her efforts in academic and extracurricular activities more frequently. Parents were also encouraged to demonstrate to Susan or in other ways reassure her of their unconditional acceptance of her. Follow-up contact with the family revealed a marked decline in the frequency of Susan's abdominal complaints.

Level II: Somatic symptom—Behaviorally based, interpersonal conflict   An abdominal complaint may serve as a defense against anxiety or interpersonal conflict which may not be readily apparent at the initial evaluation. Even careful behavioral analysis may fail to identify underlying problems unless the patient or her family willingly discloses them. The anxiety or conflict may surface if family or peer reinforcement of the symptom is removed. However, unless the clinician has planned for this outcome, symptom removal may have potentially harmful effects. Carefully used, though, symptom removal greatly aids management of the patient and her family because the previously hidden anxiety or conflict can be addressed. Most of the time referral to a mental health professional will be necessary in cases of this type.

Case example: Shirley presented at age 16 with abdominal pain, lethargy, and a history of weight loss. The medical history and physical examination were noncontributory. Initial interview indicated that she maintained her school grades adequately but did not participate in many peer-related social activities. This represented a long-term preference for solitary activities, not a recent change. Her abdominal pain did not keep her from school but it did elicit sympathy from her family and served to diminish conflict at home.

Independent interview and initial psychologic assessment indicated that both Shirley and her parents were quite reticent to discuss any interpersonal conflict. Although the family members showed little spontaneous interaction, no significant sources of excessive conflict other than typical adolescent-parent interactions were apparent. Shirley was passive and quiet during the initial interview; this trait seemed to be consistent with her father's personality. The mother was much more outgoing and verbal, both in the interview and in discussion of family interactions. Symptom checklist responses showed a defensive profile, but the checklist and interview did not identify a severe degree of depression. It was not felt that symptom removal would result in a significant depression or suicidal ideation.

Behavioral removal of the abdominal pain was planned with weekly contact to determine if other problems arose. Parents were instructed to ignore abdominal complaints and to reduce concerns about Shirley's eating habits, which had been one source of conflict. Return in 1 week revealed a decrease in the abdominal pain and no conflict was apparent. However, a return in 2 weeks did reveal a significant change: The mother complained about Shirley's increased hostility and anger, and Shirley was much more openly hostile toward her mother. Several more weeks of consultation revealed that the mother was quite jealous of Shirley's close relationship with the father, who encouraged this relationship. Furthermore, Shirley rejected the mother's dominating style in the home and verbalized these feelings over several sessions. After six sessions, there was decrease in anger-based conflict, an increase in open family communication, and no reoccurrence of the abdominal pain.

Level III: Somatic symptom—Emotionally damaging circumstances   In some cases the abdominal complaint may allow the adolescent to avoid serious emotionally damaging situations, such as those frequently found in families disrupted by physical or sexual abuse of the female adolescent by a family member, incest, parental alcoholism, or spouse abuse. In addition, serious peer involvement in drug and/or sexual activity may provoke symptoms. The adolescent may be unable to discuss these problems without assistance. Removal of a symptom which protects against damaging personal interactions may precipitate suicide. Thus, careful psychologic personality assessment is important before symptom removal when this type of case is suspected.

Case example: Betty, 13 years old, had abdominal pain and a normal physical examination. Interview revealed that she was quite socially active and had adequate school grades. There appeared to be no recent changes in eating or sleeping patterns and no apparent signs of psychologic conflict with peers. Discussion of child-parent interaction indicated that Betty was the oldest of four children, and she frequently had responsibility for caring for some of the younger children. She did not appear to resent this, and, in fact, appeared to enjoy babysitting with younger brothers and sisters. The family rejected the possibility of a psychologic interpretation for the abdominal pain, although the mother did not deny the possibility as strongly as the father. Betty revealed no sign of conflict with the parents during individual interview.

Primary concerns at this juncture were an abdominal complaint with no apparent physical or behavioral explanation. Further concern was lack of any disclosure of child-parent conflict, even those conflicts expected for normal adolescent-parent interactions. Therefore, the decision was made to avoid symptom removal and to perform more thorough psychologic investigation.

A second interview and psychologic testing revealed that Betty did admit to some transient irritable states lasting one to several hours which did not interfere with school or social functioning. The parents seemed unaware of these irritable moods. Betty's personality evaluation suggested a highly sensitive individual with no signs of thought disorder or conduct disorder. There were indications of excessive rumination and depression. At this juncture, it was determined to provide ongoing psychologic consultation in an attempt to identify underlying etiology prior to symptom removal.

After three more psychologic consultation sessions, it was revealed that Betty experienced irritability along with severe abdominal pain and headache, usually in the evening at home. After several more sessions, it was determined that the father had excessive alcohol consumption and frequently yelled at the mother and threatened physical violence. During these times, Betty frequently gathered her younger siblings in her bedroom and engaged them in play activities to divert their attention from parental conflict. Further evaluation revealed that Betty was severely depressed and that her mother was unaware of her daughter's significant depression. The mother consulted with legal and social authorities, and the father was removed from the home. Ongoing therapy with Betty occurred at the same time the mother was seeing an adult psychologist. Both worked on their significant depressive feelings, as well as underlying feelings of hostility toward the father. The mother had made a suicide attempt in the past, and Betty had thought about the possibility of suicide as a way to escape her intolerable home setting.

Because of the complexities of the psychoemotional problems which underlay this adolescent's abdominal pain, attempts to remove symptoms as discussed above would not have been appropriate. Early involvement of a psychologist was crucial to management in this case.

Summary

Evaluation and management of abdominal pain that cannot be explained by disease or dysfunction demands careful attention to the behavioral aspects of the symptom, the family and social environment, and the adolescent's psychologic status. Symptom removal can be a brief and appropriate treatment for selected patients. When conflict or emotionally damaging interpersonal interactions, previously masked by the symptom, are uncovered, careful analysis is necessary. Interpersonal counseling may be important along with symptom removal in some cases, and psychotherapy may be indicated before symptom removal in other more severe emotional conditions.

The primary physician can many times effectively deal with level I complaints when there is an obvious behavioral component. Furthermore, physicians with experience in the medical care of adolescents can many times treat level II cases when there is no apparent sign of significant depression and no concern about possible suicidal ideation. In this case, weekly sessions will allow rapid identification of underlying sources of conflict unmasked by behavioral removal of the symptom. If a level III case is suspected, that is, a case with a potentially emotionally damaging situation or an unavoidable home situation, then symptom removal should *not* be attempted. Immediate consultation for intensive psychologic and/or psychiatric assessment and therapeutic intervention is indicated.

References

Aach RD: Liver disease: Viral hepatitis. In Feigin RD, Cherry JD (eds): *Textbook of Pediatric Infectious Diseases*, ed 2. WB Saunders, Philadelphia, 1987a, pp 718–741.

Aach RD: Cholecystitis in childhood. In Feigin RD, Cherry JD (eds): *Textbook of Pediatric Infectious Diseases*, ed 2. WB Saunders, Philadelphia, 1987b, pp 741–746.

ACIP: Recommendations for protection against viral hepatitis. *MMWR* 4:313–334, 1985.

ACOG Technical Bulletin: Dysmenorrhea. Number 68, March 1983.

Adams JT, Libertino JA, Schwartz SI: Significance of an elevated serum amylase. *Surgery* 63:877–884, 1968.

Adelman A, Metcalf L: Abdominal pain in a university family practice setting. *J Fam Pract* 16:1107–1111, 1983.

Allen DM, Diamond LK, Howell DA: Anaphylactoid purpura in children (Schonlein-Henoch syndrome). *Am J Dis Child* 99:833–854, 1960.

Ament ME: Inflammatory disease of the colon: Ulcerative colitis and Crohn's colitis. *J Pediatr* 86:322–334, 1975.

American Psychiatric Association: *Diagnostic and Statistical Manual of Mental Disorders*, ed 3. American Psychiatric Association, Washington, DC, 1980, pp 69–72.

Apley J: *The Child With Abdominal Pains*. Blackwell Scientific Publications, London, 1975.

Apley J, Hale B: Children with recurrent abdominal pain and how do they grow up? *Br Med J* 3:7–9, 1973.

Apley J, Naish N: Recurrent abdominal pains: A field survey of 1000 school children. *Arch Dis Child* 33:165–170, 1958.

Ariyan S, Shessel FS, Pickett L: Cholecystitis and cholelithiasis masking as abdominal crisis in sickle cell disease. *Pediatrics* 58:252–258, 1976.

Asgeirssen G, Wientzen RL: Epidemiology and pathophysiology of Neisseria gonorrhoeae infection. *Semin Adolesc Med* 2:99–105, 1986.

Ballard HS, Eisinger RP, Gallo G: Renal manifestations of the Henoch-Schoenlein syndrome in adults. *Am J Med* 49:328–335, 1970.

Barr RG: Abdominal pain in the female adolescent. *Pediatr Rev* 4:281–289, 1983.

Barr RG: Abdominal pain. In Hoekelman RA (ed): *Primary Pediatric Care*. CV Mosby, St. Louis, 1987, pp 843–849.

Barr RG, Feuerstein M: Recurrent abdominal pain syndrome. How appropriate are our basic clinical assumptions? In McGrath PJ, Firestone P (eds): *Pediatric and Adolescent Behavioral Medicine: Issues in Treatment*. Springer, New York, 1983, pp 13–27.

Barrett-Connor E: Cholelithiasis in sickle cell anemia. *Am J Med* 45:889–898, 1968.

Bendig DW: Peptic disease. In Kelley VC (ed): *Kelley Practice of Pediatrics*. Harper & Row, Philadelphia, 1985, vol 5, ch 21, pp 1–10.

Bennett RC, Hughes ESR: Urinary calculi and ulcerative colitis. *Br Med J* 2:494–496, 1972.

Bennion LJ, Ginsberg RL, Garnick ME, Bennett PH: Effects of oral contraceptives on the gallbladder of normal women. *N Engl J Med* 294:189–192, 1976.

Bennion LJ, Grundy SM: Effects of obesity and caloric intake in biliary lipid metabolism in man. *J Clin Invest* 56:996–1011, 1975.

Berger HG, Honig PJ, Liebman R: Recurrent abdominal pain: Gaining control of the symptom. *Am J Dis Child* 131:1340–1344, 1977.

Berger PC, Kuhn JP: Computed tomography of blunt abdominal trauma in childhood. *Am J Roentgenology* 136:105–110, 1981.

Berman W: The hemolytic uremic syndrome: Initial clinical presentation mimicking ulcerative colitis. *J Pediatr* 81:275–278, 1972.

Berman M, Alter HJ, Ishak KG, et al: The chronic sequelae of non-A, non-B hepatitis. *Ann Intern Med* 91:1–6, 1979.

Bishop WP, Ulshen MH: Bacterial gastroenteritis. *Pediatr Clin North Am* 35:69–87, 1988.

Blum RW, Stark T: Cognitive development in adolescence. *Semin Adolesc Med* 1:25–32, 1985.

Bongard F, Landers DV, Lewis F: Differential diagnosis of appendicitis and pelvic inflammatory disease: A prospective analysis. *Am J Surg* 150:90–96, 1985.

Bonica JJ: *Principles and Practice of Obstetric Analgesia and Anesthesia*. FA Davis, Philadelphia, 1967, pp 98–115.

Brandborg LL: Other infectious, inflammatory, and miscellaneous diseases. In Sleisinger MH, Fordtran JS (eds): *Gastrointestinal Disease*, ed 2. WB Saunders, Philadelphia, 1978, pp 1076–1093.

Brandt ML, Pokorny WJ, McGill CW, Harberg FJ: Late presentations of midgut malrotation in children. *Am J Surg* 150:767–771, 1985.

Burbige EJ, Shi-Shung H, Bayless TM: Clinical manifestations of Crohn's disease in children and adolescents. *Pediatries* 55:866–871, 1975.

Burkitt DP, Meisner P: How to manage constipation with high-fiber diet. *Geriatrics* 34:33–40, 1979.

Burton JR, Smolev JK: Urinary Stones. In Burton JR, Barker LR, Zieve PD (eds): *Principles of Ambulatory Medicine*, ed 2. Williams & Wilkins, Baltimore, 1986, pp 532–542.

Cavanaugh RM: An approach to chronic abdominal pain in adolescents. *Compr Ther* 10:52–57, 1987.

Centers for Disease Control: Sexually Transmitted Disease Treatment Guidelines, 1985. *MMWR* 34:1–ff, 1985.

Chadwick VS, Modha K, Dowling RH: Mechanism of hyperoxaluria in patients with ileal dysfunction. *N Engl J Med* 289:172–176, 1973.

Chan CLK, Wood C: Pelvic adhesiolysis—the assessment of symptom relief by 100 patients. *Aust N Z J Obstet Gynaecol* 225:295–289, 1985.

Christensen MF, Mortenson O: Long term prognosis in children with recurrent abdominal pain. *Arch Dis Child* 50:110–114, 1975.

Coleman WL, Levine MD: Recurrent abdominal pain: The cost of the aches and the aches of the cost. *Pediatr Rev* 8:143–151, 1986.

Committee on Nutrition, American Academy of Pediatrics: Plant fiber intake in the pediatric diet. *Pediatrics* 67:572–575, 1981.

Coupet E: Ectopic pregnancy: The surgical epidemic. *J Natl Med Assoc* 81:567–572, 1989.

Crossley RB: Hospital admissions for abdominal pain in childhood. *J R Soc Med* 75:772–775, 1982.

Daniel WA Jr: Growth at adolescence: Clinical correlates. *Semin Adolesc Med* 1:15–24, 1985.

Daum F, Aigues H: Inflammatory bowel disease. In Silverberg M (eds): *Pediatric Gastroenterology*. Medical Examination Publishing Co, New York, 1983, pp 340–357.

de Dombal FT: Acute abdominal pain: An OGME Survey. *Scand J Gastroenterol* 14(Suppl):29–43, 1979.

Delp MH, Manning RT: *Major's Physical Diagnosis*, ed 9. WB Saunders, Philadelphia, 1981, pp 323–375.

Derogatis LR: *SCL-90-R, Administration, Scoring, and Procedures Manual-II for the Revised Version*. Clinical Psychometric Research, Towson, MD, 1977.

Drake DP: Acute abdominal pain in children. *J R Soc Med* 73:641–645, 1980.

Dunn DH, Williams RD, Gonzalez R: Intermittent hydronephrosis: A cause of abdominal pain. *Arch Surg* 113:329–330, 1978.

DuPont HL: Nonfluid therapy and selected chemoprophylaxis of acute diarrhea. *Am J Med* 78(Suppl 6B):81–90, 1985.

Edwards MW, Forman WM, Walton J: Audit of abdominal pain in general practice. *J R Coll Gen Pract* 35:235–238, 1985.

Eichelberger MR, Hoelzer DJ, Koop CE: Acute pancreatitis: The difficulties of diagnosis and therapy. *J Pediatr Surg* 17:244–254, 1982.

Eisenberg M: Foodborne illness. In Kelley VC (ed): *Kelley Practice of Pediatrics*. Harper & Row, Philadelphia, 1985, vol 3, ch 32, pp 1–18.

Engel GL: Psychogenic pain and the pain-prone patient. *Am J Med* 26:899–918, 1959.

Engel GL: The need for a new medical model: A challenge for biomedical science. *Science* 199:129–136, 1977.

Eschenbach DA: Acute pelvic inflammatory disease. In Sciarra JJ (ed): *Gynecology and Obstetrics*. Harper & Row, Philadelphia, 1986, vol 1, ch 44, pp 1–20.

Farmer RG: Clinical features and natural history of inflammatory bowel disease. *Med Clin North Am* 64:1103–1115, 1980.

Feighner JP, Rubin E, Guze SB, Munoz R: Diagnostic criteria for use in psychiatric research. *Arch Gen Psychiatry* 26:57–63, 1972.

Figelman AR: Understanding and recognizing the effects of Chlamydia trachomatis infections. *Semin Adolesc Med* 2:107–111, 1986.

Fihn SD, Stamm WE: Interpretation and comparison of treatment studies for uncomplicated urinary tract infections in women. *Rev Infect Dis* 7:468–478, 1985.

Filly RA: Ectopic pregnancy: The role of sonography. *Radiology* 162:661–668, 1987.

Folkman J: Appendicitis. In Ravitch MM, Welch KJ, Benson CD, Aberdeen E, Randolph JG (eds): *Pediatric Surgery*, ed 3. Year Book Medical Publishers, Chicago, 1979, pp 1004–1009.

Freij BJ: Acute pelvic inflammatory disease. *Semin Adolesc Med* 2:143–153, 1986.

Frey J: The family context of adolescence. *Semin Adolesc Med* 1:47–54, 1985.

Galler JR, Neustein S, Walker WA: Clinical aspects of recurrent abdominal pain in children. *Adv Pediatr* 27:31–53, 1980.

Gilmore OJA, Brodribb AJM, Browett JP: Appendicitis and mimicking conditions: A prospective study. *Lancet* 2:421–424, 1975.

Glasier CM, Siegel MJ, McAlister WH, et al: Henoch-Schonlein syndrome in children: Gastrointestinal manifestations. *Am J Roentgenology* 136:1081–1085, 1981.

Goldstein DP, deCholnoky C, Leventhal JM, Emans SH: New insights into the old problem of pelvic pain. *J Pediatr Surg* 14:675–680, 1979.

Greenberg M, Kangarloo H, Cochran ST, Sample WF: The ultrasonographic diagnosis of cholecystitis and cholelithiasis in children. *Radiology* 137:745–749, 1980.

Gryboski JD: Crohn's disease in children. *Pediatr Rev* 2:239–244, 1981.

Hager WD, Eschenbach DA, Spence MR, Sweet RL: Criteria for diagnosis and grading of salpingitis. *Obstet Gynecol* 61:113–114, 1983.

Hallatt JG, Steele CH, Snyder M: Ruptured corpus luteum with hemoperitoneum: A study of 173 surgical cases. *Am J Obstet Gynecol* 149:5–9, 1984.

Haller JO, Kassner G, Staiano S, Schneider M: Ultrasonic diagnosis of gynecologic disorders in children. *Pediatrics* 62:339–342, 1978.

Hamilton JR: Viral enteritis. *Pediatr Clin North Am* 35:89–101, 1988.

Harrop-Griffiths J, Katon W, Walker E, Holm L, Russo J, Hickok L: The association between chronic pelvic pain, psychiatric diagnoses, and childhood sexual abuse. *Obstet Gynecol* 71:589–594, 1988.

Hornick RB: Salmonella infections. In Feigin RD, Cherry JD (eds): *Textbook of Pediatric Infectious Diseases*, ed 2. WB Saunders, Philadelphia, 1987a, pp 673–683.

Hornick RB: Shigella infections. In Feigin RD, Cherry JD (eds): *Textbook of Pediatric Infectious Diseases*, ed 2. WB Saunders, Philadelphia, 1987b, pp 683–688.

Hricak H: MRI of the female pelvis: A review. *Am J Roentgenology* 146:1115–1122, 1986.

Jacobsen L: Differential diagnosis of acute pelvic inflammatory disease. *Am J Obstet Gynecol* 138:1006–1011, 1980.

Jastak S, Wilkinson GS: *Wide Range Achievement Test-Revised*. Psychological Corporation, San Antonio, 1984.

Jewett TC, Caldarola V, Karp MP, Allen JE, Cooney DR: Intramural hematoma of the duodenum. *Arch Surg* 123:54–58, 1988.

Johnson SR, Laube DW: Chronic pelvic pain: Evaluation and treatment. *Iowa Med* 76:572–577, 1986.

Jones PF: Acute abdominal pain in childhood, with special reference to cases not due to acute appendicitis. *Br Med J* 1:284–286, 1969.

Kaplan BS, Proesmans W: The hemolytic uremic syndrome of childhood and its variants. *Semin Hematol* 24:148–160, 1987.

Kettwich DL, Goldman RS, Woodside JR, Crawford ED, Borden TA: Flank pain and microhematuria in a young woman. *J Urol* 123:756–760, 1980.

Keusch GT: Enterotoxigenic and enteropathogenic Escherichia coli. In Feigin RD, Cherry JD (eds): *Textbook of Pediatric Infectious Diseases*, ed 2. WB Saunders, Philadelphia, 1987a, pp 660–670.

Keusch GT: Enteroinvasive Escherichia coli. In Feigin RD, Cherry JD (eds): *Textbook of Pediatric Infectious Diseases*, ed 2. WB Saunders, Philadelphia, 1987b, pp 670–673.

Kirschner BS: Inflammatory bowel disease in children. *Pediatr Clin North Am* 35:189–208, 1988.

Kleinhaus S, Hein K, Sheran M, Boley SJ: Laparoscopy for diagnosis and treatment of abdominal pain in adolescent girls. *Arch Surg* 112:1178–1179, 1977.

Kobayashi O, Wada H, Okawa K, Takeyama I: Schonlein-Henoch's syndrome in children. In Berlyne GM, Giovannetti S (eds): *Contributions to Nephrology*, vol 4. Karger, New York, 1977, pp 48–71.

Komaroff AL: Acute dysuria in women. *N Engl J Med* 310:368–375, 1984.

Kreipe RE, McAnarney ER: Psychosocial aspects of adolescent medicine. *Semin Adolesc Med* 1:33–45, 1985.

Krugman S: Viral hepatitis: 1985 update. *Pediatr Rev* 7:3–11, 1985.

Kuhn JP: Diagnostic imaging for the evaluation of abdominal trauma in children. *Pediatr Clin North Am* 32:1427–1447, 1985.

Kunin CM: *Detection, Prevention and Management of Urinary Tract Infections*, ed 3. Lea & Febiger, Philadelphia, 1979.

Lerner A, Lebenthal E: Acute pancreatitis in children—an update. In Moss AJ (ed): *Pediatrics Update: Reviews for Physicians*. Elsevier, New York, 1986, pp 241–256.

Levine MD, Rappaport LA: Recurrent abdominal pain in school children: The loneliness of the long-distance physician. *Pediatr Clin North Am* 31:969–991, 1984.

Lewin GA, Mikity V, Wingert WA: Barium enema: An outpatient procedure in the early diagnosis of acute appendicitis. *J Pediatr* 92:451–453, 1978.

Liebman WB, Thaler MM: Pediatric considerations of abdominal pain and the acute abdomen. In Sleisinger MH, Fordtran JS (eds): *Gastrointestinal Disease*, ed 2. WB Saunders, Philadelphia, 1978, pp 411–424.

Loening-Baucke V, Encopresis and enuresis. In Wolraich M (ed): *Practical Assessment and Management of Children with Disorders of Development and Learning*. Year Book Medical Publishers, Chicago, 1987.

McCarthy S, Taylor KJW: Sonography of vaginal masses. *Am J Roentgenology* 140:1005–1008, 1983.

McGrath PJ, Unruh AM: *Pain in Children and Adolescents*. Elsevier, New York, 1987a, pp 47–104.

McGrath PJ, Unruh AM: *Pain in Children and Adolescents*. Elsevier, New York, 1987b, pp 143–162.

McGrath PJ, Unruh AM: *Pain in Children and Adolescents*. Elsevier, New York, 1987c, pp 305–316.

Meadow SR, Glasgow EF, et al. Schonlein-Henoch nephritis. *Q J Med* 163:241–252, 1972.

Merskey H, Albe-Fessard DG, Bonica JF, et al: Definitions and notes on usage recommended by the IASP Subcommittee on Taxonomy. *Pain* 6:249–252, 1979.

Messer RD, Keating JP: Inflammatory bowel disease in childhood. In Moss AJ (ed): *Pediatrics Update*. Elsevier, New York, 1980, pp 103–124.

Miller FJW, Court SDM, Knox EG, Branden S: *The School Years in Newcastle-upon-Tyne*. Oxford University Press, Oxford, 1974.

Moffatt M, Embree J, Grimm P, Law B: Short-course antibiotic therapy for urinary tract infections in children. *Am J Dis Child* 142:57–61, 1988.

Moosa AR: Diagnostic tests and procedures in acute pancreatitis. *N Engl J Med* 311:639–643, 1984.

Moscicki A, Shafer M: Normal reproductive development in the adolescent female. *J Adolesc Health Care* 7:41S–64S, 1986.

Nord KS: Peptic ulcer disease in children and adolescents: Evolving dilemmas. *J Pediatr Gastroenterol Nutr* 2:397–399, 1983.

Orr D: Adolescence, stress, and psychosomatic issues. *J Adolesc Health Care* 7:97S–108S, 1986.

Orsini LF, Salardi S, Pilu G, Bovicelli L, Cacciari E: Pelvic organs in premenarcheal girls: Real-time ultrasonography. *Radiology* 153:113–116, 1984.

Oster J: Recurrent abdominal pain, headache, and limb pains in children and adolescents. *Pediatrics* 50:429–436, 1972.

Parcel JS, Nader PR, Meyer MP: Adolescent health concerns, problems, and patterns of utilization in a triethnic urban population. *Pediatrics* 60:157–164, 1977.

Pearce S, Knight C, Beard RW: Pelvic pain—a common gynaecological problem. *J Psychosom Obstet Gynaecol* 1:12–17, 1982.

Pellerin D, Bertin P, Nihow-Fekete C: Cholelithiasis and ileal pathology in childhood. *J Pediatr Surg* 10:35–41, 1975.

Philbrick JT, Bracikowski JP: Single-dose antibiotic treatment for uncomplicated urinary tract infections. *Arch Intern Med* 145:1672–1678, 1985.

Pickering LK: Antimicrobial therapy of gastrointestinal infections. *Pediatr Clin North Am* 30:373–388, 1983.

Pickering LK, Cleary TG: Approach to patients with gastrointestinal infections and food poisoning. In Feigin RD, Cherry JD (eds): *Textbook of Pediatric Infectious Diseases*, ed 2. WB Saunders, Philadelphia, 1987, pp 622–651.

Present DH, Rabinowitz JG, Banks PA, Janowitz HD: Obstructive hydronephrosis. *N Engl J Med* 280:523–528, 1969.

Pringle MLK, Butler NR, Davie R: *11,000 Seven Year Olds*. Longmans, London, 1966.

Puri P, Boyd E, Blake N, Guiney EJ: Duodenal ulcer disease in childhood: A continuing disease in adult life. *J Pediatr Surg* 13:525–526, 1978.

Quay HC, Peterson D: *Manual for the Revised Behavior Problem Checklist*. University of Miami, Coral Gables, FL, 1983.

Ramenofsky ML: Pediatric abdominal trauma. *Pediatr Ann* 16:318–326, 1987.

Rapkin AJ: Adhesions and pelvic pain: a retrospective study. *Obstet Gynecol* 68:13–15, 1986.

Rapkin AJ, Kames LD: The pain management approach to chronic pelvic pain. *J Reprod Med* 32:323–327, 1987.

Renaer M, Vertommen H, Nijs P, Wagemans L, van Hemelrijk J: Psychological aspects of chronic pelvic pain in women. *Am J Obstet Gynecol* 134:75–80, 1979.

Risser W, Mullins D, Butler PM, West MS: Diagnosing psychiatric disorders in adolescent females with abdominal pain. *J Adolesc Health Care* 8:431–435, 1987.

Ritchie WGM: Sonographic evaluation of normal and induced ovulation. *Radiology* 161:1–10, 1986.

Robb JDA, Thomas PS, Orszulak J, Odling-Smee GW: Duodenal ulcer in children. *Arch Dis Child* 47:688–696, 1972.

Rosenblum ND, Winter HS: Steroid effects on the course of abdominal pain in children with Henoch-Schonlein purpura. *Pediatrics* 79:1018–1021, 1987.

Ross DM, Ross SA: *Childhood Pain: Current Issues, Research and Management*. Urban & Schwarzenberg, Baltimore, 1988.

Sack RB, Barker LR: Acute gastroenteritis and associated conditions. In Barker LR, Burton JR, Zeive PD (eds): *Principles of Ambulatory Medicine*, ed 2. Williams & Wilkins, Baltimore, 1986, pp 324–333.

Savrin RA, Clatworthy HW Jr: Appendiceal rupture: A continuing diagnostic problem. *Pediatrics* 63:37–43, 1979.

Schrock TR: Acute appendicitis. In Sleisinger MH, Fordtran JS (eds): *Gastrointestinal Disease*, ed 3. WB Saunders, Philadelphia, 1983, pp 1268–1275.

Schuster MM: Abdominal pain. In Barker LR, Burton JR, Zeive PD (eds): *Principles of Ambulatory Medicine*, ed 2. Williams & Wilkins, Baltimore, 1986a, pp 428–437.

Schuster MM: The irritable bowel syndrome. In Barker LR, Burton JR, Zeive PD (eds): *Principles of Ambulatory Medicine*, ed 2. Williams & Wilkins, Baltimore, 1986b, pp 480–488.

Shafer MB, Irwin CE, Sweet RL: Acute salpingitis in the adolescent female. *J Pediatr* 100:339–350, 1982.

Siegel MJ, Glasier CM, Sagel SS: CT of pelvic disorders in children. *Am J Roentgenology* 137:1139–1143, 1981.

Silber TJ: Approaching the adolescent patient. *J Adolesc Health Care* 7:31S–40S, 1986.

Silverberg M: Functional gastrointestinal disorders. In Silverberg M (ed): *Pediatric Gastroenterology*. Medical Examination Publishing Co, New Hyde Park, NY, 1983, pp 270–275.

Silverberg M, Daum F: Irritable bowel syndrome in children and adolescents. *Pract Gastroenterol* 3:25, 1979.

Slocumb JC: Neurologic factors in chronic pelvic pain: Trigger points and the abdominal pelvic pain syndrome. *Am J Obstet Gynecol* 149:536–543, 1984.

Smith EI: Appendicitis and peritonitis. In Kelley VC (ed): *Practice of Pediatrics*. Harper & Row, Philadelphia, 1985, vol 5, ch 32, pp 1–13.

Speilberger CD, Gorusch RL, Lushene R: *The State-Trait Anxiety Inventory: Test Manual.* Consulting Psychology Press, Palo Alto, CA, 1969.

Spiro HM: *Clinical Gastroenterology.* MacMillan, London, 1970, pp 2–6.

Stanghellini V, Camilleri M, Malagelada J-R: Chronic intestinal pseudoobstruction: Clinical and intestinal manometric findings. *Gut* 28:5–12, 1987.

Stapleton FB: Urolithiasis in children: New perspectives. In Moss AJ (ed): *Pediatrics Update: Reviews for Physicians.* Elsevier, New York, 1986, pp 241–256.

Starfield B, Gross E, Wood M: Psychosocial and psychosomatic diagnosis in primary care of children. *Pediatrics* 66:159–167, 1980.

Stenchever MA: Significant symptoms and signs in different age groups. In: Droegemueller W, Herbst AL, Mishell DR Jr, Stenchever MA: *Comprehensive Gynecology.* CV Mosby, St Louis, 1987, pp 153–159.

Strahlman RS: Appendicitis. In Hoekelman RA (ed): *Primary Pediatric Care.* CV Mosby, St. Louis, 1987, pp 1142–1144.

Szmuness W, Dienstag JL, Purcell RH, Harley EJ, Stevens CE, Wong DC: Distribution of antibody to hepatitis A antigen in urban adult populations. *N Engl J Med* 295:755–759, 1976.

Tam PKH, Saing H, Lau TK: Diagnosis of peptic ulcer in children: The past and the present. *J Pediatr Surg* 21:129–131, 1986.

Ternberg JL, Keating JP: Acute acalculous cholecystitis. *Arch Surg* 110:543–547, 1975.

Thomson HJ: Active observation in acute abdominal pain. *Am J Surg* 152:552–555, 1986.

Wall PD: On the relation of injury to pain. *Pain* 6:253–264, 1979.

Washington AE, Arno PS, Brooks MA: The economic cost of pelvic inflammatory disease. *JAMA* 255:1735–1738, 1986.

Way LW: Abdominal pain and the acute abdomen. In Sleisinger MH, Fordtran JS (eds): *Gastrointestinal Disease*, ed 3. WB Saunders, Philadelphia, 1983, pp 207–221.

Weinstein L: Yersiniosis. In Feigin RD, Cherry JD (eds): *Textbook of Pediatric Infectious Diseases*, ed 2. WB Saunders, Philadelphia, 1987, pp 689–698.

Whitehead WE, Schuster MM: Psychological management of irritable bowel syndrome. *Pract Gastroenterol* 3:32, 1979.

Wilfert C, Gutman L: Sexually transmitted diseases. In Feigin RE, Cherry JD (eds): *Textbook of Pediatric Infectious Diseases*, ed 2. WB Saunders, Philadelphia, 1987, pp 595–621.

Wyatt RG, Kapikian AZ: Viral gastrointestinal infections. In Feigin RD, Cherry JD (eds): *Textbook of Pediatric Infectious Diseases*, ed 2. WB Saunders, Philadelphia, 1987, pp 699–717.

Yang P, Banwell JG: Dietary fiber: Its role in the pathogenesis and treatment of constipation. *Pract Gastroenterol* 10:28–32, 1986.

Yeh SC, Futterweit W, Thornton JC: Polycystic ovarian disease: US features in 104 patients. *Radiology* 163:111–116, 1987.

Index

Abdominal pain, 175–176. *See also* Pelvic
    pain
  abrupt onset, 177
  acute, 184–185
  and adolescent development, 174–175
  associated signs and symptoms, 179
  causes of, 174–175
  characteristic patterns, 178–179
  classification of, 175–176
  of constipation, 189
  differential diagnosis, 174
  dysfunctional, 175–176
  evaluation of, 173, 176–184
  with gallbladder inflammation, 196–197
  in gastrointestinal disorders, 186–194
  gradual onset, 177
  gynecologic, 174, 197–209
  history, 176–179
  imaging evaluation of, 181–184
  in inflammatory diseases of liver, 196
  with intraperitoneal fluid, 178–179
  laboratory tests with, 180
  location, 178
  nongynecologic, causes of, 186–197
  organic, 175–176
  periumbilical, 187
  physical examination with, 179–180
  presentation, 175
  psychogenic, 175–176, 214–223
    differential diagnosis, 218–219
    integration of evaluative data, 217–218
    treatment, 219–223
  rapid onset, 177
  recurrent, 177, 185–186
    behavioral analysis of, 219–223
    differential diagnosis of, clinical
      interview in, 215–216
    in irritable bowel syndrome, 191
    treatment, 219–223
  referred, 177
  relation to meals, 178
  renal/urinary tract causes of, 194–195
  timing, 177–178
Abdominal trauma, 177, 194
Abortion
  legal aspects of, 16–17
  minors' access to, 63
  parental consent or notification before,
    16–17, 63
  rate of, 1
  risk of, 29
Acetowhite reaction, 79
Acne
  nodulocystic, isotretinoin therapy, and
    amenorrhea, 151
  and oral contraceptives, 25–27, 35–36
Acquired immunodeficiency syndrome
    (AIDS), 108. *See also* Human
    immunodeficiency virus
Acute surgical abdomen, 177, 186
Acyclovir, for herpes genital infection, 96
Addison's disease, 154
Adenomyosis, 162
Adhesions
  management, 214
  pain with, 212
Adnexal disorders, 202–207
Adnexal mass, 199, 203
  ultrasound of, 183
Adnexal tenderness, 187, 199, 203
  in appendicitis, 187
  in pelvic inflammatory disease, 187
Adnexal torsion, 207
  diagnostic approach to, 199
  laboratory assessment of, 200
  ultrasound of, 182–183
Adolescent development. *See also* Breast
    development; Puberty and abdominal
    pain, 174–175
  cognitive stages of, 10
Adrenal tumors, 114
Aeromonas hydrophila, gastroenteritis caused
    by, 189
Affective disorders. *See also* Depression and
    amenorrhea, 150
AIDS. *See* Acquired immunodeficiency
    syndrome
Albright's syndrome, 114
Amastia, 117
Amazia, 117
Amebiasis, 104
Amenorrhea, 143–151, 154–155
  definition of, 144
  with oral contraceptives, 36

Amenorrhea—*continued*
  postpartum, 151
  post pill, 151
  prevalence, 144
  primary, 145–147
    causes of, 145, 147
    indications for evaluation of, 145
    reproductive prognosis in, 147
    sequential evaluation of, 147
  secondary
    causes of, 149
    definition of, 148
    differential diagnosis, 148
    sequential evaluation of, 148–149
Amenorrhea-galactorrhea syndrome, 132
Anal intercourse, 8
Anaphylactoid purpura, 194
Anaprox. *See* Naproxen sodium
Anatomic anomalies, 146
Androgen excess, 152
Androgen insensitivity, 147
Anemia, 180
Anger, 218–219
Anorexia nervosa, 146, 150
  and abdominal pain, 193
  and secondary amenorrhea, 148
Anosmia, 146
Antidepressant therapy, and chronic pain
    syndrome, 214
Antifungal agents, 88
Antiprostaglandin, to induce rapid cessation
    of uterine bleeding, 156
Anxiety, 218–219
Appendicitis, 184
  acute
    complication rate, 186
    differential diagnosis, 186
    prevalence, 186
  diagnostic approach to, 199
  history, 187
  laboratory assessment of, 187, 200
  pain of, 187
  physical examination with, 187
  ultrasound in, 183
Arrhenoblastoma, 152
Arthritis, gonococcal, 94–95
  and pregnancy, 107
Asherman syndrome, 147
Aspirin, 161
Assault and battery, 64–65
Athelia, 117
Athletic activity. *See also* Sports
  and amenorrhea, 145–146, 148–150

Bacterial vaginitis, 83
Bacterial vaginosis, 78, 86
Baird v. Bellotti, 63

Barium enema, 184, 187
Barrier contraception. *See* Contraception,
    barrier methods of
Bartholin's gland abscess, 78
Bartholin's gland duct, inflammation of, in
    gonorrhea, 91
Behavior, objective assessment of, 216–217
Behçet's disease, 104–105
Bellotti provisions, 63
Biopsychosocial model of illness, 173
Births, to teenagers, 1
Black teenagers
  rates of sexual activity and pregnancy, 5
  sexual activity, 2
Bleeding disorders, 154
Bloating, 167
Body fat, percentage of, for maintenance of
    ovulatory cycles, 150
Bowel obstruction, 193
Breast(s)
  abnormalities, psychosocial aspects,
    136–137
  abscesses, 126, 135
  aspiration, 127–128
  asymmetry, 120
  atrophy of, 119–120
  cellulitis, 126
  cutaneous scarring, 126–127
  cysts, 122–123
  dimensions, recording, 129
  ecchymosis, 135–136
  fat necrosis, 136
  fibroadenomas, 121–122, 128
  fibrocystic changes of, 122–123
  granular cell myoblastomas of, 124–125
  hematomas, 135–136
  infections, 126
  intraductal papillomas, 124
  trauma, and sports, 124, 135–136
  tuberous, 117–118
  virginal hypertrophy, 117–119
Breast budding, 113, 121
  and onset of menarche, 141
Breast cancer, 137
  in adolescents, 125–126
    treatment, 128
  in adults
    incidence of, 126
    risk factors for, 126
  and oral contraceptives, 31–32
Breast development, 113–114, 131–132, 145
  anomalies of, 114–120
  delayed and slow, 117
  onset of, 137
  in pregnant female, 131–132
  Tanner stages of, 114–115
  unequal, 119
Breast disorders, 113–137
  benign, and oral contraceptives, 33

Breast examination, 129–131, 137
Breast masses, 121–128
    benign, 121–125
    cystic, 127–128
    diagnostic tools for assessing, 127
    excisional biopsy, 127–128, 136
    inflammatory, 126
    management of, 127–128
    neoplastic, 125–126
    solid benign–appearing, 127–128
    suspicious for malignancy, 127–128
    trauma-induced, 124
    types of, 125
Breast self–examination, 130–131
Bromocriptine
    for breast symptoms, in premenstrual
        syndrome, 167
    for lowering serum prolactin, 135
Bulimia, and abdominal pain, 193
Butoconazole nitrate (Femstat), 88–89

Caffeine, and premenstrual syndrome, 165
Calymmatobacterium (Donovania)
        granulomatosis, 103
Campylobacter pylori, gastroenteritis caused
        by, 188–189
Candida albicans, 76, 79, 85
    hyphae, 88
    infection, treatment of male for, 89
    in preadolescent, 83
    spores, 88
    vaginitis
        causes, 87
        diagnostic procedures, 88
        precipitating factors for, 87–88
        symptoms and signs, 87–88
        treatment, 88–89
Candida tropicalis, 87–88
Carey v. Population Services International,
        15, 63–64
Carotenemia, and secondary amenorrhea, 148
Cefotaxime, 92
Cefoxitin, 92
Ceftriaxone, 92, 94–95
Cervical abnormalities, 77
Cervical cancer, 76, 79
    and oral contraceptives, 32
Cervical cap, 49–50
    and adolescent patient, 50
    availability, 49
    displacement during use, 50
    effectiveness, 24, 46, 49
    fitting, 49–50
    historical perspective on, 45
    insertion, 50
    odor associated with, 50
    and pap smears, 50

as protection against sexually transmitted
        disease, 49
    removal, after placement, 50
Cervical intraepithelial neoplasia, and herpes,
        97
Cervical/vaginal secretions, saline
        preparation of, 76, 78
Cervicitis, 154
    acute, 201
    chlamydial, 97–98, 201
    gonorrheal, 91–92, 201
    herpetic, 95–97
    mucopurulent
        diagnostic approach to, 199
        laboratory assessment of, 200
Cervix
    disorders of, 201
    normal, 77
Chancroid, 102
Chickenpox, 83
Childbirth, risk of, 29
Chlamydia psittaci, 97
Chlamydia trachomatis, 76, 78, 94,
        202–203. *See also* Lymphogranuloma
        venereum
    cervicitis, 97–98, 201
        diagnosis, 97–98
        symptoms and signs, 97
        treatment, 98
    infections, 90, 97–98
        in prepubertal girls, 84
    and oral contraceptive use, 32
    pelvic inflammatory disease caused by,
        98–99
    perihepatitis, 93
    protection against, with condoms, 46
    urethral syndrome, 97
Cholecystitis, 196–197
    ultrasound in, 183
Cholelithiasis, 184
    ultrasound in, 183
Cholesterol levels. *See also* Lipid profile
    and oral contraceptives, 25–27
Clear cell adenocarcinoma, of vagina, 107,
        154
Clinical interview
    in differential diagnosis of recurrent
        abdominal pain, 215–216
    with parents, 215
    with patient, 215–216
Clitoris, 76
Clonidine, in management of premenstrual
        symptoms, 167
Clotrimazole (Gyne–Lotrimin, Mycelex–G),
        88–90
Clotting. *See also* Coagulation disorder and
        oral contraceptives, 28
Clue cells, 76, 78, 86
Coagulation disorder, 154

Colposcope, 81, 83
Communication, intergenerational, problems
     in, 59–60
Computed tomography, abdominal and
     pelvic, 184
Condom dermatitis, 47
Condoms, 45–49
  and adolescent patient, 48
  advantages of, 23
  allergies to, 47
  availability, 46
  breakage, 46–47
  concerns about, 47–48
  cost of, 46
  effectiveness, 46
    theoretical vs. actual, 24
  failure
    rate of, 46
    sources of, 46–47
  historical perspective on, 45
  Hugger, 45, 47
  instructions to patients on proper use of, 48
  and male sensitivity during intercourse, 47
  Mentor, 47
  in preventing sexually transmitted disease,
     46
  sizes, 45
  with spermicidal lubricants, 45
  with spermicide, effectiveness of,
     theoretical vs. actual, 24
  storage, 49
  tearing, with oil-based lubricants, 47
  types of, 45
  use of, 9–10
Condyloma acuminata, 79, 105–106
  diagnosis of, 106
  and pregnancy, 107
  symptoms and signs, 106
  treatment, 106
Confidentiality, 13, 35. *See also* Health
     record, privacy; Privacy rights
  in adolescent health care, implementing,
     66–68
    American Academy of Pediatrics policy
       position on, 59
    breech of, 60, 72
    and confrontation with parents, 69–70
    and contraception, 60–62
    policies and practices about, establishment
       of, in office setting, 68–69
    requirement of adolescents for, 59–60
    securing parents' agreement to, 69
Congenital adrenal hyperplasia, 146, 152
Constipation, 189–190
  causes, 189
  diagnosis of, 210
    physical examination in, 190
  disimpaction, 190
  high fiber diet for, 191

laboratory and radiographic evaluation of,
     190, 211
  laxative therapy, 190–191
  management, 190
  outcome, 191
Constitutional rights, minors', 62–63
Contraception
  barrier methods of, 45–56
    failure of, and intercourse frequency, 25
    historical perspective on, 45
    pregnancy rates of, 45–46
  confidentiality issues for minor adolescents
       obtaining, 60–62, 66–67
  failure to use, explanations for, 10–11
  legal aspects of, 15–16, 65
  postcoital, 38–39
Contraceptive practices, teenage, 8–13
Contraceptives, 1. *See also* Cervical cap;
     Condoms; Diaphragm; Oral
     contraceptives
  effect on sexual activity, 12–13
  physician willingness to prescribe, 13–14
  use of, 9–10
Contrast studies, of gastrointestinal and
     urinary tracts, 184
Corpus luteum cyst, 205–207
Corynebacterium vaginale, 86
Cotton undergarments, 82, 84, 86, 101
Craniopharyngioma, 132
Crohn disease, 192
Cryptococcus, 87
Culdocentesis, 100
Cullen sign, 197
Cushing's disease, 152
Cushing's syndrome, 146
Cystitis
  diagnostic approach to, 199
  laboratory assessment of, 200
Cystosarcoma phyllodes, 124
Cytomegalovirus, protection against, with
     condoms, 46

Danazol
  for breast symptoms, in premenstrual
     syndrome, 167
  as treatment for fibrocystic breast disease,
     123
Dancers, amenorrhea in, 149
Department of Health and Human Services.
     See Squeal rule
Depo-Provera, to induce reversible
     amenorrhea, 156
Depression, 214, 218–219, 222–223
Dermatitis, gonococcal, 94–95
Dermatitis medicamentosa, 86, 101
Dermatophytids, 88
DES. *See* Diethylstilbestrol
Desogestrel, 27

DGI. *See* Gonococcal infections,
  disseminated
Diabetes mellitus, 154
Diaphragm, 51
  and adolescent patient, 53
  advantages of, 23–24
  allergy to, 53
  availability of, 51
  contraindications to, 53
  disadvantages of, 24
  effectiveness of, 46, 51
    theoretical vs. actual, 24
  embarrassment with insertion, 52
  failure of, 51
  fitting, 51–52
  historical perspective on, 45
  as protection against sexually transmitted
    disease, 51
  readjustment, 52
  refitting, 52
  sizes, 51
  timing of use, 52
  urinary tract infection associated with, 53
  usage rates, 23
Diet, in management of premenstrual
  symptoms, 165–166
Diethylstilbestrol, 75, 77, 154
  as postcoital contraceptive, 38
  vaginal clear cell adenocarcinoma induced
    by, 107, 154
Diethylstilbestrol-induced vaginal adenosis,
  107
Diiodohydroxyquinoline–hydrocortisone, 91
Direct fluorescent antibody test, 76, 78
Diuretic therapy, in premenstrual syndrome,
  167
Doe v. Bolton, 63
Doe v. Irwin, 15
Doxycycline, 100
Drug use, and earlier onset of sexual
  intercourse, 5
Duodenum, intramural hematoma of, 194
Dysfunctional gynecologic pain, 186
Dysfunctional uterine bleeding, 151–157
  definition of, 152
  diagnosis of, 153
  differential diagnosis, 154
  etiology, 153–155
  laboratory evaluation of, 155
  management, 155
  prognosis, 156–157
Dysmenorrhea, 153, 157–162, 207–209
  associated symptoms, 208
  congestive, 158
  etiology, 158–160
  and gynecologic age, 157–158
  incidence of, 157–158
  management, 160–161
  prevalence of, 142, 157–158

  primary, 158, 207–208
    definition of, 158
    diagnosis, 199, 208
    laboratory assessment of, 200
  secondary, 161–162, 207
    characteristics of, 162
    with pelvic inflammatory disease, 212
  severity of, 157–158
  spasmodic, 158
  treatment, with oral contraceptives, 33–35
Dysuria-pyuria syndrome, 194

Eating disorders
  and abdominal pain, 193
  and amenorrhea, 148, 150
Ectopic pregnancy, 100, 186, 198–201,
  206–207
  diagnostic approach to, 199
  laboratory assessment of, 200
  ultrasound image in, 181
Ectropion, 77
EIA. *See* Enzyme immunoassay
Emancipation, for adolescent, 59–60
Emergency care, of minors, 64, 71
Empty sella syndrome, 132
Endocarditis, gonococcal, 95
Endometrial cancer, lowered risk of, with
  oral contraceptives, 31, 33
Endometrial polyps, 162
Endometriosis, 146, 154, 162
  chronic pain of, 209
  diagnostic approach to, 199
  laboratory assessment of, 200
  management, 214
  pain of, 209
Endometritis
  chronic, 209–212
    diagnosis, 210
    laboratory assessment with, 211
  nonpuerperal, 209–212
Endomyces albicans. See Candida albicans
β-Endorphin, and premenstrual
  symptoms, 165
Enemas, 190
Entamoeba histolytica
  proctitis, 94
  vulvar ulcerations, 104
Enterobius vermicularis, 104
Enuresis, 195
Enzyme immunoassay, 76, 78
Erythrocyte sedimentation rate, 180, 203
Escherichia coli, enteropathogenic, 188
Estranes, 38
Estrogen
  and atrophic vaginitis, 150
  conjugated, as postcoital contraceptive, 38
  deficit, and osteoporosis, 150
  effect on genital tract, 84

Estrogen—*continued*
exogenous, long-term exposure to, 114
and premenstrual symptoms, 165
topical, for prepubertal nonspecific
vaginitis, 84
Ethinyl estradiol, 25
as postcoital contraceptive, 38
Exercise, in management of premenstrual
symptoms, 165–166

Family
communication within, and contraceptive
use, 10–11
and early sexual relationships, 5
as topic of clinical interview, 216
Family practitioners, willingness to treat
teenagers, 13–14
Femstat. *See* Butoconazole nitrate
Ferrous sulfate supplementations, 156
Fever
of acute appendicitis, 187
of acute pelvic inflammatory disease, 203
Fibroadenomas
of breast, 121–122, 128
juvenile giant, 124
Fibrocystic breast disease. *See* Fibrocystic
mastopathies
Fibrocystic mastopathies, 122–123, 127
and breast cancer, 123–124
therapy for, 123
Fitz-Hugh-Curtis syndrome, 93, 100, 204
Flunidazole, 91
Fluorescent antibody test, for *G. vaginalis*,
86
Follicle cysts, 205–206
Follicle-stimulating hormone, 144
Folliculitis, 77
Forbes-Albright syndrome, 132
Foreign bodies, in vagina, 81–83, 154

Galactoceles, 122
Galactorrhea, 131–135, 146, 151, 155
definition of, 131
drugs associated with, 133–134
etiology, 132–134
evaluation, 134–135
idiopathic, 134
management, 135
neurogenic causes of, 134
prevalence of, 131
Gardnerella vaginalis, 78, 85
bacteremia, 86
in prepubertal girl, 83
vaginitis, 78, 86
diagnostic procedures, 86
symptoms and signs, 86
treatment, 87

Gastrocolic reflex, 191
Gastroenteritis, 187–189
acute, 186
Aeromonas, 188–189
Campylobacter, 188–189
Giardia, 189
Salmonella, 188
Shigella, 188
viral, 188
Yersinia, 186, 188–189
Genital tract obstruction, 146
Gestodone, 27
Giardia lamblia, gastroenteritis, 189
Giardiasis, 104
Glucose metabolism, and oral contraceptives,
32
Gonadal dysgenesis, 145
Gonadotropin-releasing hormone, 144
Gonadotropin-releasing hormone agonist, in
management of premenstrual
symptoms, 167
Gonococcal arthritis dermatitis syndrome, 92,
94
Gonococcal infection, 77–78
disseminated, 78, 92, 94
and oral contraceptive use, 32
Gonorrhea, 90. *See also Neisseria
gonorrhoeae*
and chlamydia, 92
pelvic inflammatory disease in, 99
treatment, 92–93
Gram stain, 82
Granular cell myoblastomas, of breast,
124–125
Granuloma inguinale, 103–104
Grey-Turner sign, 197
Growth, after menarche, 141
Guarding, 187, 197
Gynecologic exam
equipment for, 75
of young girl, 81–82
Gynecologists, willingness to treat teenagers,
13–14
Gyne-Lotrimin. *See* Clotrimazole

Haemophilus ducreyi, 102
Haemophilus vaginalis, 86
Headache, premenstrual, 142
Health insurance, 72
Health record
documentation, 70–71
privacy, 67–69, 72–73
Hematocolpometra, 146
Hematocolpos, 146
Hematuria, 180
Hemolytic-uremic syndrome, 195
Hemoperitoneum, 162
Henoch-Schoenlein purpura, 194–195

Hepatitis, 196
    carrier state, 196
    chronic, 196
    signs and symptoms, 196
    types of, 196
Hepatitis B, protection against, with
    condoms, 46
Herpes simplex, 76, 79, 94
    carcinogenic risk with, 97
    infection, 90
    type I, 83, 95
    type II, 83
        cervicitis, 95–97
            complications, 96
            diagnostic procedures, 96
            symptoms and signs, 96
            treatment, 96–97
Hidradenitis suppurativa, 77
Hidradenoma, 107
HIV. *See* Human immunodeficiency virus
HMO, confidential care under, 72
Hodgeson v. Minnesota, 63
Homosexuality, 8
HPV. *See Papillomavirus*
Huffman speculum, 81–83
Human chorionic gonadotropin assay, 181,
    201, 206–207
Human immunodeficiency virus
    and oral contraceptives, 32
    protection against, with condoms, 46, 48
Hydrometrocolpos, ultrasound detection of,
    181
Hydronephrosis, 192, 195
21–Hydroxylase deficiency, 152
Hymen, imperforate, 77, 146
Hypergonadotropic hypogonadism, 145
Hyperprolactinemia, 132, 151, 155
    and primary amenorrhea, 146
Hypertension, 28
    risk of, with oral contraceptives, 31
Hyperthyroidism, and amenorrhea, 154
Hypogonadotropic hypogonadism, 145–146
Hypomastia, 117–118
Hypothyroidism, 134, 146
    and galactorrhea, 133
    management, 135
    and menorrhagia, 154

Ibuprofen, for dysmenorrhea, 160–161
Idiopathic thrombocytopenic purpura, 154
Imidazole drugs, 88–89
Inflammatory bowel disease, 180, 186, 192
Informed consent, ability of minor to give,
    64–66, 71
Ingraham v. Wright, 63
In re Gault, 62
Insecurity, 218–219

Intercourse
    first
        age at, 3
        contraceptive use at, 9, 12
    rate of
        by age, 3–4
        among teenagers, 2–3
Intestinal pseudoobstruction, 193
Intrauterine device(s)
    disadvantages of, 24, 154
    and dysmenorrhea, 162
    effectiveness of, theoretical vs. actual, 24
    as postcoital contraceptive, 38
    use of, 9
Irritable bowel syndrome, 191–192
    treatment, 192
Isotretinoin therapy, for nodulocystic acne,
    and amenorrhea, 151
IUD. *See* Intrauterine device(s)

Jarisch-Herxheimer reaction, 102
Juvenile giant fibroadenoma, 124

Kallman syndrome, 146
Ketoconazole, 89
KOH. *See* Potassium hydroxide
Koilocytes, 79–80

Lactation, 132
Laparoscopy, 203
    for patient with chronic pelvic pain,
        213–214
Law
    and care of teenagers, 14–17
    and contraception, 65
    implementing, in clinical practice, 68–69
    knowledge of, required for physician, 68
    state, and minors' consent to treatment,
        64–66
Laxatives, 190–191
Leukoplakia, 107
Leukorrhea, 77
    in *Candida* vaginitis, 87
    physiologic, 82, 85–86
        diagnostic procedures, 86
        symptoms and signs, 85
        treatment, 86
Levonorgestrel, 25
Lice, pubic, 80, 107
Lichen sclerosis et atrophicus, 107
Lipid profile, effect of oral contraceptives on,
    25–27, 38
Lipschutz cells, 105
Liver cancer, and oral contraceptives, 31
Luteal phase deficiency, 163
    in female athletes, 148

Luteinizing hormone, 144
Lymphogranuloma venereum, 94, 102–103

Macromastia, 117–119
Magnetic resonance imaging, abdominal and
    pelvic, 184
Males, sexual activity of, 2–3
Marijuana, and earlier onset of sexual
    intercourse, 5
Mastitis, 126
Masturbation, 81–82
Maturation index, 76
Mature minor
    consent to abortion, 17
    legal concept of, 15, 33, 59, 62–64
Meckel diverticulum, 193
Medicaid, 71
Mefenamic acid (Ponstel)
    for dysmenorrhea, 160–161
    in management of dysfunctional uterine
        bleeding, 156
    for PMS symptoms, 166
α-Melanocyte-stimulating hormone, and
        premenstrual symptoms, 165
Menarche
    age at, and reproductive performance, 142
    delayed, 145
    mean age of, 141–142
    and mean weight, 141
    occurrence of, by Tanner stage, 141
Meningitis, gonococcal, 95
Menometrorrhagia, 153
Menorrhagia, 153–155
    management, 155
Menstrual blood loss, 153
Menstrual calendar, 143–144
Menstrual cycles, anovulatory
    after menarche, 153
    in female athletes, 148
Menstrual disorders, 141–167
    drug-induced, 155
    in female athletes, 148
    and gynecologic outcomes, 143
Menstrual history, 143, 213
Menstrual patterns
    irregular, causes, 142
    normal, 141–142
Menstruation
    after oral contraceptive discontinuation, 32
    hygiene, 143
    knowledge and beliefs about, 143
    symptoms related to, 142
Mesenteric adenitis, 186
Metronidazole, 100
    in trichomoniasis, 90–91
Metrorrhagia, 153

Miconazole nitrate (Monistat), 88–89
Migraine, 28
Mini-pill, 26, 28, 38
    contraceptive action, 38
    pregnancy rate with, 38
Minors' consent laws, benefits of, 73
Mittelschmerz, 162, 205
Molluscum contagiosum, 80, 83
    diagnostic procedures, 105
    symptoms and signs, 105
    treatment, 105
Monilia albicans. See Candida albicans
Monilial vaginitis, 79, 87–88, 101
    and pregnancy, 107
Moniliasis, protection against, with condoms,
    46
Monilids, 88
Monistat. See Miconazole nitrate
Mosaicism, 145–146
Mycelex-G. See Clotrimazole
Mycoplasma hominis, pelvic inflammatory
        disease caused by, 98–99

Naprosyn. See Naproxen
Naproxen (Naprosyn), in management of
        dysfunctional uterine bleeding, 156
Naproxen sodium (Anaprox), for
        dysmenorrhea, 160–161
Negligence, 64
Neisseria gonorrhoeae, 76, 85
    carrier state, 91
    cervicitis, 91–92, 201
    diagnostic procedures, 92
    isolation, 77
    pelvic inflammatory disease caused by,
        98–99
    penicillinase–producing, 92–95
    perihepatitis, 93
    in prepubertal girls, 84
    prevalence, 91
    proctitis, 94
    protection against, with condoms, 46
    transmission, 91
    vaginitis, 91
Nephrolithiasis
    in Crohn's disease, 192
    in ulcerative colitis, 192
Nipples
    absence of, 117
    accessory, 114, 116
    cold injury to, 136
    inverted, 119
    minor injuries to, 136
Nipple secretion. See Galactorrhea
Nonoxynol-9, 45, 51, 55
    in vaginal sponge, 54

Nonspecific vaginitis, 78
  in prepubertal girl, 81–84
  treatment of, 82–83
Nonsteroidal antiinflammatory drugs, for
    dysmenorrhea, 160–161
Norgestimate, 27
Norplant, 24
Norwalk agent, gastroenteritis, 188
Nystatin vaginal tablets, 89

Occult blood, in stool, 180
Octoxynol-9, 55
Oidium albicans. See Candida albicans
Oligomenorrhea, 143–144
  clinical aspects, 151–152
  definition of, 144, 151–152
  prevalence, 144
Oral contraceptives
  advantages of, 23
  amenorrhea after, 151
  amenorrhea with, 36
  beneficial effects of, 33
  choice of pill, 35–36
  clotting propensity with, 28
  combination, 25
  compliance rates with, 35
  contraindications, 28
  cost of, 35
  death related to, 29–31
  depression with, 36
  drugs that may interfere with, 29
  effectiveness of, theoretical vs. actual, 24
  effect on lipid profile, 25–27, 38
  estrogen dose, 35
  follow-up, 37
  formulation, 25–27
  and galactorrhea, 36, 132–133
  headaches with, 36–37
  hypertension with, 36
  laboratory changes in patients taking,
      28–29
  low-dose, 26, 36
    breakthrough bleeding with, 35–36
  in management of dysfunctional uterine
      bleeding, 156
  mechanism of action, 27–28
  multiphasic, 25, 36–38
  nausea or vomiting with, 36
  pain with, 36–37
  and pelvic inflammatory disease, 32
  and premenstrual syndrome, 166
  prescribing, 33–35
  for primary dysmenorrhea, 160
  problems with, management of, 36
  progesterone-only, 38
  progestin dose, 25, 35
  and prolactinomas, 132

  and risk of cancer, 31–32
  safety, 23, 28–31
    during first trimester of pregnancy, 36
  screening exam for, 33–35
  screening history for, 33–35
  side effects, 25
    management, 36
  teenagers' sources of information about,
      33–34
  starting, 37
  to treat and prevent fibrocystic
      mastopathies, 123
  to treat dysmenorrhea, 208–209
  use of, 9–10
  vascular risks of, 31
  weight gain with, 36
Oral sex, 8
Osteomyelitis, gonococcal, 94
Otoscope, 81, 83
Ovarian cancer, lowered risk of, with oral
      contraceptives, 31, 33
Ovarian cyst, 162
  functional, 205
    recurrent, 209
  recurrent, management, 214
  ruptured, 198, 205
    diagnostic approach to, 199
    laboratory assessment of, 200
    ultrasound identification of, 181
Ovarian failure, 146
Ovarian teratoma, ultrasound identification
      of, 181
Ovarian tumors, 114
  ultrasound identification of, 181
Ovral, as postcoital contraceptive, 38
Ovulation, 141–142
  after oral contraceptive discontinuation, 32
  pain of, 162, 205
    diagnosis, 210
    laboratory assessment with, 211

Pain. *See also* Abdominal pain; Pelvic pain;
      Referred pain
  chronic, evaluation of, 174
  definition of, 173
  experience, factors affecting, 176
  reactivity to, 173
  recurrent, evaluation of, 174
Pancreatitis, 197
  ultrasound in, 183
Papillomavirus, 76, 79, 105
  carcinogenic risk, 97
Pap smear, 75–76, 79–80
  abnormal, and cervical cap, 50
  in trichomoniasis, 90
Paraguard T380, 24
Paralytic ileus, 193

Parametritis, 202
Parasitic gynecologic diseases, 104
Parental consent or notification, 15
   for contraceptive care, 35, 65–66
   mandatory, perceived impact on family
      planning clinic use, 60–61
   before a minor's abortion, 16–17, 63
   for treatment of minor, legal basis of, 64
Parental interview, in assessment of
      psychosomatic factors, 215
Parents
   relationships with, of sexually active
      teenagers, 5
   role in sex education, 18
Parietal pain, 175
Payment for services, 13–14, 71
Pediatricians, willingness to treat teenagers,
      13–14
Pediculosis pubis, 80, 107
Peer relationships, as topic of clinical
      interview, 216
Pelvic examination
   basic, 76–77
   in evaluation of abdominal pain, 179
   fear of, 14
   for oral contraceptive user, 37
   for patient with chronic pelvic pain, 213
Pelvic inflammatory disease, 77–78, 98–100,
      162
   vs. appendicitis, 186–187
   bacterial agents of, 98–99
   causes of, 98, 202
   chronic, 212
   clinical aspects, 99
   complications of, 100–101
   definition of, 202
   diagnosis, 99–100, 199, 203–204, 210
   diagnostic criteria for, 203
   differential diagnosis, 99, 203
   with gonorrhea, 92
   hospitalization for, 100, 204–205
   incidence of, 14, 98
   infertility after, 100
   laboratory assessment of, 200, 211
   morbidity, 202
   and oral contraceptives, 32
   pain in, 212
   prevalence, 202
   risk factors for, 98, 202
   sequelae, 204–205
   treatment, 100–101, 204–205
   ultrasound in, 183
Pelvic pain
   acute
      in adolescents, 198–199
      laboratory assessment of, 200
      pregnancy-related causes of, 198
   chronic, 161–162, 209–214
      clinical approach to, 209–210

differential diagnosis, 210
emotional/functional
      diagnosis, 210
   laboratory assessment with, 211
evaluation, 213
history, 213
imaging tests, 213
laboratory assessment of, 211, 213
management, 214
in pelvic inflammatory disease, 99
psychoemotional component, 212
   management, 214
Penicillin, treatment of syphilis, 102
Peptic ulcer disease, 186, 192–193
Perihepatitis, gonococcal, 93
Peritoneal pain, 178
Phthirus pubis, 80, 107
Physician
   and adolescent, clinical interaction,
      174–175
   attitudes toward teenage patients, 13–14
   and law, 14–17
   role of, in adolescent sexuality, 13–18
   teenagers' perceptions of, 13
Pinworm, 104
Pituitary microadenoma, 132, 134, 151
Pituitary tumor, and galactorrhea, 132
Plain radiographs, of abdomen, 184
Planned Parenthood of Central Missouri v.
      Danforth, 63
Platelet defect, 154
Pneumonia, 186, 197
Podophyllin, 106
Poland's syndrome, 117
Polycystic ovary, 145, 151–152, 154–155,
      181
   ultrasound image in, 181–182
Polymastia, 114–116
Polythelia, 114, 116
Ponstel. *See* Mefenamic acid
Potassium hydroxide, 75–76, 78–79, 82, 86
Povidone-iodine, 91
Precocious puberty, 114, 121
Pregnancy
   and amenorrhea, 148
   risk of, 29
      from single episode of sexual intercourse
         at mid–cycle, 38
   teenage
      and contraceptive use, 8
      prevention, 1, 18
      rate of, 1
         factors affecting, 1
   ultrasound image in, 181
Pregnancy tests. *See also* Human chorionic
      gonadotropin assay
   urine, 76
Premarin, to induce rapid cessation of uterine
      bleeding, 156

Premenstrual syndrome, 158, 162–167
    and daily consumption of
        caffeine–containing beverages, 165
    definition of, 162–163
    diagnostic criteria, 162–163
    etiology, 164
    management, 165–167
    and psychopathology, 164
    response to hormonal therapy, 164
    role of neuropeptides in, 165
    symptoms, 162–164
    treatment, with oral contraceptives, 33
Premenstrual tension, 163–164
Privacy rights, 15, 59, 61, 67
    and womens' reproductive rights, 63
Proctitis, 94
    gonococcal, 91, 94
Progestasert, disadvantages, 24
Progesterone
    bioavailability, 166–167
    for premenstrual syndrome, 166
Progesterone-only pill. *See* Mini-pill
Progestins, 38
    estrogenic and antiestrogenic or androgenic
        effects, 25, 27
    in oral contraceptives, 25, 35
        relative potencies of, 25, 27
Prolactin, 131–132. *See also*
        Hyperprolactinemia
    levels
        and galactorrhea, 132
        normal, 134
        with tumor, 134
    suppression and stimulation tests, 135
Prolactin inhibitory factor, 132
Prolactinoma, 132–133
    diagnosis, 134–135
    management, 135
Prostaglandin
    in etiology of dysmenorrhea, 158–159
    synthesis, in uterus, 159
Prostaglandin synthetase inhibitors
    in management of dysmenorrhea, 157,
        160, 208–209
    in reducing menstrual blood loss, 155–156
Provera, 156
Pruritus ani, 107
Pruritus vulvae, 107–108
Pseudoprecocious puberty, 114
Pseudostupidity, 10
Puberty, 113–114, 174
    normal, 144–145
    onset of, 113
Pubic hair, development, 145
Pyelonephritis, 194
Pyridoxine therapy, and premenstrual
        syndrome, 166

Rebound tenderness, 197, 199
Reduction mammoplasty, 119
Referral
    to gynecologist, 68, 75, 108
    to subsidized or low–cost resource, 72
Referred pain, 175, 177–178
Regional enteritis, 146
    ultrasound in, 183
Reiter's syndrome, 107
Religion, and rates of sexual activity, 5–6
Renal vein thrombosis, acute, 195
Reporting
    legal requirements for, 72
    of sexually active minor, 61
Respiratory pathogens, genital infections
        with, 81–83
Revised Behavior Problem Checklist, 217
Rhythm method, use of, 9
Right upper quadrant pain, 93, 178, 197, 202
Risks
    of contraception and pregnancy, 30
    voluntary and involuntary, in everyday
        life, 29–30
Roe v. Wade, 17, 63
Rokitansky-Kuster-Hauser syndrome, 146
Rotavirus, gastroenteritis, 188
Runners, amenorrhea in, 148–149
    and eating and affective disorders, 150

Saccharomyces, 87
Salmonella, gastroenteritis, 188
Salpingitis, 154, 198, 202
    diagnostic approach to, 199
    laboratory assessment of, 200
Salpingoophoritis, 202
Sarcoma botryoid, 107
Sarcoptes scabiei var. *hominis*, 106
SBHCs. *See* School-based health clinics
Scabies, 106–107
School, as topic of clinical interview, 216
School-based health clinics, 18
    contraceptives dispensed from, 9
    number of, 9
    and teenage pregnancy rates, 8–9
Scleroderma, involving breast, 119
SCL-90-R, 217
Self-esteem, and sexual activity, 6
Septicemia, 92
    with gonorrhea, 94
Serositis, 162
Serotonin, and premenstrual symptoms, 165
Sex education
    and contraceptive use, 10–11
    effects of, 12
    parental, 18
    school-based, 18
    state policies on, 11–12
    television as source of, 6–7, 19

Sexual abuse, 61–62, 81, 213
    and pelvic pain, 212
Sexual activity
    as risk-taking or transitional behavior, 5
    teenage, 2–4
        explanations for, 4–7
        rates of, 3
Sexual history, obtaining, 14
Sexual intercourse. *See* Intercourse
Sexuality, adolescent, 2–13
Sexually transmitted disease, 77–80
    agents, in adolescent, 85
    mixed, 92, 101
    and pregnancy, 107
    prevention, 23–24
    protection against
        with cervical cap, 49
        with condom, 46
        with condoms, 48
        with diaphragm, 51
        with vaginal contraceptive sponge, 54
        with vaginal spermicidal agents, 55
Sexual partners, number of, before and after
        obtaining oral contraceptives, 12–13
Sexual practices, teenage, 7–8
Shigella, 83, 94
    gastroenteritis, 188
Shigellosis, 104
Shoulder pain, referred, 178
Sickle cell anemia, 180, 186
    and gallstones, 196
Sick role, 218–219
Sitz baths, 83–84, 89
Skeletal growth, and oral contraceptives, 32
Skene's glands, inflammation of, in
        gonorrhea, 91
*Slaby v. Akron Center for Reproductive
        Health*, 63
Smoking, 35
    and oral contraceptives, 28
Society, and teenage sexual activity, 18–19
Socioeconomic level, and sexual activity, 6
Specula, 75, 81–83, 213
Spermicide
    allergic reaction to, 56
    and birth defects, 56
    disadvantages of, 24
    effectiveness of, theoretical vs. actual, 24
    vaginal insert, 55–56
        and adolescent patient, 56
        effectiveness, 46, 55
        historical perspective on, 45
        insertion, 56
        need for repeated use, 56
Spontaneous abortion, 198
    diagnostic approach to, 199
    laboratory assessment of, 200
Sports. *See also* Athletic activity
    trauma to breast during, 124, 135–136

Squeal rule, 15–16, 60–61
Staphylococcal food poisoning, 188
State–Trait Anxiety Inventory, 217
Statutory rape, 61–62
STD. *See* Sexually transmitted disease
Strawberry marks (spots), 78, 90
Streptococcus, β–hemolytic, 94
Stress
    and abdominal pain, 176, 214–223
    and amenorrhea, 148
    and galactorrhea, 134
    and psychogenic pain, 176
Stroke, 28
    thrombotic, risk of, with oral
        contraceptives, 31
Subarachnoid hemorrhage, risk of, with oral
        contraceptives, 31
Suicide, 219, 223
Surgical abdomen, 177, 186
Syphilis, 79, 101–102
    diagnosis, 101–102
    protection against, with condoms, 46
    secondary, 101–102
    treatment, 102

Tampons, 143
Television
    and adolescent sexual behavior, 6–7
    sex education from, 6–7, 19
Terconazole, 88–89
Testicular feminization, 147
Thelarche, 113, 121
    premature, 114, 121
Thinking, developmental stages of, in
        teenagers, 10
Third-party payment, 71–72
Thrombocytopenia, 154
Thyroid function tests, 134
Thyrotropin-releasing hormone, 133
Tinea globrata, 88
*Tinker v. the Des Moines Independent School
        District*, 62–63
Tort law, 64
Torulopsis glabrata, 87
Toxic shock syndrome, 143
    and vaginal contraceptive sponges, 54
Transverse vaginal septum, 146
Traveller's diarrhea, 188
Treponema pallidum, 79, 94, 101
Trichomonas vaginalis, 76, 78, 83–85
    in prepubertal girl, 83–84
    vaginitis, 89–91
Trichomoniasis
    carrier state, 90
    diagnostic procedures, 90
    incubation period, 89
    postpartum, 90
    spread, 89

symptoms and signs, 90
treatment, 90
Tuboovarian abscess, 198
Turner syndrome, 145
Tzanck prep, 79

Ulcerative colitis, 146, 192
Ultrasonography. *See* Ultrasound
Ultrasound, 100, 187
   breast, 127
   pelvic, 76
   transabdominal, 181–184
   transvaginal, 181
Ureterocele, ultrasound detection of, 181
Urethritis, gonococcal, 91
   treatment of, 93
Urinalysis, 180, 194–195
Urinary incontinence, 189
Urinary tract abnormalities, 195
   ultrasound detection of, 181
Urinary tract infection, 184, 186
   abdominal pain in, 194
   associated with diaphragm use, 53
   diagnosis of, 194
   treatment, 194
Urinary tract obstruction, ultrasound in, 183
Urinary tract stones, 195
Uterine evacuation, by suction curettage, 198
Uterine fibroids, 162
Uterine synechiae, 147

Vagina
   abnormalities, 77
   clear cell adenocarcinoma, 107, 154
   normal, 77
   normal flora, 85, 92
   pH, 82, 84
Vaginal adenosis, 77
Vaginal agenesis, 77
Vaginal contraceptive sponge, 53–55
   and adolescent patient, 55
   allergic reaction to, 54
   availability, 53
   disadvantages of, 24
   and discomfort during intercourse, 54
   effectiveness, 46, 53–54
   historical perspective on, 45
   odor with, 55
   as protection against sexually transmitted
      disease, 54
   retention, 54
   tearing, 54
   and toxic shock syndrome, 54

Vaginal duplication, ultrasound detection of,
   181
Vaginal epithelium
   desquamation of, 77
   estrogen response of, 75
   nonestrogenized, 77, 81
Vaginal insert spermicides. *See* Spermicide,
   vaginal insert
Vaginal lacerations, 154
Vaginitis, 154. *See also* Nonspecific
   vaginitis; Vulvovaginitis
   bacterial, 83
   Candida albicans, 87–89
   Gardnerella vaginalis, 78, 86
   monilial, 79, 87–88, 101, 107
   prepubertal, 81–84
   pubertal, 84–85
   Trichomonas vaginalis, 89–91
Vaginocervical ecchymosis, 78, 90
Venous thromboembolism, risk of, with oral
   contraceptives, 31
Verapamil, in management of premenstrual
   symptoms, 167
Vesicles, on labia or vulva, 83
Visceral pain, 175, 178
Vitamin B_6, side effects, 166
Vitamin E, and premenstrual syndrome, 166
Vitamins, in management of premenstrual
   symptoms, 165–166
von Willebrand's disease, 154
Vulvar sarcoma or carcinomas, 107
Vulvitis, 81, 100–101
   causes of, 101
Vulvovaginitis, 81–98
   causes of, 81–82
   in adolescent, 85

Webster v. Reproductive Health Services, 17,
   63
Weight loss
   and primary amenorrhea, 146
   and secondary amenorrhea, 148
Whiff test, 79, 86
White blood cell count, 180, 197
Wide Range Achievement Test–Revised, 217
Withdrawal
   effectiveness of, theoretical vs. actual, 24
   use of, 9–10

Yeast infection, 79
Yersinia enterocoliticus, 83
   gastroenteritis, 186, 188–189